INTEGRATED CARDIOPULMONARY PHARMACOLOGY

D1637475

INTEGRATED CARDIOPULMONARY PHARMACOLOGY

BRUCE J. COLBERT
MS, RRT
Director of Allied Health
University of Pittsburgh at Johnstown

BARB J. MASON
Pharm. D.
Professor and Vice Chair
Idaho State University College of Pharmacy

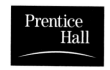

Prentice
Hall

Upper Saddle River, New Jersey 07458

Library of Congress Cataloging-in-Publication Data

Colbert, Bruce J.
   Integrated cardiopulmonary pharmacology / Bruce J. Colbert,
Barb J. Mason.
      p.   cm.
   Includes bibliographical references and index.
   ISBN 0-13-030518-9
   1. Pulmonary pharmacology.   2. Cardiovascular pharmacology.
3. Respiratory agents.   4. Cardiovascular agents.
5. Cardiopulmonary system—Effect of drugs on.   I. Mason, Barb J.
II. Title.

RM388 .C635   2001
615'.71—dc21   2001036164

Publisher: *Julie Levin Alexander*
Acquisitions Editor: *Mark Cohen*
Assistant Editor: *Melissa Kerian*
Marketing Manager: *David Hough*
Director of Production & Manufacturing: *Bruce Johnson*
Managing Production Editor: *Patrick Walsh*
Manufacturing Buyer: *Pat Brown*
Production Liaison: *Julie Li*
Production Editor: *Sharon Anderson*
Creative Director: *Cheryl Asherman*
Cover Design Coordinator: *Maria Guglielmo*
Cover Designer: *Gary J. Sella*
Composition: *BookMasters, Inc.*
Printing and Binding: *Courier Westford*

Pearson Education LTD.
Pearson Education Australia PTY, Limited
Pearson Education Singapore, Pte. Ltd
Pearson Education North Asia Ltd
Pearson Education Canada, Ltd.
Pearson Educación de Mexico, S.A. de C.V.
Pearson Education,—Japan
Pearson Education Malaysia, Pte. Ltd
Pearson Education, Upper Saddle River, New Jersey

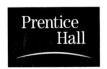

10 9 8 7 6 5

ISBN 0-13-030518-9

To my parents, Robert and Josephine Colbert, who taught me the importance of family, and to my loving wife, Patty, and two wonderful children, Jeremy and Joshua, who continue to teach me its importance.

Bruce Colbert

To my daughter, Stacia, and to my parents, Charlie and Evelyn Repschlaeger, who instinctively taught me the definition of support and have actively provided it on a daily basis, through all my personal and professional endeavors.

Barb Mason

Contents

List of Tables

Preface

Pharmacology is often perceived as one of the more difficult subjects in a medical curriculum. There are several possible explanations. First, there are difficult concepts and terms that are inherent to this subject. Second, there is a massive amount of information, often presented in a dry and highly technical manner. Finally, once a text is printed, it is practically out of date because of all the recent breakthroughs, new drugs, and new delivery devices that have been developed before it even hits the bookstores. We took all these factors into account as we developed and pilot-tested this innovative project. So what makes this book unique and able to address these concerns?

First and foremost, this truly is an *integrated project* at several levels and not just a "buzz word" thrown into the title. The authors and publisher took very seriously the integrated aspect of this project and first sought the interdisciplinary perspective offered by both pharmacists and respiratory therapists. In addition, pharmacology was integrated and linked to physiology and pathology to give a total understanding and enhance connectional and relevant learning. The authors also took very seriously the concept of writing in a style that did not distance the student from the material and encouraged "learning and relating" the material versus massive memorization.

Finally, there are some things we did not take so seriously. While we were serious about the contents, relevancy, and accuracy of the material, we had fun writing, researching, and collaborating on this project. We utilized splashes of humor within this textbook, with the underlying idea that what is learned with humor is not readily forgotten. While humor will make the learning easier, never take lightly your responsibilities as a health care professional.

SPECIAL TEXTBOOK FEATURES

Our goal is to produce a truly introductory and interactive pharmacology text that students can connect with and learn pharmacology. Several features will be incorporated into the textbook to help accomplish that goal; they include the following:

Get Connected to the Web Site: This special text feature will connect the student to a managed companion Web page with current updates, new drugs, animations, videos, audio glossary and drug pronunciation, sample tests, and references.

Learning Hints and Controversies: These special features will be contained in each chapter to ensure understanding of difficult concepts and to stimulate further thought.

Clinical Pearls: Instances of this special feature will also be interspersed throughout the chapters to connect the knowledge and show the relevancy of learning the material. In addition, numerous clinical applications will be demonstrated to give a "real world" connection.

Key Terms: Key terms will be boldfaced and included in a glossary. In addition, an audio glossary and drug name pronunciation will be provided on the Web site. Symbols, units, and abbreviation or medical terms will be defined in the chapter opener for easy reference.

Chapter Questions: Periodic "Stop and Review" problems within each chapter will help to ensure concept understanding before a student can move on and get really lost. Comprehensive questions will also be included at the end of the chapter; they will build from multiple choice and matching questions to higher-level critical thinking and case-study questions. An interactive chapter exam will also be provided on the Web site.

THE INTEGRATED WEB SITE

Further proof of the commitment to integration lies in a unique and interactive web site that fully supports the text. While the textbook can certainly stand on its own, the web site is a powerful adjunct that can greatly facilitate learning and keep both faculty and students up on the "latest and greatest" in pharmacology. One of the difficult aspects of teaching pharmacology is that by the time a textbook is produced, there is a wealth of new information, some theories are challenged, and new drugs or types of therapies are beginning to emerge. We have developed a managed companion Web site in conjunction with the textbook that will add new information for each specific chapter on a semi annual basis. For each chapter, the following "buttons" can be engaged:

Animations: Highly visual representations of complex concepts can be demonstrated and reinforced via animations. For example, protein binding is not only discussed in the text, but visual animations of protein binding and displacement can also be viewed to enhance learning.

Videos: Clinical procedures, drug preparations, and delivery devices can be viewed on quality videos. For example, various oxygen therapy delivery techniques and devices are shown, along with proper monitoring techniques.

Updates: New information that continually surfaces after the book goes into production, such as new drugs and/or treatments, will be posted semi annually to the pertinent chapter.

Glossary and Drug Pronunciation: Pharmacological terms and especially drug names are very difficult to pronounce. A very bright student can be wrongly judged in clinical owing to poor pronunciation of drug names. Therefore, each chapter will have an audio glossary and drug names section.

Extended Concepts: Additional information concerning topics within each chapter can be expanded upon within the Web site. This can allow students to further pursue knowledge in their own areas of interest.

Chapter Quiz: A sample chapter test can be taken and scored for feedback.

References and Additional Readings: These are listed per chapter.
The Web site can be accessed at www.prenhall.com/colbert

DRUG COMPANION GUIDE

A separate concise pocket drug companion guide is integrated with the textbook. This guide will give further details concerning drug actions, uses, and interactions, along with specific routes and pediatric and adult dosages. In addition, more detailed pharmacokinetics, contraindications, and side effects will given, along with additional pertinent information. Removing some of this information that can easily be looked up from the textbook allows focus to be placed on "learning" pharmacologic principles and mechanisms of actions of specific drug classifications to facilitate optimal disease management. All drugs that are bolded and designated with Rx symbol are in the companion guide.

ACKNOWLEDGMENTS

The authors would like to acknowledge the following people who have contributed to this integrated project.

Mark Cohen, editor from Prentice Hall, whose tremendous persistence, assistance, and enthusiasm has led to the development of this project.

The contributing authors whose expertise truly added to the text. They are Carla Frye (Chapters 13 and 14), Roger Hefflinger (Chapter 11), Terri Price (Chapters 5, 6, and 15) and Catherine Hitt (Chapter 8).

Sharlene Hetrick, administrative assistant extraordinaire for whom one author is immensely grateful and indebted.

University of Pittsburgh at Johnstown's Respiratory Care Class of 2001 who gave input into the concept of this project and evaluated original sample chapters for readability. They helped with the vision of this integrated project. They are:

Kristin Angelo	Susan Robinson
Michael Becker	Cheri Roudabush
Carla Boast	Derek Shilcosky
Jill Brant	Erica Stiffler
Tara Jerz	Hazel Weighly
Jesse Kirkpatrick	Julie Wiancko
Yvonne Mumma	

University of Pittsburgh at Johnstown's Respiratory Care Class of 2002 who pilot tested the book by reading copies of the raw manuscript and scribbled drawings for their Pharmacology class. Their comments added much to this project. They are:

Amy Bennet	Kristy Kerrigan
Lisa Chandler	Jennifer Sirko
Keri-Ann Christie	Lisa Smith
Rebecca Fodor	Christopher White

The reviewers for their careful analysis and insightful comments. They are:

Lynn Walter Capraun, MS, RRT
Program Director
Respiratory Care
Valencia Community College
Orlando, Florida

Joseph S. DiPietro, Ph.D., RRT
Professor and Director
Respiratory Care and
Polysomnography Programs
Southwest Virginia Community College
Richlands, Virginia

Charles S. Cornfield, MS, RRT
Program Director
Respiratory Therapist Program
Gannon University
Erie, Pennsylvania

Christine G. Fitzgerald, M.H.S., RRT
Director of Clinical Education
Department of Cardiopulmonary Science
Quinnipiac University
Hamden, Connecticut

Douglas G. Gibson, BA, RRT
Program Director
Respiratory Care
McLennan Community College
Waco, Texas

Joy Reed, RN, MSN
Assistant Professor of Nursing
Indiana Wesleyan University
Marion, Indiana

Richard A. Patze, M.Ed., RRT
Dean, Health Related Health Professions
Pima Community College
Tucson, Arizona

Thomas Schaltenbrand, MBA, RRT
Director of Clinical Education
Certified Respiratory Therapist Program
Kaskasia College
Belleville, Illinois

Charles Vincent Preuss, Ph.D., R.Ph.
Assistant Professor
College of Pharmacy
Ferris State University
Big Rapids, Michigan

April Hershberger, the animator for the Web site, who made our "blurry artistic vision" a quality reality.

Rick Povich, the videographer, whose quality camera work developed instructional videos to complement the text.

CHAPTER 1

General Pharmacological Principles

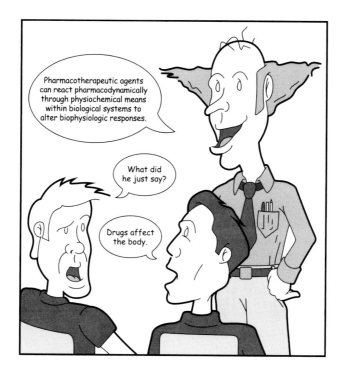

OBJECTIVES

Upon completion of this chapter you will be able to

- Define key terms related to pharmacological principles
- Utilize drug-reference sources of information
- Discuss advantages and disadvantages of different routes of administration
- Describe the processes of drug absorption, distribution, metabolism, and elimination
- Explain differences in pharmacokinetics, pharmacodynamics, and adverse effects of drugs in pediatric, geriatric, pregnant, and breast-feeding patients
- Discuss factors that may alter a patient's response to a drug
- Discuss principles of drug poisonings, adverse drug reactions, and interactions
- Discuss responsibilities in drug administration

ABBREVIATIONS

CNS	central nervous system	COPD	chronic obstructive pulmonary disease
DNA	deoxyribonucleic acid		
FDA	Food and Drug Administration	IV	intravenous
HIV	human immunodeficiency virus	PO	by mouth (Latin *per os*)
AHFS	American Hospital Formulary Service	SL	sublingual
		NG	nasogastric
PDR	Physicians' Desk Reference	NPO	nothing by mouth
USAN	United States Adopted Name Council	IM	intramuscular
		GI	gastrointestinal
USP	United States Pharmacopeia	Vd	volume of distribution
ADR	adverse drug reaction	$T_{1/2}$	half-life
ACE	angiotensin-converting enzyme	TI	therapeutic index
OTC	over the counter		

INTRODUCTION

For the healthcare professional, medication administration carries with it many responsibilities. With the vast array of drugs currently used in the practice of medicine, and new ones constantly being tested and developed, it is an impossible task to know every detail about every drug. However, if one is well grounded in basic pharmacologic principles, one will know where to look and be able to understand the medical language that describes drugs and their interactions within the human organism.

This chapter discusses fundamental principles of pharmacology and strives to provide you with a healthy respect for drugs and knowledge that you can apply daily in pharmacotherapy decision-making. After reading this chapter, you will understand the language of pharmacology and the important concepts in safe and effective drug administration.

BASIC TERMS

Drugs are one of the most important aspects of clinical medicine. **Pharmacology,** or the "study of drugs and their action on the body," is a discipline that hinges on basic and clinical science. Pharmacology has a very long history. Ancient civilizations used plants containing ephedrine for breathing disorders, the Native American Indians used wild mint for stomach disorders, and the list could go on and on. There has also been a darker side, when drugs were manufactured for nonmedical reasons. Examples include the infamous opium dens of the past and, in modern times, dangerous designer drugs that have killed many people.

Although pharmacology is the broad term to describe the study of drugs in general, **therapeutics** is defined as the "study of drugs used to cure, treat, or prevent disease." Often the terms pharmacology and therapeutics are combined into the term **pharmacotherapy.** Another recent term that relates to these concepts is **disease management.** Disease management refers to the collective management of all aspects of the patient's disease and is not just isolated to pharmacotherapy. Pharmacotherapy usually is one of the main components of disease management.

Drugs with similar characteristics are grouped together as a pharmacological classification or class. One can predict how drugs in a class will act. For example, drugs in the xanthine class can stimulate the central nervous system (CNS) and have a diuretic effect (i.e., they increase urine output), among other things. Caffeine found in coffee and the prescribed drug theophylline are both in this class and have similar effects, which you would be aware of if you ever drank large amounts of coffee. This text will focus on understanding the individual pharmacological classes and avoid emphasis on massive memorization of individual drugs. This is important because new drugs are released every day, and the need for knowledge of pharmacology and therapeutics is something that grows constantly. The accompanying Web site will provide you with continual updates on new drugs in the various classes discussed as you journey through this textbook.

Drugs can also be classified by their therapeutic category such as bronchodilators. A therapeutic category can have several different pharmacological classes and Chapters 5 through 11 are organized by therapeutic categories. For example, the class of xanthines will be discussed in the bronchodilator chapter, along with other classes of drugs (beta adrenergics and anticholinergics) that are also used as bronchodilators.

DRUG DEVELOPMENT

Tylonol= Brand name

Acetaminophen.

Generic name

Drugs actually are derived from a variety of sources, such as plants, animals, minerals, chemicals, and recombinant deoxyribonucleic acid (DNA). Chemicals can be made into drugs synthetically or can be genetically bio-engineered. Most drugs are now synthetic, but it is predicted that in the future many will be bioengineered.

The Food and Drug Administration (FDA) is the federal agency that regulates drug testing and approves new drugs on the market. Much to the discontent of animal activists, drugs are first tested on animals. Then each drug must pass four phases of human testing. The phases proceed through testing in healthy volunteers (frequently starving healthcare professional students), to testing in people with the disease against which the drug is expected to work, to large multicenter trials, and finally to post-marketing surveillance. The FDA has to constantly balance the need to get a medically useful drug on the market quickly with the realization that the safety of the consumer is at stake. A good example of this is the testing and approval of new drugs for the treatment of the Human Immunodeficiency Virus (HIV).

< CONTROVERSY >

The cost of development of a new drug to the pharmaceutical industry is between $100 million and $500 million. The relationship between drugs and high healthcare costs is a topic of frequent public and political debate. High pharmaceutical costs cause some patients to make questionable cost-saving decisions to take veterinary-quality medication or drugs produced in other countries, available at a lower price.

STOP & REVIEW

Describe the process a new drug must undergo for approval. There are several ethical, moral, and legal issues implied in the previous section on drug development. Can you expand upon them? Can you think of others?

---

www.prenhall.com/colbert

Recombinant DNA technology allows us to produce biologically active substances that are normally in the body and market them commercially. Go to the Web site to learn more about this emerging technology.

HERBALS

Herbal product use is growing in popularity. Frequently herbal use is the result of patient self-medication, and healthcare professionals aren't aware of it unless they ask. Although it is true that many drugs that have been used for years are from plants and have been the fore-runners of many of our current medications, there is little scientific evidence available at this time supporting product benefits. This is because the FDA treats herbals as dietary supplements, and standards for supplements are different than those for drugs. The long and short of it is that with herbal products, there is currently little control for dosage and contaminants.

www.prenhall.com/colbert

More scientific data becomes available every day on herbal use. This Web site has some examples of herbal product use, both therapeutic and toxic.

DRUG INFORMATION SOURCES

All health professionals must recognize their knowledge limitations and know where to find drug information. Depending on your workplace, there should be a variety of different drug reference books accessible to you. Good drug references and sources, in the authors' opinion, include the *American Hospital Formulary Service* (AHFS), *Drug Information*, by the American Society of Health System Pharmacists, and *Drug Facts and Comparisons*, by the Wolters Kluwer Company. *Drug Facts and Comparisons* has useful tables comparing drugs within a class. AHFS provides more information than drug package inserts. For example, it lists unapproved medical indications.

The PDR or *Physicians' Desk Reference* published yearly by Medical Economics Company is useful if you are looking for product information required by the FDA. The PDR is very useful, because it includes photos of drugs. This is useful for tablet or capsule identification in, for example, emergency room overdose situations. The PDR contains the same information as a package insert supplied with the bottle of medication provided by the manufacturer. It will include drug name, clinical pharmacology, indications, contraindications, drug interactions, adverse drug reactions, dosage, and administration.

As technology changes and newer drugs are developed, you have a responsibility to update your knowledge. No one would deny that this is a formidable task. All you need to do is look at the size of the old PDRs compared with today's. The drug information you learn in school is frequently replaced with new concepts once you are out in practice. This requires that you devise a method of updating your knowledge though self-directed learning and continuing education.

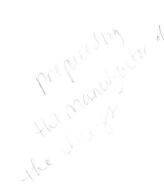

CONTROVERSY

Prescribing patterns and treatments can change daily in response to new research published in medical journals, especially for drug therapy. What would you do if the prescriber is not incorporating the latest research findings into patient treatment?

www.prenhall.com/colbert

On the Web site, you will see some of the latest results of evidence-based medicine research studies related to cardiopulmonary pharmacotherapy.

INTERPRETING DRUG INFORMATION

CLINICAL PEARL
The United States Pharmacopeia (USP) is the official organization that is responsible for establishing drug standards.

Finding a good valid source of drug information is the first step. Understanding and interpreting the information presented is the next step before one can apply this knowledge in drug administration and evaluation. Some of the typical information presented will include the drug name(s), the clinical pharmacology of how it works, indications and usage, contraindications, drug interactions, adverse reactions, and dosage and administration. Let's discuss each of these categories by elaborating upon the specific sections contained in a drug package insert.

Drug Names

LEARNING HINT
Many drugs in a class have generic names that end in the same syllable, e.g., beta blockers: propranolol, metoprolol, atenolol. Traditionally, generic names are written in all lowercase letters.

One of the most complicating factors for students encountering a drug for the first time is that it has not one name but at least two and frequently more. Drugs have chemical names that describe the structure. An example is [4S-(4α,4aα,5aα,6β,12aα,)]-4-(Dimethylamino)-1,4, 4a,5,5a,6,11,12a-octahydro-3,6,10,12,12a-penthydroxy-6-methyl-1,11-dioxo-2-naphthacenecarboxamide. Imagine asking for that at your local pharmacy! The chemical name is important as a point of reference to manufacture the drug, but has little practical use for the practitioner or consumer. Minor chemical changes in a drug can greatly change pharmacological activity. This lesson has been learned the hard way by drug abusers in home labs creating designer drugs that turn out to have dangerous side effects.

Drugs are also assigned generic names by the United States Adopted Name (USAN) Council. The generic name for the previous chemical name is tetracyline hydrochloride. Generic names are not owned by any particular pharmaceutical company and therefore are considered the nonproprietary name.

LEARNING HINT
Trade names are traditionally capitalized and may contain a registered trademark (®).

Once a drug is approved, a particular pharmaceutical company can produce and market it under their brand or trade name. The company that originally discovered the drug owns the trade name, which is derived with the help of creative marketing people. The trade name often relates to some aspect of either the generic name or the drug itself. For example, Sudafed is the trade name for the generic drug pseudoephedrine. Some other examples of some innovative names are Theobid, Respbid, and Slo-Bid. Seeing "Bid" in the name, you can guess the dosage frequency, because bid means twice a day. From "Slo" in the name, you can hypothesize that the drug is a slow-release product. Names frequently give clues to drug indications, e.g., Flovent, for increasing air flow and ventilation. See Figure 1-1 for a portion of a drug package insert related to drug names for the bronchodilator Proventil.

CLINICAL PEARL
Drugs may have more than one name. This is because after the patent on the registered trademark expires, a generic drug product containing the same drug and dosage form can be developed by different drug companies. This is why we have both generic and brand names for many drugs.

Clinical Pharmacology

provide

In this section, you will learn about the mechanism of action of the drug and its specific classification. More on these topics will be covered in the upcoming pharmacokinetics section and in each specific chapter covering the various categories of drugs. See Figure 1-2 for the clinical pharmacology section of the drug package insert for Proventil.

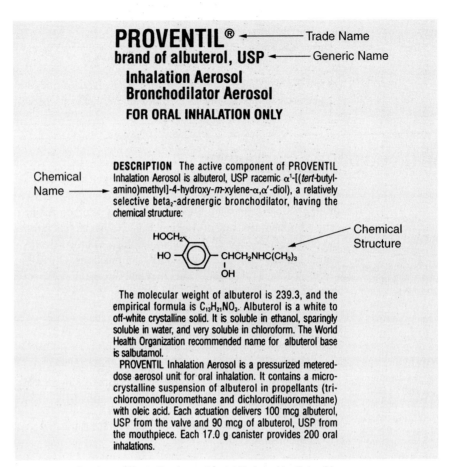

Figure 1-1 Portion of Drug Package Insert Related to Drug Names

Source: Reprinted with permission of Schering Corporation, Kenilworth, NJ. Copyright © 1986, 1993, 1995, 1999, Schering Corporation.

CLINICAL PHARMACOLOGY The primary action of beta-adrenergic drugs, including albuterol, is to stimulate adenyl cyclase, the enzyme which catalyzes the formation of cyclic-3´,5´-adenosine monophosphate (cyclic AMP) from adenosine triphosphate (ATP) in beta-adrenergic cells. The cyclic AMP thus formed mediates the cellular responses. Increased cyclic AMP levels are associated with relaxation of bronchial smooth muscle and inhibition of release of mediators of immediate hypersensitivity from cells, especially from mast cells.

In vitro studies and *in vivo* pharmacologic studies have demonstrated that albuterol has a preferential effect on beta₂-adrenergic receptors compared with isoproterenol. While it is recognized that beta₂-adrenergic receptors are the predominant receptors in bronchial smooth muscle, data indicate that there is a population of beta₂-receptors in the human heart existing in a concentration between 10% and 50%. The precise function of these receptors has not been established.

In controlled clinical trials, albuterol has been shown to have more effect on the respiratory tract, in the form of bronchial smooth muscle relaxation than isoproterenol at comparable doses while producing fewer cardiovascular effects. Controlled clinical studies and other clinical experience have shown that inhaled albuterol, like other beta-adrenergic agonist drugs, can produce a significant cardiovascular effect in some patients, as measured by pulse rate, blood pressure, symptoms, and/or ECG changes.

Albuterol is longer acting than isoproterenol in most patients by any route of administration because it is not a substrate for the cellular uptake processes for catecholamines nor for catechol-*O*-methyl transferase.

The effects of rising doses of albuterol and isoproterenol aerosols were studied in volunteers and asthmatic patients. Results in normal volunteers indicated that the propensity for increase in heart rate for albuterol is ½ to ¼ that of isoproterenol. In asthmatic patients similar cardiovascular differentiation between the two drugs was also seen.

Figure 1-2 Portion of Drug Package Insert Related to Clinical Pharmacology for the Drug Proventil

Source: Reprinted with permission of Schering Corporation, Kenilworth, NJ. Copyright © 1986, 1993, 1999, Schering Corporation.

Indication and Usage

This section will inform you of the clinical indication, i.e., why you would consider using this particular medication. The official clinical indication shows for what diseases the FDA has reviewed the research and approved scientific drug use. However, one should note that sometimes drugs are prescribed for uses not listed as an indication in the drug package insert. See Figure 1-3 for the indication and usage section of the drug package insert for Proventil.

Contraindications

This section contains warnings as to particular patients or situations in which you should not use this medication. This section may also give you precautions to follow when administering this drug, or situations that may warrant closer patient monitoring. See Figure 1-4 for the contraindication section of the drug package insert for Proventil.

STOP

& REVIEW

What is the difference between a generic and a brand name? What is the difference between an indication and a contraindication?

Drug Interactions

Often the patient is receiving more than just a single drug, and the potential for two or more drugs to interact exists. Drugs can interact in many ways to change the effects of one or more of the drugs involved. Drugs can interact with each other, as in the case of psyllium and digoxin given concurrently. The digoxin will bind together with the psyllium within the stomach and not be absorbed systemically to the same expected extent as if digoxin were administered separately. Therefore, you may see a reduced effect from the digoxin than anticipated. Another example would be the drug cimetidine, which is known for inhibiting the liver enzymes that metabolize some other drugs. Therefore, patients on cimetidine may show increased effects of other drugs they may be taking, because these drugs may now not be broken down or metabolized as readily.

Drug interactions usually carry a negative connotation among health professionals, but they are not always bad. When two drugs are given together and the result of those two can be summed up by the equation $1 + 1 = 2$, the interaction is **additive.** Additive means that the sum of the effects of two drugs given together is equal to each of them given separately but at the same time. This can be beneficial when, for example, you are treating a patient with high blood pressure and you want to avoid the side effects that may occur with high doses of one drug. By giving lower doses of two drugs and relying on the additive hypotensive effects being equal to the single drug at a higher dose, side effects can sometimes be avoided.

In some cases, giving two drugs together can result in a greater effect than would be expected by giving them together. When two drugs are given together and interact to equal $1 + 1 = 3$, then **synergism** occurs. While mathematically incorrect, this describes the summation of each drug activity exceeding the sum of the two individual drugs. This can be very beneficial in the case of treatment of an infection with combination antibiotics. If you really want to drive mathematicians

INDICATIONS AND USAGE PROVENTIL Inhalation Aerosol is indicated in patients 12 years of age and older, for the prevention and relief of bronchospasm in patients with reversible obstructive airway disease, and for the prevention of exercise-induced bronchospasm.

Figure 1-3 Portion of Drug Package Insert Related to Indications and Usage for the Drug Proventil

Source: Reprinted with permission of Schering Corporation, Kenilworth, NJ. Copyright © 1986, 1993, 1995, 1999, Schering Corporation.

CONTRAINDICATIONS PROVENTIL Inhalation Aerosol is contraindicated in patients with a history of hypersensitivity to albuterol or any of its components.

WARNINGS Deterioration of Asthma: Asthma may deteriorate acutely over a period of hours, or chronically over several days or longer. If the patient needs more doses of PROVENTIL Inhalation Aerosol than usual, this may be a marker of destabilization of asthma and requires re-evaluation of the patient and the treatment regimen, giving special consideration to the possible need for anti-inflammatory treatment, eg, corticosteroids.

Use of Anti-inflammatory Agents: The use of beta-adrenergic agonist bronchodilators alone may not be adequate to control asthma in many patients. Early consideration should be given to adding anti-inflammatory agents, eg, corticosteroids.

Paradoxical Bronchospasm: PROVENTIL Inhalation Aerosol can produce paradoxical bronchospasm, which may be life threatening. If paradoxical bronchospasm occurs, PROVENTIL Inhalation Aerosol should be discontinued immediately and alternative therapy instituted. It should be recognized that paradoxical bronchospasm, when associated with inhaled formulations, frequently occurs with the first use of a new canister or vial.

Cardiovascular Effects: PROVENTIL Inhalation Aerosol, like all other beta-adrenergic agonists, can produce a clinically significant cardiovascular effect in some patients as measured by pulse rate, blood pressure, and/or symptoms. Although such effects are uncommon after administration of PROVENTIL Inhalation Aerosol at recommended doses, if they occur, the drug may need to be discontinued. In addition, beta-agonists have been reported to produce electrocardiogram (ECG) changes, such as flattening of the T wave, prolongation of the QT_c interval, and ST segment depression. The clinical significance of these findings is unknown. Therefore, PROVENTIL Inhalation Aerosol, like all sympathomimetic amines, should be used with caution in patients with cardiovascular disorders, especially coronary insufficiency, cardiac arrhythmias, and hypertension.

Immediate Hypersensitivity Reactions: Immediate hypersensitivity reactions may occur after administration of albuterol, as demonstrated by rare cases of urticaria, angioedema, rash, bronchospasm, anaphylaxis, and oropharyngeal edema.

Figure 1-4 Portion of Drug Package Insert Related to Contraindications for the Drug Proventil

Source: Reprinted with permission of Schering Corporation, Kenilworth, NJ. Copyright © 1986, 1993, 1995, 1999, Schering Corporation.

crazy, **potentiation** can be numerically described as $1 + 0 = 3$. This means that one of the drugs, having no direct effect, increases the response of the other drug, which normally has a lesser effect. You can see how this could be confused with synergism, yet it is not synonymous. See Figure 1-5, which shows the drug interaction section of the drug package insert.

Some drugs are at higher risk for causing drug interactions, and some patients are at higher risk of having drug interactions. There are certain drugs known to be at high risk for causing drug interactions and are even considered to be "red flag drugs." Please see Table 1-1, which lists some major red flag drugs.

Adverse Drug Reactions (ADRs)

Not only can drugs interact with each other, but what about the unintended interactions within the human body? Contrary to the Hippocratic Oath, which says, "First do no harm," at least 5% of reported hospitalizations are the result of an adverse drug reaction (ADR). When patients have unintended side effects from medication, they are having an ADR. Such reactions also occur in patients already in the hospital, which can then result in an increased length of stay. Adverse drug reactions can range from a side effect that is mild and goes away with repeated use or discontinuation to a more severe or life-threatening reaction.

One can easily confuse the terms ADR and drug allergy and use the terms synonymously. ADRs include many things, such as tremors, bronchospasms, headaches, changes in laboratory results of renal function, photosensitivity, etc. An allergy or hypersensitivity is but one example of an ADR, but not all ADRs are allergies. Drug allergies induce a hypersensitivity reaction. This reaction can vary in severity and can be thought of as a continuum. Allergies can be acute and life threatening, as for example in anaphylactic shock, or can be found on the milder end of the continuum, e.g., in the form of a dermatological rash. See Figure 1-6 for the ADR section of the drug insert for Proventil.

CLINICAL PEARL
Just because these common drugs are considered red flag drugs doesn't mean they should not be administered. It simply means more attention should be paid to the potential for their interaction with other drugs the patient may have been prescribed.

STOP & REVIEW

What is the difference between an allergy and an ADR?

Drug Interactions: Other short-acting sympathomimetic aerosol bronchodilators should not be used concomitantly with albuterol. If additional adrenergic drugs are to be administered by any route, they should be used with caution to avoid deleterious cardiovascular effects.

Beta Blockers: Beta-adrenergic receptor blocking agents not only block the pulmonary effect of beta-agonists, such as PROVENTIL Inhalation Aerosol but may produce severe bronchospasm in asthmatic patients. Therefore, patients with asthma should not normally be treated with beta-blockers. However, under certain circumstances, eg, as prophylaxis after myocardial infarction, there may be no acceptable alternatives to the use of beta-adrenergic blocking agents in patients with asthma. In this setting, cardioselective beta-blockers could be considered, although they should be administered with caution.

Diuretics: The ECG changes and/or hypokalemia that may result from the administration of nonpotassium-sparing diuretics (such as loop or thiazide diuretics) can be acutely worsened by beta-agonists, especially when the recom-mended dose of the beta-agonist is exceeded. Although the clinical significance of these effects is not known, caution is advised in the coadministration of beta-agonists with nonpotassium-sparing diuretics.

Digoxin: Mean decreases of 16% to 22% in serum digoxin levels were demonstrated after single dose intravenous and oral administration of albuterol, respectively, to normal volunteers who had received digoxin for 10 days. The clinical significance of this finding for patients with obstructive airway disease who are receiving albuterol and digoxin on a chronic basis is unclear. Nevertheless, it would be prudent to carefully evaluate the serum digoxin levels in patients who are currently receiving digoxin and albuterol.

Monoamine Oxidase Inhibitors or Tricyclic Antidepressants: Albuterol should be administered with extreme caution to patients being treated with monoamine oxidase inhibitors or tricyclic antidepressants, or within 2 weeks of discontinuation of such agents, because the action of albuterol on the vascular system may be potentiated.

Figure 1-5 Portion of Drug Package Insert Related to Drug Interactions for the Drug Proventil

Source: Reprinted with permission of Schering Corporation, Kenilworth, NJ. Copyright © 1986, 1993, 1995, 1999, Schering Corporation.

CLINICAL PEARL

With a recent push to get drugs approved faster and on the market sooner, ADRs are frequently not detected until post-marketing surveillance. Enrolling enough patients in research studies to detect all ADRs before FDA approval is not feasible, so rare ADRs may not be detected until widespread use of a drug in a large population.

Knowledge of ADRs in select populations such as pregnant women would be especially useful. However, enrolling pregnant patients in research is not always ethical. Consequently, information on how drugs adversely affect the fetus is not always known or reported. Absorption, as one of the concepts of pharmacokinetics, to be discussed later in this chapter, needs to be considered when discussing pregnancy and ADRs. When you think of drug absorption for women of child-bearing age, it is safest to assume that any drug given to a pregnant woman may also be given to the baby and may be crossing the fetal placental barrier. The same would apply to lactating women, with drugs passing from breast milk to the baby.

Teratogenicity refers to a drug's potential to damage a fetus in utero when administered to a pregnant woman. The teratogenicity of drugs has a classification system based on risk and limited data available. For example, drugs that have evidence of fetal risk that outweighs any possible benefit are considered "category X" and are absolutely contraindicated. For other drugs, including some for asthma and chronic diseases like epilepsy, the risks to the baby of the mother of not having her disease controlled with a drug can outweigh the risks of drug exposure for the baby. Decisions about drug use in pregnant women need to be made mutually by the patient and healthcare provider.

One of the most serious ADRs with cardiopulmonary implications is a hypersensitivity reaction that can present as acute pulmonary edema, bronchial asthma, pulmonary fibrosis, or respiratory muscle impairment affecting the patient's ability to ventilate. These reactions may have a direct cytotoxic effect on alveolar endothelial cells and can severely impair the vital process of gas exchange. Over 150 drugs have been shown to have pulmonary ADRs, and Table 1-2 lists some examples of drug-induced pulmonary adverse reactions.

Table 1-1 Red Flag Drugs

Drug Name
warfarin
cimetidine
aspirin
phenytoin
theophylline

ADVERSE REACTIONS The adverse reactions of albuterol are similar in nature to those of other sympathomimetic agents, although the incidence of certain cardiovascular effects is less with albuterol.

Percent Incidence of Adverse Reactions in Patients ≥ 12 Years of Age in a 13-Week Clinical Trial* (n=147)

Adverse Event	PROVENTIL Inhalation Aerosol	Isoproterenol Inhaler
Tremor	< 15	< 15
Nausea	< 15	< 15
Tachycardia	10	10
Palpitations	< 10	< 15
Nervousness	< 10	< 15
Increased Blood Pressure	< 5	< 5
Dizziness	< 5	< 5
Heartburn	< 5	< 5

*A 13-week, double-blind study compared albuterol and isoproterenol aerosols in 147 asthmatic patients.

Cases of urticaria, angioedema, rash, bronchospasm, hoarseness, oropharyngeal edema, and arrhythmias (including atrial fibrillation, supraventricular tachycardia, and extrasystoles) have also been reported after the use of inhaled albuterol. In addition, albuterol, like other sympathomimetic agents, can cause adverse reactions such as hypertension, angina, vomiting, vertigo, central nervous system stimulation, insomnia, headache, unusual taste, and drying or irritation of the oropharynx.

Figure 1-6 Portion of Drug Package Insert Related to Adverse Reactions for the Drug Proventil

Source: Reprinted with permission of Schering Corporation, Kenilworth, NJ. Copyright © 1986, 1993, 1995, 1999, Schering Corporation.

There are other pulmonary complications. Angiotensin-converting enzyme (ACE) inhibitors for the heart, as discussed further in Chapter 9, cause cough in up to 15% of patients treated. Plain aspirin you can buy over the counter (OTC) without a prescription can cause bronchospasms in 4% to 20% of patients with asthma. Even topical beta blocker eye drops can be absorbed enough to aggravate chronic obstructive pulmonary disease (COPD).

Dosage and Administration

This section will discuss the standard dose for the medication. In addition, it should elaborate on how the medication is supplied and whether any special treatment or care should be given to preserve its effectiveness. This section describes the route of administration of the drug. The route of administration is such an important topic that it will be discussed separately in the upcoming section. Please see Figure 1-7 for the dosage and administration section of the drug package insert for Proventil.

ROUTES OF ADMINISTRATION (Portal of entry)

One of the first mysteries of pharmacology is the simple and common question of why some drugs are given orally and others are given by a shot or even by other means. Routes of administration of drugs are selected according to the rate of onset of drug activity desired and physiochemical factors that affect drug absorption. For example, some drugs given by mouth undergo what is called a **first-pass effect.** After being absorbed, drugs with a first-pass effect do not go directly into the systemic circulation, but instead go through the liver. In the liver, the drug undergoes a metabolic change. The liver enzymes inactivate some of the drug before it reaches the blood circulation. For this reason, the dosage of an orally administered drug may need to be higher then when it is administered by a route that bypasses

Table 1-2   Drug-Induced Pulmonary ADRs

ADR	*Drug*
Pulmonary edema	heroin
	IV fluids
	epinephrine
	hydrochlorothiazide
	salicylates
Pulmonary fibrosis	amiodarone
	busulfan
	paraquat
Respiratory muscle impairment	alcohol
	narcotics
	sedatives
	penicillamine
Bronchospasm	ACE inhibitors *treats BP*
	beta blockers
	nonsteroidal anti-inflammatory drugs (NSAIDs)

(handwritten margin note: ACE Converting)

the liver, such as the intravenous route. Drugs given **parenterally** (via injection) can avoid the first-pass effect, which explains why doses of the same drug vary depending on the route of administration, e.g., oral propranolol 80 mg versus 1 mg of the drug intravenously (IV). These two routes with very different dosages will produce about the same response.

Drugs' routes are also selected based on how compliant the patient is in regularly taking prescribed medication. For example, depot formulations of drugs given intramuscularly for noncompliant schizophrenic patients every two weeks can keep their disease controlled, whereas they may not consistently take their prescribed oral medications. Depot formulations are drugs that are slowly released once administered, so they only need to be given every week or so, depending on the drug. Some depot drugs are formulated in oil, which allows for slow release into the bloodstream. Depot birth control is an alternative for women who do not wish to get pregnant but may be less compliant with other forms of birth control.

Enteral Routes

Enteral routes of drug absorption are via the gastrointestinal tract for systemic purposes and include the oral (PO), sublingual (SL), nasogastric (NG) tube, and rectal routes. The oral route is usually considered the most common and convenient route. **Sublingual** drugs are absorbed quickly, owing to the rich vasculature under the tongue, which explains why this route is used for quick relief of cardiac chest pain with nitroglycerin. Rectal drug administration can be very effective for those patients ordered "nothing by mouth" (NPO) or those who are vomiting or unable to swallow oral medications. Patients who are receiving enteral nutrition via the gastric tube will frequently be given drugs through that tube as well, as long as drug stability and compatibility in mixing with foods and liquids are taken into consideration.

Parenteral Routes *any route other than the intestine*

Parenteral routes include the injectable routes. This can be through central lines, intra-arterial, intravenous (IV), intramuscular (IM), and subcutaneous routes. Drugs given parenterally go right into the blood stream, and absorption is rapid, so this route is desirable for emergency situations when an immediate response is needed. Drugs that are insoluble and cannot be dissolved cannot be given intravenously. Some drugs cannot be administered together intravenously because of physical incompatibilities. There are thick

(handwritten note: Not all drug can be mixed.)

DOSAGE AND ADMINISTRATION   *Treatment of acute episodes of bronchospasm or prevention of asthmatic symptoms:* The usual dosage for adults and children 12 years of age and older is 2 inhalations repeated every 4 to 6 hours; in some patients, 1 inhalation every 4 hours may be sufficient. More frequent administration or a larger number of inhalations is not recommended. For maintenance therapy or prevention of exacerbation of bronchospasm, 2 inhalations, 4 times a day should be sufficient.

The use of PROVENTIL Inhalation Aerosol can be continued as medically indicated to control recurring bouts of bronchospasm. During this time most patients gain optimal benefit from regular use of the inhaler. Safe usage for periods extending over several years has been documented.

If a previously effective dosage regimen fails to provide the usual response, this may be a marker of destabilization of asthma and requires re-evaluation of the patient and treatment regimen, giving special consideration to the possible need for anti-inflammatory treatment, eg, corticosteroids.

Exercise-Induced Bronchospasm Prevention: The usual dosage for adults and children 12 years and older is 2 inhalations, 15 minutes prior to exercise. For treatment, see above.

It is recommended to "test spray" PROVENTIL Inhalation Aerosol into the air before using for the first time and in cases where the aerosol has not been used for a prolonged period of time.

HOW SUPPLIED   PROVENTIL Inhalation Aerosol, 17.0 g canister contains 200 metered inhalations, box of one (NDC 0085-0614-02). Each actuation delivers 100 mcg of albuterol from the valve and 90 mcg of albuterol from the mouthpiece. Each canister is supplied with a yellow plastic actuator with orange dust cap, and Patient's Instructions.

PROVENTIL Inhalation Aerosol REFILL canister, 17.0 g, contains 200 metered inhalations, with Patient's Instructions; box of one (NDC 0085-0614-03).

The correct amount of medication in each inhalation cannot be assured after 200 actuations from the 17.0 g canister even though the canister is not completely empty. The canister should be discarded when the labeled number of actuations have been used.

Store between 15° and 30°C (59° and 86°F). Failure to use the product within this temperature range may result in improper dosing. For optimal results, the canister should be at room temperature before use. Shake well before using.

PROVENTIL Inhalation Aerosol canister should be used only with the actuator provided. The yellow actuator should not be used with other aerosol medication canisters.

Note: The indented statement below is required by the Federal government's Clean Air Act for all products containing or manufactured with chlorofluorocarbons (CFCs).

Warning: Contains dichlorodifluoromethane (CFC-12) and trichloromonofluoromethane (CFC-11), substances which harm public health and the environment by destroying ozone in the upper atmosphere.

A notice similar to the above WARNING has been placed in the "Patient's Instructions for Use" portion of this package insert under the Environmental Protection Agency's (EPA's) regulations. The patient's warning states that the patient should consult his or her physician if there are questions about alternatives.

Schering®

Schering Corporation
Kenilworth, NJ 07033 USA

Rev. 5/00   19529339

Copyright © 1986, 1993, 1995, 1999, Schering Corporation. All rights reserved.

Figure 1-7 Portion of Drug Package Insert Related to Dosage and Administration for the Drug Proventil

Source: Reprinted with permission of Schering Corporation, Kenilworth, NJ. Copyright © 1986, 1993, 1995, 1999, Schering Corporation.

reference books dedicated to describing which drugs are compatible with each other in solution.

The rate for IM drug absorption depends on the formulation used. Clear or water-based solutions have a rapid effect. Suspensions that are cloudy or oil-based have a slower rate of absorption. Parenteral administration carries with it the risk of infection, pain, or local irritation.

Other Routes

Topical drugs are administered onto the skin or mucous membranes. Examples include nitroglycerin ointment and skin creams. Inhalation drug delivery is a form of topical delivery to the lungs that helps avoid systemic side effects. Inhalation drug therapy or medicated aerosol therapy delivers micron-sized aerosol particles through the bronchial tree to the lungs, providing for rapid absorption. Local administration of a drug to the lungs is advantageous because of their large surface area and location close to the pulmonary circulation. It is also so important in cardiopulmonary pharmacotherapy that it deserves a whole chapter (Chapter 4) on the subject.

LEARNING HINT

Parenteral is a term derived from the Greek *para,* "apart from," plus *enteron,* "intestine," and technically means any route outside of the oral and intestinal tract. Clinically, it refers to the injectable routes.

Table 1-3 Administration Routes

Route	Major Points	Examples
Oral (PO)	May be enteric coated, sustained release, tablet, capsule, some crushable, some lose their potency when crushed—most convenient and economical	most prescribed drugs and over-the-counter (OTC) medications
Sublingual (SL)	Quick onset with good salivary flow	nitroglycerin
Rectal	Can be more convenient when patients can't swallow (nausea/NPO)	anti-nausea medications
NG tube	Careful of drug stability and clogging up the tube	nutritional feedings
Intravenous (IV)	Quick onset, emergency situations, and long-term infusions	emergency meds
Intramuscular (IM)	Once it's injected, it's there to stay, even if side effects occur	iron
Transdermal	Easier to remember, because dosing is less frequent	nicotine or nitroglycerin patches
Inhalational	Less systemic side effects, requires coordination	metered dose inhalers (MDIs)

Transdermal delivery of drug occurs through a skin patch that allows the drug to be released slowly; this provides for sustained blood levels throughout the day without the patient having to remember to take medications. In the busy lives of people, drugs need to be dosed so they will not interfere with lifestyle, which may enhance compliance and keep drugs effective. See Table 1-3 for a summary of administration routes.

PHARMACOKINETICS

Pharmacokinetics means the movement (kinesis) of the drug throughout our body. Pharmacokinetics is the study of what happens to the drug from the time it is put into the body until it has left the body. Pharmacokinetic principles help determine drug dosage in terms of amount, duration, and frequency. Pharmacokinetics includes the following processes: absorption, distribution, metabolism, and elimination of a drug. Absorption occurs when the drug passes from its administration site into plasma. Distribution determines where the drug goes once it is within the body. For any drug to work, it must be absorbed and distributed to an active site. Metabolism refers to biotransformation, in which drugs are converted to a water-soluble form for elimination. Elimination of a drug occurs by hepatic metabolism or renal excretion. We will break each of these components of pharmacokinetics down and talk about each in a different section.

LEARNING HINT

Pharmacokinetics is often confused with pharmacodynamics. Pharmacokinetics is what the body does to the drug. Pharmacodynamics, on the other hand, is what the drug does to the body and will be discussed shortly.

Absorption

A drug must first be disintegrated or dissolved before it can be absorbed into the systemic circulation. The rate-limiting step in absorption is disintegration. If a drug doesn't have to disintegrate and is already in a solution, it will work quicker. Injections of drugs (IM, subcutaneous and intradermal) are absorbed from body tissues, with only intravenous injections completely bypassing the step of absorption.

But not all of the drug may reach the bloodstream. **Bioavailability** measures the amount of drug that has been absorbed into the circulation. Bioavailability is influenced by drug solubility, dosage form, route of administration, pH values, and salt form, to name a few. One example of this concept is how the pH (measure of the acidity or alkalinity) of different parts of the gastrointestinal (GI) tract can affect the absorption and thus bioavailability of the drug. Some drugs are permanently charged, but most are weak acids or bases whose ionization is affected by pH. In other words, the drug can exist in either its ionized or its nonionized form depending upon the pH values of surrounding fluids. The important aspect of ionization is that the nonionized (no charge or neutral) drug is absorbed through membranes where it can be active, and the ionized (charged) form of the drug is not. The stomach is very acidic at pH 1 to pH 2, whereas the intestines are about pH 4 to pH 5, and further along the tract, the alkalinity increases. This means that drugs such as aspirin, which are more in their non-ionized form at acidic pHs, would be better absorbed in acidic environments such as the stomach. Alkaline drugs such as quinidine become more nonionized in alkalinic environments and are therefore better absorbed as they progress through the GI tract.

Ultimately drugs must be absorbed through membranes to reach their action site. Drugs can pass through some membranes but not all. Different mechanisms of drugs passing through membranes include passive diffusion, facilitated diffusion, active transport, and passage through ion channels. These transfer processes will be discussed in chapters where they are pertinent.

CLINICAL PEARL

Specially coated (enteric) tablets are designed to resist being absorbed in the stomach, where they may be irritating to the stomach lining.

STOP & REVIEW

If you were in pain, would you rather have a codeine tablet or solution, and why?

CLINICAL PEARL

The rate of absorption can be proportional to rate of blood flow at the site. Sometimes drugs are administered in combination with epinephrine, which is a vasoconstrictor. When epinephrine is given with a local anesthetic, such as lidocaine, the decreased blood flow from vasoconstriction keeps much of the drug at the desired site and may therefore decrease the risk of side effects systemically when just a local effect is desired.

IV drug absorption differs if the drug is given as a continuous infusion (IV drip) or as an intermittent dose (injected IV shot or bolus). A continuous infusion gives a regulated consistent dosage over time, often referred to as a **steady state** in drug concentration in the plasma. An intermittent intravenous dose would have more peaks and troughs in drug concentrations (see Figure 1-8).

For some drugs, blood-level lab testing is available to tell us whether an individual patient has the appropriate amount of drug in the blood to be effective or toxic. The effective blood level is considered the therapeutic blood level and has a defined **therapeutic range.** Below this level, the drug is likely less effective, and above this level, toxicity may result (see Table 1-4, which lists common drugs that have blood-level lab testing available).

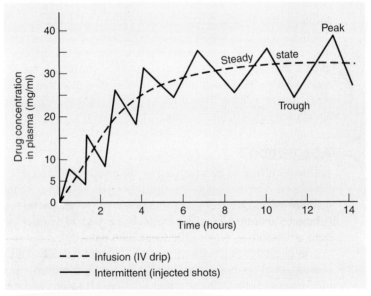

Figure 1-8 Intermittent and Infusion Dosing

Table 1-4 Drugs with Blood-Level Tests
and Therapeutic Ranges

Drug Name
theophylline
digoxin
phenytoin
lithium
carbamazepine
gentamicin
vancomycin

Distribution

After absorption, the drug is distributed in the body. The major vehicle for distribution is via the bloodstream. As mentioned in the absorption section, the drug must also distribute through membranes to reach certain active pharmacologic sites called receptors. Different drugs are able to distribute to different locations. The blood flow, fat or water solubility of the drug, and **protein binding** influence drug distribution.

Protein binding occurs when portions of the drug are bound to proteins within the bloodstream, such as albumin, and are thus unable to bind with active pharmacologic sites to have a desired effect. For example, if a person has low serum albumin (i.e., malnourishment), there is not as much protein for the drug to bind to; therefore, much of the drug will be free within the bloodstream. Since free unbound drug is active drug, patients with low albumin may have higher blood levels of free active drug than someone with normal albumin and will show a greater drug response.

Drugs differ in their percentage of protein binding. The PDR includes information on protein binding percentages. Knowledge of protein binding is important, because protein binding displacement is one mechanism of how drugs interact with each other. If there are only so many proteins for a drug to bind to and another drug is added to a patient whose proteins are already bound by a previous drug, the drugs will compete for placement on the protein. The one that is not bound is going to be free to find an active receptor site.

www.prenhall.com/colbert

A picture is worth a thousand words. By seeing proteins being displaced, you will be able to understand drug binding. Go to the Web to see animations of this protein binding and displacement.

Volume of distribution (Vd) describes the areas in the body where drugs can be distributed. Fat-soluble (lipophilic) drugs pass through fat easier than water. Fat-soluble drugs have an increased effect in patients with more fat, and water-soluble drugs have an increased effect in those with larger water compartments. Fat and water compartments change with age and are one explanation for why different doses may be needed in young and elderly. For example, the sedative diazepam (Valium) is a fat-soluble drug. Obese patients could be sedated longer on a given dose of diazepam than lean patients.

Metabolism

After a drug has been absorbed and distributed, metabolism occurs, because the body works to get rid of anything foreign. Before a drug can be excreted, it usually has to be metabolized so that it becomes more water soluble and more able to leave the body via urine, feces, or sweat. The drug gets broken down into several components or metabolites. Some metabolites of a drug are active and others are not. Metabolism may be by any of the following examples of chemical reactions: oxidation, conjugation, acetylation, or glucuronidation, to name a few.

One of the major organs for drug metabolism is the liver. The liver has a microsomal drug oxidation system called the cytochrome P-450 system, which is responsible for metabolizing many drugs. These enzymes can be induced (increased in activity) or inhibited (decreased in activity). This is a common mechanism for drug interactions. Enzyme induction may explain why patients who frequently drink alcohol are more tolerant of alcohol effects, because the alcohol may be metabolized quicker.

Drug doses can change depending on whether the liver enzymes are inducing or inhibiting, and there is no easy way to know other than to be aware of drugs that affect enzymes. See Table 1-5 for drugs that affect liver enzymes.

There is no good way to predict the liver's ability to metabolize drugs in a patient. Some patients genetically lack enzymes to metabolize certain drugs. In addition, liver-function lab tests do not correlate with the body's ability to metabolize a drug, and liver drug elimination cannot be quantitatively assessed. Liver disease may indicate that a particular drug should not be used or should be dosed differently. Because the liver is a site of drug metabolism, it is also an organ susceptible to drug-induced liver toxicity. Over 600 drugs have been associated with drug-induced liver toxicity. Alcohol and acetaminophen are two common ones, especially when used in combination.

Elimination

The last component of pharmacokinetics is elimination. Some drugs are eliminated after they are metabolized, and others are excreted unchanged in the urine. Yet others are eliminated in feces or even through the skin or pulmonary system. Inhalational anesthesia requires that the gas pass from inspired air to the blood and brain. Drug action is terminated when it is eliminated in the lungs.

Renal excretion rate is affected by glomerular filtration, tubular secretion, and tubular reabsorption. Impaired renal function can prolong the effects of drugs, because they will not be readily eliminated and remain longer within the system.

Because drugs can be excreted in the urine, urine testing is becoming more commonly used in the workplace. Urine testing can be used to screen patients for drug abuse or for poisoning identification. Depending on whether the drug is fat or water soluble can influence how long after ingestion it is detected in the urine. Urine testing and even saliva testing are useful to monitor patients in drug rehabilitation programs. Tests differ in sen-

CLINICAL PEARL

Some races have an increased frequency of a genetic deficiency of the enzyme that metabolizes alcohol and are therefore more susceptible to its effects. The topic of research that studies genetic differences in drug response is called pharmacogenetics.

CLINICAL PEARL

The alcohol breath test is used to assess intoxication because ethanol is excreted in expired air. Drug urine screens in the workplace are used to detect past and current medication use on the basis of excretion of drug metabolites (breakdown products) in the urine.

Table 1-5 Drugs That Affect Liver Enzymes

Inducers	Inhibitors
Barbiturates	Cimetidine
Phenytoin	Disulfuram
Carbamazepine	Allopurinol
Rifampin	Influenza vaccine

sitivity and specificity. False positives can occur or tests can become positive for inhalants if the person tested has simply been present in a room where others were inhaling a drug.

Why would patients with kidney disease or decreased kidney function, as in the elderly, be prescribed lower doses of a medication?

Now that we have completed the discussion of pharmacokinetics, see Figure 1-9, which relates its four phases.

PHARMACODYNAMICS

how the drug moves throughout the body

As stated earlier, **pharmacodynamics** is what the drug does to the body. Once a drug is absorbed and distributed, the drug action requires drug presence at a particular type of **receptor.** Receptors are targets for drugs; they are molecules located on the cell surface. This is where the action takes place. They are not, however, the only target for drugs, because drugs also bind to carrier molecules and ion channels, for example, and each of these will be discussed in upcoming chapters.

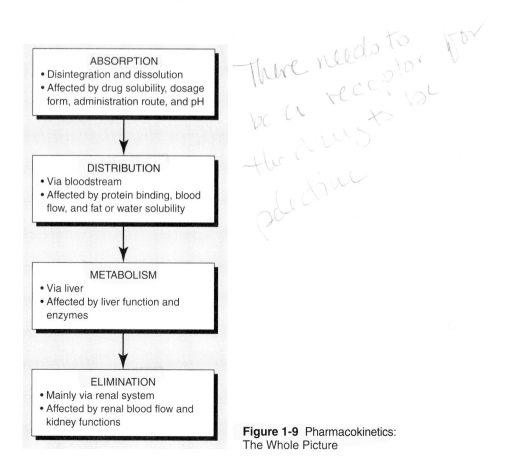

There needs to be a receptor for the drug to be effective

ABSORPTION
• Disintegration and dissolution
• Affected by drug solubility, dosage form, administration route, and pH

DISTRIBUTION
• Via bloodstream
• Affected by protein binding, blood flow, and fat or water solubility

METABOLISM
• Via liver
• Affected by liver function and enzymes

ELIMINATION
• Mainly via renal system
• Affected by renal blood flow and kidney functions

Figure 1-9 Pharmacokinetics: The Whole Picture

Selectivity

There are only so many receptors per cell and only certain kinds of receptors on different cells. Since most drugs produce several effects, **selectivity** refers to the extent to which a drug acts at one specific site or receptor. The more specific a drug can be on a particular cell or tissue, the more useful it is. Unfortunately no drug acts with complete selectivity, which is why side effects occur. If you give a drug that kills a microorganism but it's not selective enough to avoid killing the patient, then the drug is not selective enough to be useful. Another example is the search for drugs that kill only cancer cells but not all living cells.

A drug produces a particular effect by combining chemically with a receptor upon which it acts. When a drug binds to a receptor, one of the following can happen:

(1) an ion channel is opened or closed
   example: calcium-channel blockers to inhibit excess calcium from entering myocardial tissue
(2) biochemical messengers are activated that initiate chemical reactions
   example: beta adrenergic bronchodilators increasing levels of cyclic 3,5-AMP, which causes smooth muscle relaxation
(3) a normal cellular function is turned on or off
   example: antibiotics that inhibit specific cellular functions that result in cellular death

Lock-and-Key Receptor Theory

A simplified description of interactions between drugs and receptors is the lock-and-key analogy. If the drug doesn't fit the receptor, no activity can occur. For example, current pain medications that have been derived from chemical variations of opium capitalize on this theory. Scientists worked with the lock-and-key theory to identify what parts of the chemical structure fit the receptor to cause analgesia and what parts cause side effects and dependence and adjusted the chemistry to make more useful drugs. See Figure 1-10, which demonstrates the lock-and-key theory.

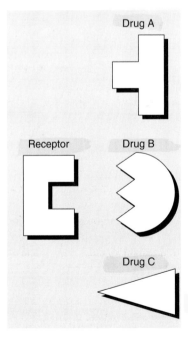

Figure 1-10 The Lock-and-Key Receptor Theory

Racemic Mixtures

Some drugs are commercially available as a **racemic** mixture, meaning one that contains two different isomers. Isomers have the exact same chemical components, only bonded differently, and can be thought of as chemical mirror images. In essence, this means there are two chemical components, even though we consider the mixture as only one drug. Each isomer may have different activity. An example is racemic epinephrine, which is made up of an L and a D isomer. The L isomer of epinephrine is 15 times more active than the D isomer. Having two isomers in one drug makes it harder to predict drug response than having an isolated isomer. Racemic epinephrine is about half as potent as the commercial preparation of epinephrine and results in less physiologic effect. Isomer isolation is the target of a lot of pharmaceutical research, and the bronchodilator racemic mixture of levalbuterol will be further discussed in Chapter 5.

Agonists Versus Antagonists

The lock-and-key receptor theory explains effects of chemicals on the biological system. Drugs bind to cellular receptors, which starts biochemical reactions that can change the cells' physiology. The same explanation applies whether chemicals are endogenous (physiologically produced) or exogenous (pharmacologically administered). However, drugs can bind with the receptor site and activate *or* block a response.

For example, both **agonists** and **antagonists** can bind to a receptor; however, they are different in what they do once combined. Agonists are drugs with affinity for a receptor that cause a specific response. Affinity is the strength of binding between a drug and a receptor. Antagonists are also drugs with affinity for a receptor but have very little or no response when combined. Agonists activate the receptors. Antagonists combine at the same site but don't cause activation of the receptor. Drug antagonism can occur when the effect of one drug is lessened or blocked completely in the presence of another. An example of chemical antagonism is when protamine is used to neutralize the anticoagulant effects of heparin by forming an inactive heparin–protamine complex. This is desirable in cases of hemorrhage due to heparin overdoses for treatment of blood clots.

Drugs within a class differ in their affinity or likelihood of interacting with a receptor. If all drugs had to do were to occupy a receptor to produce a pharmacological effect, then all drugs acting on a receptor would produce the same effect. The explanation for why this isn't true is intrinsic activity, which can best be explained with numbers. Intrinsic activity is a measure of a drug's effectiveness at causing a response, or efficacy of the drug at the receptor. For example, a drug with an intrinsic activity of 1 is a full agonist. A drug with an intrinsic activity of 0.5 is a partial agonist. An antagonist has intrinsic activity of 0 but does have affinity to bind. Both full and partial agonists want to bind to the receptor and thus have affinity, but a full agonist would be more efficacious and cause a greater response.

Potency

Drug potency refers to the amount of drug required to produce the response desired. When the response is measured against drug concentrations, dose–response relationship can be seen (please see Figure 1-11). Dose–response relationships are important in understanding how to titrate drugs to reach maximum efficacy. The lower the dose required to provide a certain effect, the more potent the drug is. Notice in Figure 1-11, drug A and drug C are more potent (require less of a dose for the desired response) than drugs B and D, respectively.

Efficacy refers to the maximum effect a drug can produce. Unfortunately, the assumption that responses produced are directly proportional to occupancy at receptors is not valid. Just because you are sitting in class occupying a chair doesn't mean you'll learn something. Likewise, just because a drug is occupying a receptor doesn't mean it will produce a therapeutic

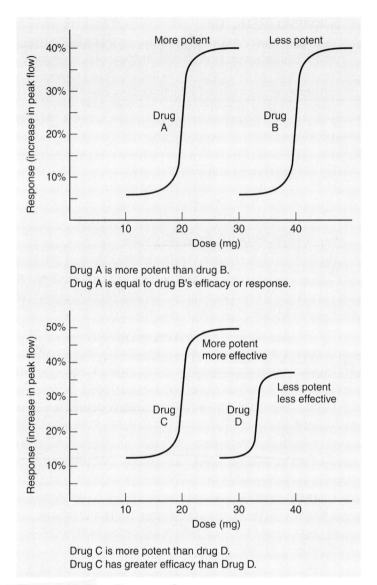

Drug A is more potent than drug B.
Drug A is equal to drug B's efficacy or response.

Drug C is more potent than drug D.
Drug C has greater efficacy than Drug D.

Figure 1-11 Dose-Response Curves

effect. Notice in the figure that drugs A and B have equal efficacy, whereas drug C has greater efficacy than drug D.

Tolerance

A common question of patients is "Will this drug wear out in effectiveness?" The relationship between concentration and effect can change over time. Drugs can lose effectiveness because receptors change, are lost, are more readily degraded, or simply adapt. Receptor adaptation can be good and may explain why people get tolerant to side effects of drugs. However, receptor **tolerance** will mean that an increased amount of a drug is needed to produce the same effect.

After a cell or tissue has been exposed to a drug for a time period, it may become less responsive to further stimulation by that agent. This is called **densensitization.** An example of a drug class with which this occurs is the sympathomimetic drugs discussed in Chapter 5. The clinical significance is that desensitization may limit therapeutic response to sympathomimetic drugs when they are needed. There are several mechanisms involved in desensitization, one of which is downregulation. Downregulation of beta receptors is a well-known phenomenon that will be discussed in Chapter 5.

Drug **dependence** is a related topic and can be physiological or psychological. Do you need your coffee in the morning or do you "need!" your coffee in the morning? If a patient has withdrawal symptoms when a drug is discontinued, they are dependent. Even laxatives can cause dependence so that normal bowel movements may not occur after chronic stimulant laxative use.

Half-Life

Once a drug is absorbed, attaches to a receptor and is distributed it's important to know how long it will be in the body. By definition, the **half-life** ($T_{1/2}$) is the amount of time it takes for the concentration of the drug to decrease by half once administered within the body. Some drugs have short half-lives, meaning they will not stay in the body long. Some drugs have long half-lives and remain in the body for longer periods of time. Dosing frequency may be different for drugs with short or long half-lives, and therefore half-life is also used to determine when a drug administered over time has reached **steady state,** or its maximum concentration in the body. Liver disease can increase the half-life of some drugs, thereby causing them to "stay around longer" and have greater than expected effects. Table 1-6 lists some common drug half-lives to show you the variability that exists.

Because it can take a while to reach steady state and the patient may need immediate drug levels, **loading doses** of drugs such as the antibiotic gentamicin or the antiseizure medication phenytoin are frequently used. Loading doses are given at a higher dose than a **maintenance dose** to more quickly achieve desired blood concentrations. Loading doses are used if a patient hasn't been on a drug before or when the receptors need to be saturated quickly for a quick response. After the initial loading dose is administered, smaller doses (maintenance doses) are needed to maintain adequate therapeutic levels.

Poisonings/Toxicity

All healthcare professionals need to be aware of drug overdoses and poisonings. The study of drugs as they relate to poisonings and environmental toxins is called **toxicology.** Estimates are 2 to 5 million poisonings a year, with the majority occurring in children less than 6 years old. Adult poisoning may be intentional or occupational. Since reporting of poisonings is voluntary, the frequency of the problem is unknown.

Poison Control Centers operate regionally to provide information on poisonings with drugs, chemicals, household products, personal care products, and plants, as well as food poisonings and animal toxins. Information is usually provided on a 24-hour basis and includes management protocols. Childproof medication containers are one way to avoid

Table 1-6 Drug Half-Lives

Drug	Half-Life
Digoxin	30–60 hrs
Aminoglycosides	2–4 hrs
Theophylline	7–9 hrs
Albuterol	2–5 hrs
Warfarin	0.5–3 days
Heparin	1–2 hrs

(handwritten annotations: "Comiclen - Bloodthinner", "Heparin - Levinox", "Zopenex 6-8 hrs")

poisonings. Since timing after ingestion can affect outcome, all families should have one ounce of ipecac syrup (an emetic) to promote vomiting if indicated in a poisoning emergency.

Emetics (agents that induce vomiting) may be absolutely contraindicated, as in the case of ingestions of caustic agents, so they should not be used until advised by a medical professional. If a product such as a drain cleanser is caustic on ingestion, it can cause even more damage as it is brought back up through the esophagus or aspirated into the lungs. Another treatment of poisoning may include decreasing absorption by giving an adsorbent to bind with the toxic agent and inducing catharsis (bowel movements).

Activated charcoal is used to prevent absorption of some drugs, such as theophylline overdoses. While emesis can remove theophylline from the stomach if induced within one hour of ingestion, activated charcoal is effective any time after theophylline exposure. Other drugs have specific antidotes to antagonize the effects of poisoning, e.g., n-acetyl-cysteine for acetaminophen (Tylenol) poisoning and naloxone (Narcan) for narcotic overdoses presenting as respiratory depression.

A term commonly used when discussing drug safety and toxicity is **therapeutic index** (TI). The therapeutic index of a drug is the ratio between the minimum effective dose and the average maximum tolerated dose. Therapeutic index gives you a quantitative measure of a drug's safety. It does not take into account the variability in drug response among individuals and is based on animal toxicity data. A drug with a low therapeutic index (ratio near 1) would potentially be able to cause more adverse effects than a drug with a high therapeutic index, because the minimum effective dose is very close to the maximum tolerated dose. The therapeutic index is not really a useful guide to drug safety in clinical use and is rarely cited as a number.

PRESCRIPTION ORDERS

All drugs require a properly authorized prescription order. Hospitals may have protocols, standing orders, or established therapy guidelines for treating a particular disease. These protocols or guidelines may exist for cost containment reasons or for quality-of-care issues. This kind of medication order requires just as much monitoring for adverse reactions and efficacy as any order, if not more. Please see Figure 1-12 for the components of a medication order.

Frequently, medical abbreviations are used within medication orders. You must familiarize yourself with these abbreviations. For a review of common medical abbreviations pertinent to drug therapy, see Table 1-7.

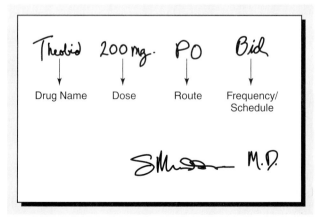

Drug Name   Dose   Route   Frequency/Schedule

Figure 1-12 Sample Medication Order

Table 1-7   Abbreviations

Abbreviation	Meaning	Abbreviation	Meaning
ac	before meals	prn	as needed
bid	twice daily	q.	every
caps	capsule	q.h.	every hour
cc	cubic centimeter	qid	four times daily
dil	dilute	qod	every other day
fl or fld	fluid	q.d.	every day
hs	at bedtime	q.2h.	every 2 hours
IM	intramuscular	q.3h.	every 3 hours
IV	intravenous	q.4h.	every 4 hours
L	liter	sig	directions
ml	milliliters	stat	immediately
NPO	nothing by mouth	tab	tablet or tablets
pc	after meals	tid	three times daily
PO	by mouth	ut dict	as directed

Many pharmacies have formularies. This means that they only stock or dispense select drugs from pharmacological classes. A **formulary** is a list of the drugs available at a particular healthcare system. Committees that make decisions on what drugs to stock may also be involved in deciding what drugs should be prescribed and when.

COMMON SENSE RULES

Medication
patient
dose
route
time

There are some classic safeguards that should be used to ensure accurate medication administration. The basics are known as the five "rights"—the right drug, dose, patient, time, and route. Before administering a drug, tell the patient the name and use of the drug. This is good patient education but also allows you to double-check the medication order if the patient gives you an unexpected response. The right dose may require calculations, or with the widespread use of unit dose, medications may be individually wrapped and labeled as a single dose. Although the right patient may seem obvious in the inpatient setting, the authors have seen confused patients in the wrong bed or answering yes to someone else's name. Therefore, *always check the patient's wrist tag*. Medication timing may be routine at some institutions but sometimes may need to be individualized for patient response and application of pharmacological principles. Route is important, because not all products have the same stability, and dose is influenced by route as well as speed of onset. Giving an IV injection of a product that is not soluble and was intended for IM route only can be very dangerous.

It is wise to administer only medications prepared personally or by the pharmacist. Always check the drug stability and expiration date. Check for allergies and chart administration and results as promptly as possible. In this day and age, it's also important to be aware of your legal responsibilities in drug administration at the state and local or institutional level.

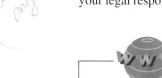

Don't trust anyone

www.prenhall.com/colbert

"To err is human," but to err in drug administration can be very dangerous. Go to the Web site to learn more about drug medication errors and what causes them.

Can you describe the five "rights" of medication administration?

SUMMARY

This chapter has two major goals. The first goal is to help you begin to feel comfortable reading drug information literature and to understand the organization and meaning of its content. The second goal is to familiarize you with what the body does when a drug is introduced (pharmacokinetics) and what the drug does to the body (pharmacodynamics).

The earlier you are introduced to general principles of pharmacology, the more time you will have to apply them to drug classifications in the chapters that follow. It's never too soon to understand the risks of drugs and the responsibility that goes with drug administration. By being able to explain the rationale for drug use and possible side effects, you can be an effective member of the healthcare team. This chapter has provided you with a sense of the need for life-long learning with the dynamic topic of pharmacotherapy.

REVIEW QUESTIONS

1. The drug name Proventil is a *(Albuterol) Brand Name*
   (a) chemical name
   (b) generic name
   (c) trade name
   (d) semi-official name

2. The process of absorption, distribution, metabolism, and elimination in the body is called:
   (a) disintegration
   (b) bioavailability
   (c) pharmacokinetics
   (d) pharmacotherapy

3. A 42-year-old patient is in the hospital recovering from an asthma exacerbation. When the nurse brings him his oral medication, he says that it looks different than his white pill at home. What could explain this?
   (a) different manufacturer of the drug
   (b) drug error
   (c) patient confusion
   (d) change in dose
   (e) all of the above

4. After a drug is absorbed, which factors can affect drug distribution?
   (a) protein binding
   (b) fat solubility
   (c) water solubility
   (d) all of the above
   (e) none of the above

5. Match the following prescription abbreviations with their definition.
   (a) qid 5 (1) as needed
   (b) prn 1 (2) intramuscular
   (c) IM 2 (3) nothing by mouth
   (d) hs 4 (4) bedtime
   (e) NPO 3 (5) four times daily

6. Define and explain the importance of the half-life of a drug.

7. Which route(s) of administration would you recommend in the following scenarios?
   (a) A home care patient has severe nausea.
   (b) A rapid onset is needed to treat an emergency in the hospital.
   (c) A patient is NPO.
   (d) Patient has a chronic respiratory inflammatory disease that requires corticosteroids that have many systemic side effects.
   (e) An executive smoker is trying to quit and needs nicotine replacement therapy.

8. Explain the relationship between pH and drug absorption.

9. Contrast agonists and antagonists.
10. What are the four phases of new drug testing and approval by the FDA?
11. Contrast the drug interactions of synergism, additive and potentiation.
12. Explain this statement: "All allergies or hypersensitive reactions are ADRs, but not all ADRs are allergies."

GLOSSARY

additive   two drugs whose sum effect when given together is equal to the effect from each given separately but at the same time.

agonist   drug that activates its receptor upon binding.

antagonist   drug that binds to its receptor without activating it.

bioavailability   fraction of drug dose that reaches the systemic circulation.

dependence   drug use that would result in withdrawal symptoms on discontinuation; can be psychological or physiological.

desensitization   loss of tissue responsiveness that can occur with drug exposure.

disease management   all inclusive management of a patient's disease.

enteral route   the route comprising oral, sublingual, nasogastric, or rectal routes of drug absorption.

first-pass effect   elimination of drug that happens after administration but before it reaches the systemic circulation.

formulary   list of drugs stocked by the pharmacy.

half-life   time it takes for the drug concentration to fall to 50% in the body.

loading dose   dose that is first administered to rapidly achieve a therapeutic concentration.

maintenance dose   doses given to keep a drug at a therapeutic level in the blood.

parenteral route   the route comprising routes that bypass the alimentary tract; injectable.

pharmacodynamics   actions of the drug on the body.

pharmacokinetics   actions of the body on the drug.

pharmacology   study of drugs and their action on the body.

pharmacotherapy   application of drug therapy to disease treatment.

potentiation   the effect of two drugs given together when one drug has no effect but increases the response of the other drug, which normally has a lesser effect.

protein binding   refers to sites such as albumin where the drug is connected or bound and inactive; influences drug distribution.

racemic   refers to drugs that contain two chemical components that may have different activity.

receptor   target for drugs to act on.

selectivity   extent to which a drug acts on one specific site or receptor.

steady state   state reached when input of the drug is equal to the output of drug over the dosing interval.

sublingual   refers to drug absorption under the tongue.

synergism   the result when two drugs are given together and their effect is greater than the effect from each given separately.

teratogenic   having an effect on prenatal development that results in abnormal structure or function.

therapeutic index   quantitative measure of a drug's safety.

therapeutic range   range of drug concentration in the body in which the drug produces the desired response.

therapeutics   study of drugs used to cure, treat, or prevent disease.

tolerance   decrease in susceptibility to a drug's effect from continued use.

toxicology   study of drugs as it relates to poisonings and environmental toxins.

transdermal   delivered through the skin.

www.prenhall.com/colbert

Use the address above to access the free, interactive Companion Web site created specifically for this textbook. Enhance your studying by viewing videos and animations, answering practice quiz questions, and reviewing an audio glossary and much more concerning Chapter 1.

CHAPTER 2

The Metric System and Drug Dosage Calculations

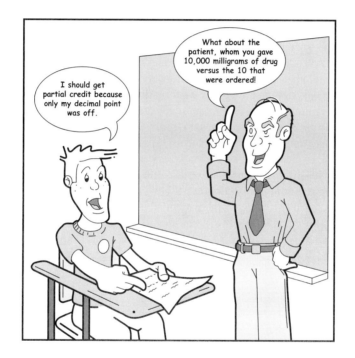

OBJECTIVES

Upon completion of this chapter you will be able to

- Define key terms relevant to drug dosage calculations
- Perform conversions of units of measurement within the Metric System
- Perform conversions between units of measurements in the Metric and English System
- Calculate strength of solutions in percentage and ratio forms
- Perform drug dosage calculations

ABBREVIATIONS

BSA	Body surface area	d	deci
c	centi	g	gram
cc	cubic centimeter	gtts	drops

K	kilo	SI	Système International
l	liter	U	units
μ	micro	USCS	United States Customary
m	meter		System
m	milli	w/v	weight/volume
mg	milligram	v/v	volume/volume
ml	milliliter		

INTRODUCTION

Whereas Chapter 1 gave you the basics of "pharmacology language," this chapter will give you the "mathematical language" of medicine. Many respiratory drugs form aerosols from various percentage strength or ratio solutions that are then administered via the inhalation route. In addition, many of the dosages are in milligrams, and some conversions are necessary to other metric units. Therefore, you need knowledge of strengths of solution and the Metric System to effectively perform drug dosage calculations.

Although most respiratory medications are packaged in single unit dosages and are already premixed at a standard dose for you to aerosolize, occasions may arise when you will need to deviate from that standard premixed dose. You may have to adjust the dosage because of factors such as patient size or age, or the concentration of the medication on hand may be different than what is ordered. For example, a particular drug may be ordered to be given at 5 milligrams/kilogram of body weight. To find the right amount to administer, you must be able to convert the patient's body weight in pounds to kilograms and then calculate how many milligrams are needed to be delivered from the strength of solution you have on hand. While it may seem complicated, it really isn't if you have a basic understanding of the following concepts:

- Exponential powers of 10
- Systems of measurements
- The Metric System
- Strengths of solution

This chapter will give you a solid understanding of each these concepts in order to solve drug dosage calculations. Make sure you completely understand each section and the example calculations before you move on, as each section builds upon the next.

EXPONENTIAL POWERS OF TEN

Exponents

The **Metric System of Measurement** is based upon the powers of 10. Therefore, understanding the powers of 10 gives us a thorough understanding of the basis of the Metric System.

To understand the powers of 10, we need to review some terminology. Consider the expression b^n, where **b** is called the **base** and **n** the **exponent.** The **n** represents the number of times that **b** is multiplied by itself. Please see Figure 2-1.

$(exponent)$

$b^n \longrightarrow 3^2 = 3 \times 3 = 9$

(base)   (base 3)

$10^3 = 10 \times 10 \times 10$

(base 10)

Figure 2-1 The Exponential Expression

If we use 10 as the base, we can develop an exponential representation of the powers of 10 as follows:

$10^0 = 1$ (Mathematically, any number that has an exponent of $0 = 1$.)

$10^1 = 10$

$10^2 = 10 \times 10 = 100$

$10^3 = 10 \times 10 \times 10 = 1,000$

$10^4 = 10 \times 10 \times 10 \times 10 = 10,000$

$10^5 = 10 \times 10 \times 10 \times 10 \times 10 = 100,000$

$10^6 = 10 \times 10 \times 10 \times 10 \times 10 \times 10 = 1,000,000$

Thus far we have discussed positive exponents that result in numbers equal to or greater than 1. However, small numbers that are less than 1 can also be represented in exponential notation. In this case we will use negative exponents. A negative exponent can be thought of as a fraction. For example:

$$10^{-1} = \frac{1}{10} = .1$$

$$10^{-2} = \frac{1}{10} \times \frac{1}{10} = .01$$

$$10^{-3} = \frac{1}{10} \times \frac{1}{10} \times \frac{1}{10} = .001$$

$$10^{-4} = \frac{1}{10} \times \frac{1}{10} \times \frac{1}{10} \times \frac{1}{10} = .0001$$

$$10^{-5} = \frac{1}{10} \times \frac{1}{10} \times \frac{1}{10} \times \frac{1}{10} \times \frac{1}{10} = .00001$$

$$10^{-6} = \frac{1}{10} \times \frac{1}{10} \times \frac{1}{10} \times \frac{1}{10} \times \frac{1}{10} \times \frac{1}{10} = .000001$$

www.prenhall.com/colbert

Scientific Notation: In medicine, we often use numbers that are extremely large (there are about 25,000,000,000 blood cells circulating in an adult's body) and extremely small (.0000005 meters is the size of some microscopic organisms). It is often useful to write these numbers in a more convenient (or shorthand) form based on their powers of 10. This abbreviated form is known as **scientific notation** and is explained on the Web page.

SYSTEMS OF MEASUREMENT

United States Customary System (USCS)

There are two major systems of measurement in our world today. The United States Customary System is used in the United States and Myanmar (formerly Burma), and the Système International (SI) is used everywhere else and especially in health care. The SI system is also known as the International or **Metric System.** The Metric System is also the system used by drug manufacturers.

The USCS system is based on the British Imperial System and uses several different designations for the basic units of length, weight, and volume. We commonly call this the **English System.** For example, in the English System volumes can be expressed as ounces, pints, quarts, gallons, pecks, bushels, or cubic feet. Distance can be expressed in inches, feet, yards, and miles. Weights are measured in ounces, pounds, and tons. This may be the system you are most familiar with, but it is not the system of choice used throughout the world and within the medical profession. That is because the English System is very cumbersome to use, since it has no common base. It is very difficult to know the relationships among each of these units, because they are not based in an orderly fashion according to the powers of 10, as in the Metric System. For example, how many pecks are in a gallon? Just what is a peck? How many inches are in a mile? These all require extensive calculations and memorization of certain equivalent values, whereas in the Metric System you simply move the decimal point to the appropriate power of 10.

The Metric System

Most scientific and medical measurements use what is commonly referred to as the Metric System. The Metric System utilizes three basic units of measure for length, volume, and mass; these are the **meter, liter,** and **gram,** respectively. While the term "mass" is commonly used for weight, mass refers to the actual amount of matter in an object, while weight is the force exerted on a body by gravity. In space or zero gravity, all objects have mass but are indeed weightless. However, since current health care is mostly confined to earthly gravitational forces, we will use the term "weight." Table 2-1 gives you the metric designations for the three basic units of measure, along with an approximate English System comparison.

Again, notice that there are only three basic types of measure (meter, liter, and gram), and the Metric System has only one base unit per measure. Because the Metric System is a base-10 system, prefixes are used to indicate different powers of 10. Conversion within the Metric System simply involves moving the decimal point the appropriate direction and power of 10 according to the prefix before the unit of measure. For example, the prefix kilo- means $1000x$ or 10^3. Therefore one kilogram is equal to 1000 grams. See Table 2-2 for the common prefixes and their respective powers of 10.

CLINICAL PEARL

The Apothecary System developed in the 1700s had measurements still used today. For example, the pint, quart, and gallon were derived from this system. Apothecary measurements for calculating liquid doses of drugs include the minim and the fluid dram. Solids are measured in grams, scruples, drams, ounces, and pounds. Two unique features of the Apothecary System are use of Roman numerals and the placement of the unit of measure before the Roman numeral. However, the Metric System is now used to calculate drug dosages, because the Apothecary System is less precise.

LEARNING HINT

Try to visualize the physical comparison between the Metric and English Systems. For example, a meter is a little more than a yard, a kilometer is less than a mile, and a liter is a little more than a quart. This visual comparison becomes important if, for example, you are ordered to immediately withdraw an endotracheal tube 2 centimeters.

Table 2-1   Metric and English System Comparison

Type	Unit	English System Comparison (approximate size)
length	meter	slightly more than a yard
volume	liter	slightly more than 1 quart
mass/weight	gram	about 1/40 of an ounce

Table 2-2 Common Prefixes of the Metric System

thousands	hundreds	tens	base units			tenth	hundredth	thousandth
kilo-	hecto-	deca-	liter, meter, or gram			deci-	centi-	milli-
(k)	(h)	(da)	(l)	(m)	(g)	(d)	(c)	(m)
10^3	10^2	10^1		10^0 or 1		10^{-1}	10^{-2}	10^{-3}

LEARNING HINT

Deci- is associated with "decade," meaning 10 years; centi- is associated with cents, there being a hundred cents in a dollar; and milli- is associated with a millipede, the bug with a thousand legs. Biological note: Millipedes don't actually have a thousand legs; it just looks like they do.

LEARNING HINT

You should know the common prefixes in Table 2-2 and the micro- prefix in Table 2-3, since they may be used frequently in medicine. Always check your answer to see if it makes sense. For example, a common mistake is moving the decimal point in the wrong direction. If you had done that in Example Calculation 1, you would have erroneously said that 500 milliliters is equal to 500,000 liters. If you visualize this, you would know that 500 comparatively very small units (milliliters) in no way can equal 500,000 comparatively larger units (liters).

It can be seen from Table 2-2 that a kilometer would be 1000 or 10^3 meters. A centigram would be .01 or one-hundredth or 10^{-2} of a gram. The ease of working with the Metric System is that to change from one prefix to another, you simply move the decimal point to the correct place. In other words, to convert within the system, simply move the decimal point for each power of 10 according to the desired prefix. For example, to convert grams to kilograms, you would move the decimal point three places to the left. Therefore, 1000 grams would be equal to 1 kilogram.

Example Calculation 1

In drug dosage calculations, you often need to convert between grams and milligrams or liters and milliliters. A common conversion may be something like "500 milliliters is equal to how many liters?" We know from Table 2-2 that 500 milliliters (mls) would be equal to .5 liters, because you would simply move the decimal point 3 spaces (or powers of 10) to the left to find the equivalent value, since you are starting with milliliters and going to the base unit of liters.

3 spaces to Left

Example Calculation 2

How many grams are equal to 50 kilograms? Again, knowing the prefixes and powers of 10, you would move the decimal point three places (powers of 10) to the right to give an equivalent answer of 50,000 grams.

Refer to Table 2-3 for a more complete listing of prefixes that can be used in the Metric System. This knowledge of the Metric System will prove invaluable to you as you work within the medical profession and even just if you travel outside of the United States. That is, of course, unless you go to Myanmar.

Table 2-3 Metric System Prefixes and Abbreviations

Prefix	Power of 10		Abbreviation
giga-	10^9	one billion	g
mega-	10^6	one million	M
kilo-	10^3	one thousand	k
hecto-	10^2	one hundred	h
deca-	10^1	ten	da
deci-	10^{-1}	one tenth	d
centi-	10^{-2}	one hundreth	c
milli-	10^{-3}	one thousandth	m
micro-	10^{-6}	one millionth	μ
nano-	10^{-9}	one billionth	n

Note: Remember that the base units of liters, meters, and grams are equal to 10^0 or 1.

1,500 mls of an IV solution is equal to how many liters?

One final note before leaving the Metric System. It has been determined that one cubic centimeter (cc) would hold the approximate volume of one milliliter (ml). Therefore, 1 cc = 1 ml. You may hear someone say you have a 500-cc IV solution on hand, while someone else may say you have a 500-ml solution; either way, they are both saying the same thing. See Figure 2-2.

What are some of the advantages of the Metric System?

www.prenhall.com/colbert

Intravenous solutions infused over time employ a specific calculation to determine the flow rate that should be set on the IV delivery device. To learn how to calculate IV flow rates, go to this chapter on the Web site.

Conversion of Units

You should now be able to work comfortably within the Metric System, but what if we need to take an English unit and convert it to a metric unit? For example, in the introduction of this chapter, we said that a certain drug's schedule was 5 milligrams per kilogram of body weight. What is the relationship between pounds in the English System and kilograms in the Metric System?

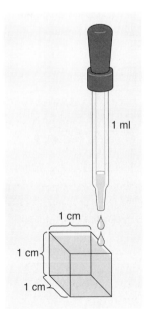

Figure 2-2 1 cc = 1 ml

The following is a method for changing units or converting between the English and Metric system. This method is sometimes referred to as the **factor-label method** or **fraction method.** This method allows your starting units to cancel or divide out until you reach your desired unit. There are two basic steps. First, write down your starting value with units over the number 1. This places it in a form of a fraction, but since 1 is in the denominator, it does not change the numerical value.

The second step involves placing the units you started with in the denominator of the next fraction to divide or cancel out, and placing the unit you want to convert to in the numerator, along with the corresponding equivalent values. The quantities in the numerator and denominator must be equivalent values but in different units! Because the values are equivalent, this is the same as multiplication by 1, which does not change the value of the mathematical expression. This allows you to treat the units as in the multiplication of fractions and "**cancel**" them out. Notice that by carefully placing the units so that canceling is possible, the units can be converted.

Example Calculation 3

How many inches are there in 1 mile?

First put down what value is given as a fraction over 1.

$$\frac{1 \text{ mile}}{1}$$

Next put miles in the denominator and the desired unit in the numerator with equivalent values. You know that 1 mile = 5,280 feet, so:

$$1 \text{ mile} = \frac{5,280 \text{ ft}}{1 \text{ mile}}$$

You've canceled out miles, but need to go to inches. Just carry the process out until you reach your desired unit.

$$1 \text{ mile} \times \frac{5,280 \text{ ft}}{1 \text{ mile}} \times \frac{12 \text{ inches}}{1 \text{ ft}} = 63,360 \text{ inches}$$

Example Calculation 4

How many seconds are there in 8 hours?

$$\frac{8 \text{ hours}}{1} \times \frac{60 \text{ minutes}}{1 \text{ hour}} \times \frac{60 \text{ seconds}}{1 \text{ minute}} = 28,800 \text{ seconds}$$

Factor-Label Method for Conversion Between Systems

One can attempt to memorize the hundreds of conversions between the English and Metric Systems, but that would be nearly impossible. All that is needed is to memorize one conversion in each of the three units of measure. This will allow a "bridging of the systems." These conversions are:

1 inch = 2.54 cm	used for units of length
2.2 lbs = 1 kg	used for units of mass or weight
1.06 qt = 1 liter	used for units of volume

Example Calculation 5

One foot is equal to how many centimeters? There is an equivalency somewhere for feet and centimeters, but you don't need to know that as long as you know the factor-label method and the conversion for distance.

Now to answer the question of how many centimeters there are in one foot:

$$\frac{1 \text{ \sout{foot}}}{1} \times \frac{12 \text{ \sout{inches}}}{1 \text{ \sout{foot}}} \times \frac{2.54 \text{ cm}}{1 \text{ \sout{inch}}} = 30.48 \text{ cm}$$

Example Calculation 6

If an individual weighs 150 pounds and the drug dosage order is 10 mg/kg, how much drug should they receive? First, you must change pounds to kilograms; therefore, write the given weight as a fraction over 1. Then place the unit you want to cancel (pounds) in the denominator and the unit you want to convert to (kilograms) in the numerator of the next fraction.

$$\frac{150 \text{ \sout{pounds}}}{1} \times \frac{\text{kilograms}}{2.2 \text{ \sout{pounds}}} = 68.18 \text{ kilograms}$$

Because the dose read 10 mg/kg, this patient should receive 10 × 68.18 kg, or 681.8 mg of the drug. You then have to be practical, working with dosage unit availability, and round the dose appropriately, i.e., 682 mg.

A quart of blood is equal to how many cc?

www.prenhall.com/colbert

Another system of measure commonly used "around the house" for cooking and to give some oral liquid medications is the Household System, which compares teaspoons, tablespoons, ounces, cups, etc. Go to the Web site for coverage of this system.

DRUG DOSAGE CALCULATIONS

Solutions

Many drugs are given in **solution** form. A solution is a chemical and physical homogeneous mixture of two or more substances. The solution will contain a **solute** and a **solvent.** A solute is either a liquid or solid that is dissolved in a liquid to form a solution. A solvent is the liquid that dissolves the solute. For example, you can make the solution hot coffee by dissolving granules of coffee (solute) in hot water (solvent).

Drug solutions can be made by dissolving either a liquid or a solid solute, which represents the active drug, in a solvent such as sterile water or normal saline solution to form a solution that is delivered to the patient through various routes of administration. If the solute being dissolved is a solid, such as a powder, the resulting solution is termed a **weight/volume (w/v)** solution, where the w represents weight or amount of solute and the v represents the total amount of solution. One can also have a **volume/volume (v/v) solu-**

LEARNING HINT

The SOLVEnt is the one that disSOLVEs the solute.

tion, where the first v represents the volume of the liquid solute and the second v represents the volume of the solution. A delicious nondrug example of this would be mixing liquid chocolate syrup (solute) in hot milk (solvent) to form the solution of hot chocolate. Don't ask about the marshmallows. See Figure 2-3.

Percentage Solutions

One way the potency of a drug can be described is by stating its **percentage of solution.** This tells the strength of the solution as parts of the solute (drug) per 100 ml of solution. After all, that is what a percent is, some number related to 100. Remember that the solute can be either a solid or a liquid. If the solute is dissolved in a solid form, it will be expressed in grams per 100 ml of solution (w/v solution). If the solute is liquid, it will be expressed in milliliters (v/v solution).

For example, a 20% salt water or saline solution would contain 20 grams of salt (solid solute) dissolved in enough water (solvent) to create 100 ml of solution. We can use this information coupled with proportions to begin to solve drug dosage problems. The majority of drug dosage calculations can be solved by setting up simple proportions. A **proportion** is a statement that compares two ratios.

In general, the proportion

$$\frac{a}{b} = \frac{c}{d}$$

is equivalent to the equation ad = bc. Sometimes it is said that the product of the means (b and c) equals the product of the extremes (a and d). This is also known as "cross-multiplying," so that

$$\text{if } \frac{a}{b} = \frac{c}{d}, \text{ then ad} = \text{bc.}$$

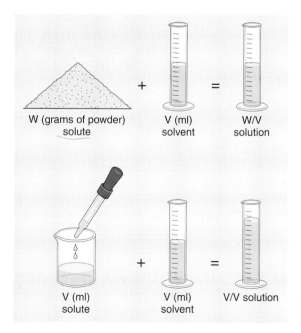

Figure 2-3 W/V and V/V Solutions

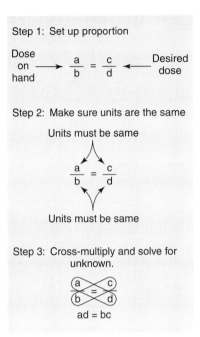

Figure 2-4 Steps to Solve
Drug Dosage Calculations

Setting Up Proportions

Armed with the previous knowledge in this chapter, you can solve drug dosage calculations with proportions in two basic steps. First, set up a proportion of the *dose on hand* related to the *desired dose*. Second, make sure all units are equal, then cross-multiply and solve the equation. See Figure 2-4, which illustrates these steps.

Several different calculation examples follow. Notice how they may all contain different information, but can be solved with the three-step solution.

Example Calculation 7

How much salt is needed to make 1,000 ml of a 20% solution?

First, put down what you know, or your dose on hand:

$$20\% \text{ solution} = \frac{20 \text{ g salt}}{100 \text{ ml of solution}}$$

Now place this into a proportion and relate to your desired dose.

Dose on hand   :   Desire dose

$$\frac{20 \text{ g salt}}{100 \text{ ml of solution}} = \frac{x \text{ g of salt}}{1{,}000 \text{ ml of solution}}$$

The *x* grams represent the "how much salt" is needed. The left side of the equation is what is known, or the dose on hand, and the right side is the unknown amount of the solute (in this case salt) needed to make the final solution.

Solving by cross-multiplying:

$$\frac{20 \text{ g salt}}{100 \text{ ml of solution}} = \frac{x \text{ g of salt}}{1{,}000 \text{ ml of solution}}$$

$$20 \times 1{,}000 = 100x$$

$$20{,}000 = 100x$$

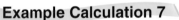

Divide both sides of the equation by the amount on the x side to find out what x is by itself:

$$\frac{20,000}{100} = \frac{\cancel{100}x}{\cancel{100}}$$

$$200 = x$$

$$x = 200$$

So to make 1,000 ml of a 20% salt solution, you would take 200 grams of salt and add enough water to fill a container to the 1,000-ml mark.

In this example, 1,000 ml could have been given as the equivalent 1 liter. When that is the case, before cross-multiplying, you must make sure all your units in the numerator and denominator are the same.

CLINICAL PEARL

Normally the drug Proventil will be mixed with a diluent such as normal saline solution or sterile water to allow it to be nebulized over a longer period of time. This diluent does not decrease the amount of drug or weaken the amount of drug given to the patient. In this example, there are 5 mg of the active drug Proventil in the solution, regardless of whether 3 cc or 5 cc of diluent are added. Only the nebulization or delivery time is increased. More on this in Chapter 4, where we will discuss aerosol delivery devices.

Example Calculation 8

The bronchodilator drug Proventil is ordered to be given 5 mg per aerosol dose. You have a .5% solution on hand. How many milliliters of drug solution should you deliver?

What is known: $\dfrac{0.5 \text{ g of Proventil}}{100 \text{ ml of solution}}$

Proportion set up to what is needed: $\dfrac{0.5 \text{ g of Proventil}}{100 \text{ ml of solution}} = \dfrac{5 \text{ mg of Proventil}}{x \text{ ml of solution}}$

But before solving, convert the .5 g to 500 mg, so your units are the same in the denominator.

$$\frac{500 \text{ mg of Proventil}}{100 \text{ ml of solution}} = \frac{5 \text{ mg of Proventil}}{x \text{ ml of solution}}$$

$$500x = 500$$

$$x = 1$$

Therefore, we would need to draw up and deliver 1 ml of our drug solution to our patient.

LEARNING HINT

After setting up the proportion, always ask yourself the catchy phrase, "Are my units congruent?" This habit will help to ensure proper results.

Example Calculation 9

Even if a drug such as heparin, insulin, or penicillin is given in units (U) rather than grams, milligrams, etc., you still solve the problem the same way. If a solution of penicillin has 2,000 U/ml, how many milliliters would you give to deliver 250 U of the drug?

CLINICAL PEARL

Some drugs have special systems developed by the manufacturer for measuring their doses. For example, there are many types of insulin available, but they are all measured in units (U).

Dose on hand   :   Desired dose

$$\frac{2,000 \text{ U of penicillin}}{1 \text{ ml}} = \frac{250 \text{ U of penicillin}}{x \text{ ml}}$$

$$2,000x = 250$$

$$x = .125 \text{ ml}$$

Therefore, .125 ml of the 2,000-U solution would be given to deliver 250 U of penicillin to the patient.

STOP

& REVIEW

You have a 10% drug solution on hand and the order states to deliver 100 milligrams of drug. How many milliliters would you deliver?

$\langle$ CONTROVERSY $\rangle$

It has been shown that many medication errors happen each year. Controversy exists over how many mistakes go unreported or unnoticed and what factors lead to these errors. What if you make a medication delivery or calculation error? What steps should you take? Whom should you notify? How can medication errors be prevented?

Ratio Solutions

Another means of expressing the strength of solution is by using a ratio instead of a percentage. The **ratio solution** represents the parts of the solute related to the parts of the solution. For example, a 1:200 solution of isoproterenol (v/v) would contain 1 ml of isoproterenol (liquid solute) in 200 ml of a solution.

We can solve word problems involving ratios with the same system used for percentage solutions. First, put down the dose on hand. Second, relate this to the unknown or desired solution. Third, make sure all units in the numerator and denominator are the same. Last, solve for x by cross-multiplying the proportion.

Example Calculation 10

How many ml of isoproterenol are in 1 ml of a 1:100 solution?

$$\text{Given:} \quad 1{:}100 \text{ solution} = \frac{1 \text{ ml isoproterenol}}{100 \text{ ml sterile water}}$$

$$\text{Relate:} \quad \frac{1 \text{ ml isoproterenol}}{100 \text{ ml sterile water}} = \frac{x \text{ ml of isoproterenol}}{1 \text{ ml sterile water}}$$

Cross-multiply:

$$1 = 100x$$

$$.01 \text{ ml} = x$$

Therefore, there is .01 ml of isoproterenol in 1 ml of a 1:100 solution of isoproterenol.

Example Calculation 11

How many milliliters of 1:200 Proventil solution would you deliver if the order were for 2.5 mg of Proventil?

$$\text{Given:} \quad 1{:}200 \text{ solution} = \frac{1 \text{ g Proventil}}{200 \text{ ml solution}}$$

Relate "on hand" to "desired" with a proportion:

$$\frac{1 \text{ g Proventil}}{200 \text{ ml solution}} = \frac{2.5 \text{ mg of Proventil}}{x \text{ ml solution}}$$

Before solving, convert grams to milligrams in the numerator so the units are the same.

$$\frac{1{,}000 \text{ mg Proventil}}{200 \text{ ml solution}} = \frac{2.5 \text{ mg Proventil}}{x \text{ ml solution}}$$

Cross-multiply:

$$1000x = 500$$
$$x = .5 \text{ ml}$$

Therefore, you would draw up .5 milliliters of a 1:200 solution of Proventil in order to deliver 2.5 milligrams to your patient.

www.prenhall.com/colbert

There are times when dosages need to be adjusted for infants and children. For a discussion of this topic, along with sample problems, please go to this chapter on the Web site.

Drug Orders in Drops

Some orders for respiratory solutions to be nebulized may come in the form of number of drops to be mixed with normal saline or distilled water. The Latin word for drops is *guttae* and is abbreviated gtt. It is helpful to know the following: gtts = drops, and 16 gtts = 1 ml = 1 cc. However, it should be noted that not all droppers are standardized and this equivalency may change according to the properties of the liquid and the orifice size of the dropper.

Example Calculation 12

A physician's order reads, "Give 8 gtts of racemic epinephrine with 3 cc of sterile water qid." How many cc of drug would be delivered per treatment? Logically, if you knew that 16 gtt = 1 cc, than 8 gtts must be equal to .5 cc. However, the numbers may not always be that easy, and problems of this nature can be solved by using the factor-label method, because it involves a known equivalency (16 gtts = 1 cc).

First put down what is given.

$$\frac{8 \text{ gtts}}{1}$$

Next place the unit you wish to cancel in the denominator and the unit you desire in the numerator, along with the equivalent values:

$$\frac{8 \text{ \cancel{gtts}}}{1} = \frac{1 \text{ ml}}{16 \text{ \cancel{gtts}}} = .5 \text{ ml}$$

www.prenhall.com/colbert

What if an order reads to give .3 cc of a drug but your medicine dropper is calibrated in .25-cc increments? How do you solve this? Go to the Web site to see an animation that shows the solution to this dilemma.

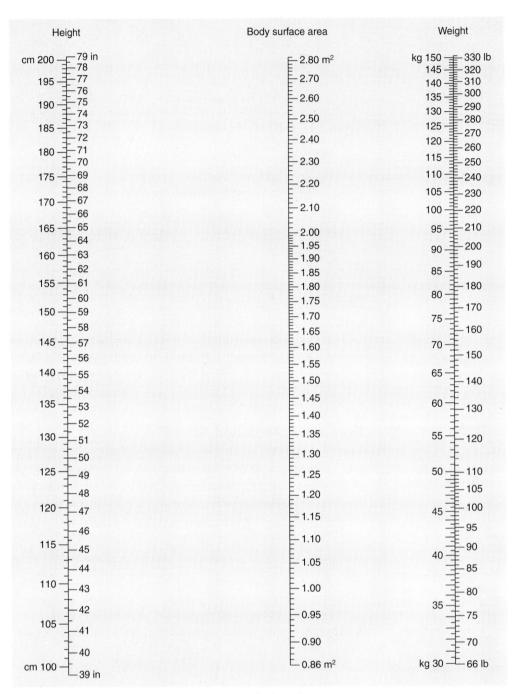

Figure 2-5 Nomogram for Determining Body Surface Area
Source: From Tiger, Steven, Julienne K. Kirk, and Robert J. Solomon, *Mathematical Concepts in Clinical Science,* Prentice Hall, Inc., 2000, p. 6.

SUMMARY

This chapter contained vital information necessary to understand the Metric System and to calculate accurate drug dosages. You should feel comfortable making conversions between different systems of measurement and working within the Metric System. Dosage measurements and calculations are a major responsibility, because giving the wrong dose can be very dangerous to the patient.

REVIEW QUESTIONS

1. The Metric System is based on the exponential powers of
   (a) 100
   (b) 10
   (c) 2
   (d) 15
2. Which of the following is <u>not</u> a basic unit of measure in the Metric System?
   (a) liter
   (b) gram
   (c) pound
   (d) meter
3. A cubic centimeter (cc) is equal to
   (a) 1 ml
   (b) 1 liter
   (c) 1 mg
   (d) 10 kg
4. The body surface nomogram compares what two units of measure?
   (a) weight and sex
   (b) height and sex
   (c) surface area and length
   (d) height and weight
5. Which type of drug solution represents a powdered drug mixed in solution?
   (a) v/v
   (b) w/v *weight + volume*
   (c) w/w
   (d) v/w
6. If a patient voids 3.2 liters of urine in a day, what is the amount in cc?

   3200 cc

7. Convert 175 lbs to kilograms.   *80kg*
8. How many ml of a 1:200 solution of drug would equal 15 mg?
9. If an order reads to deliver 5 mg of a drug and you have a 1:200 solution on hand, how many ml would you administer to your patient? How many gtts? *drop*
10. If you give 6 ml of a 0.1% strength solution, how many mg are in the dose?
11. How many ml of a 1:1000 epinephrine solution are needed for a 5-mg dose?
12. Methylprednisolone 4 mg is equivalent to 20 mg of hydrocortisone. Your patient is on 40 mg of hydrocortisone daily and the doctor wants to switch to methylprednisolone. What would be the equipotent methylprednisolone dose?
13. If beclomethasone inhaled corticosteroid is available in a device that delivers 42 μg/puff, how many puffs per day would the patient need to get a dose of 336 μg?
14. A patient is not controlled on 300 mg twice daily of Theodur. The doctor wants him to take 1200 mg daily. How many tablets should the patient take per day?
15. How many mg of active ingredient are there in 4 cc of 1:200 albuterol?

   $$\frac{1000}{200} = 5m \quad \begin{array}{l} 4ml \\ DD \end{array}$$
   $$M \quad \begin{array}{l} 4ml \\ 20\,mg/ml \end{array}$$

GLOSSARY

base   the number being multiplied in an exponential expression.

canceling units   method of changing starting units to the desired units.

English System of measurement   the common household system of measurement using miles, feet, ounces, pounds, etc.

exponent   the number of times the base is multiplied in an exponential expression.

Factor-label method or fraction method   method for changing units or converting between the English and Metric Systems.

gram (g)   a basic unit of mass in the Metric System.

liter (l)   a basic unit of liquid measure in the Metric System.

meter (m)   a basic unit of length in the Metric System.

Metric System of Measurement   a system of measurement based on powers of 10.

percentage solution   strength of solution as parts of solute per 100 ml of solution.

proportion   a statement that compares two ratios.

ratio solution   a method of expressing the strength of solution as a ratio that represents parts of solute related to parts of solution.

scientific notation   a means of representing very large or very small numbers or the scribblings of Albert Einstein.

solute   a liquid or solid that is dissolved in a liquid to form a solution.

solution   a physically homogeneous mixture of two or more liquids.

solvent   the liquid that dissolves the solute.

units   a method of measuring a dose.

v/v drug solution   a solution represented by the volume of the liquid solute in the volume of solution.

w/v drug solution   a solution in which the solute being dissolved is a solid.

www.prenhall.com/colbert

Use the address above to access the free, interactive Companion Web site created specifically for this textbook. Enhance your studying by viewing videos and animations, answering practice quiz questions, and reviewing an audio glossary and much more related to Chapter 2.

CHAPTER 3

Pharmacology of the Autonomic Nervous System

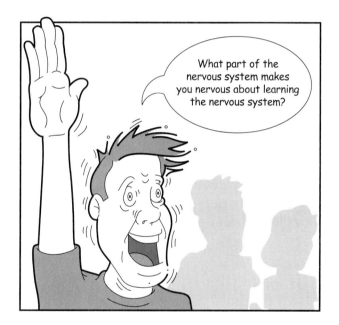

OBJECTIVES

Upon completion of this chapter you will be able to

- Describe the divisions of the central and peripheral nervous systems
- Define key terms relative to pharmacology of the autonomic nervous system
- Describe the anatomy, neurotransmitters, and receptors of the autonomic nervous system
- State four classifications of autonomic nervous system drugs on the basis of how and where they work
- Relate the pharmacology of the autonomic nervous system to the "specific chapters" and drug classifications that are relevant

ABBREVIATIONS

ANS	autonomic nervous system	ACh	acetylcholine
CNS	central nervous system	ACLS	advanced cardiac life support
CPU	central processing unit	MAO	monoamine oxidase
GI	Gastrointestinal	COMT	catechol-o-methyltransferase
PNS	peripheral nervous system	AChE	acetylcholinesterase
NE	norepinephrine		

INTRODUCTION

The nervous system and endocrine system represent the control systems of the body. These systems coordinate complex activities to maintain day-to-day functioning and a stable internal homeostatic environment. In times of stress, these systems must quickly integrate complex activities to combat the stress and maintain survival. The endocrine system will be discussed in Chapter 7 under the steroid classification of drugs.

This chapter will discuss in general terms how the **central** and **peripheral nervous systems** (**CNS** and **PNS**) receive and process information and how drugs can affect this activity. The nervous system is responsible for day-to-day functioning of both voluntary and involuntary activities throughout the body, and only by understanding how it works will you have the basis for understanding drug effects on various skeletal and smooth muscles, glands, and organs.

The pharmacology of drugs affecting the nervous system is admittedly difficult to understand. The majority of drugs discussed in this chapter work on the PNS. Only the basics of the PNS and CNS will be presented in this chapter, with specifics discussed later, in appropriate chapters. For example, drugs that work on the CNS such as skeletal muscle relaxants and narcotic medications for pain are discussed later, in Chapter 11. PNS drugs affecting the heart rate and respiratory airway tone will be further addressed in the relevant chapters on bronchodilators and cardiovascular drugs. This chapter is simply laying the foundation for understanding nervous system drug pharmacology; we will build upon it in upcoming chapters.

NERVOUS SYSTEM DIVISIONS

The nervous system consists of the **central nervous system** (CNS) and the **peripheral nervous system** (PNS). The CNS is comprised of the brain and spinal cord. The brain is analogous to the central processing unit (CPU) of a computer, which handles information from a variety of sources. The spinal cord is the main branch that transmits messages to and from the brain.

LEARNING HINT

The flow of information into your brain, or sensory (afferent) input, is what helps you read this book. The output from the brain that controls the muscles (motor) is what helps you turn the pages in this book.

The PNS is comprised of all the nerves "outside" of the brain and spinal cord. PNS anatomy and physiology is more pertinent to cardiopulmonary pharmacotherapy than that of the CNS, so this chapter will emphasize the PNS. The PNS basically mediates between the CNS and the external and internal body environments. Peripheral system nerves carry sensory information along **afferent nerves** from all parts of the body to the brain for processing. Therefore, "afferent" and "sensory" are used as synonymous terms. Likewise, the brain can send information along **efferent nerves** or motor pathways via the PNS to have "effects" on various parts of the body. See Figure 3-1.

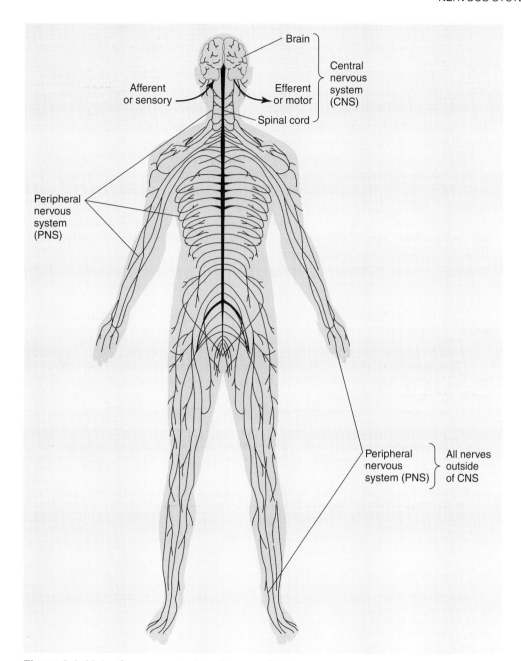

Figure 3-1 Major Components of the Nervous System

PNS Divisions

The peripheral nervous system is what connects the rest of your body, neurologically speaking, to your brain and spinal cord. The PNS is divided into two main divisions, the **somatic nervous system** and the **autonomic nervous system (ANS).** The somatic nervous system controls skeletal muscles during voluntary movement and therefore represents the voluntary portion of the PNS. An example of the somatic nervous system is the control of the muscles in your hand to turn the page of this book. We will focus on the somatic nervous system in the chapter on skeletal muscle relaxants. The somatic nervous system also conducts sensory information such as pain and touch back to the brain via afferent nerves.

The ANS is the involuntary or automatic part of the PNS—we have little or no control over its action. An example of involuntary control is the reaction of the pupil to light on the retina: In bright light conditions, your pupil constricts to protect the retina from too much light exposure, which could be damaging. You do not consciously tell your pupil to constrict, and therefore this is an autonomic response of the PNS.

Other major organ systems in the body regulated by the ANS include the cardiopulmonary and digestive systems. While you may consciously decide to eat a hamburger, using your voluntary or somatic system for this process, the rest of the digestive process is under autonomic control and goes on with little or no thought. In addition to glands and organs, the involuntary muscles controlled by the autonomic nervous system include the specialized cardiac muscle controlling the heart and the smooth muscle found in the airways, blood vessels, reproductive tract, and GI tract.

STOP
& REVIEW

What branch of the nervous system controls digestive actions?

The autonomic system is further divided into the **sympathetic** and **parasympathetic** branches. The parasympathetic branch is concerned with daily body upkeep and maintaining a homeostatic environment. The sympathetic system represents the alert system for stressful situations and is often referred to as the "fight or flight" system. Because the balance between these two systems is what controls our normal heart rate and the smooth muscle tone of our airways, this balance becomes of major pharmacologic importance. Please see Figure 3-2, which demonstrates the divisions of the nervous system.

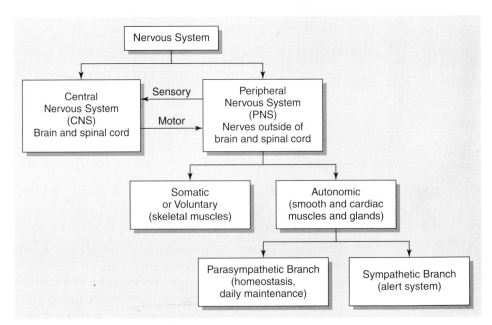

Figure 3-2 Nervous System Divisions

Table 3-1   Effects of the Parasympathetic and Sympathetic Nervous Systems

Organ or System	Parasympathetic Effect	Sympathetic Effect
Heart	decreases rate and contractile force	increases rate and contractile force
Lungs	bronchoconstricts	bronchodilates
Eyes	pupil constriction	pupil dilation
Hair muscles	relaxes	contracts and causes hair to stand on end (piloerection)
Gastrointestinal	increases digestion	decreases digestion
Urinary	constricts bladder	relaxes bladder

It is important to note that the parasympathetic and sympathetic systems usually work in a coordinated but opposing fashion to regulate autonomic control. For example, if you were confronted by a stranger with a knife in a dark alley, several physiologic changes would occur, because the sympathetic system would be alerted. Your pupils would dilate to bring in more light for the situation at hand. Your heart rate and force of contraction would increase to get much-needed oxygen to muscles for the impending "fight or flight." Your respiratory system would be stimulated to increase ventilation to bring in more oxygen. Certain vascular changes would occur to provide more blood flow to essential areas and constrict blood flow to nonessential areas such as the GI tract.

However, you cannot maintain this hypermetabolic state for long periods of time, and once the danger was removed (hopefully by peaceful police intervention), you would eventually have to return to a homeostatic state and then wonder why you were ever in the dark alley in the first place. The parasympathetic system would become dominant and bring your heart rate and respirations back toward normal resting levels.

What was just described is a physiologic response to stress and a return to homeostasis via the two branches of the autonomic nervous system. The activity of each of these branches can also be altered by pharmacological means. This is good, since some pathological conditions of the organs can be treated pharmacologically by capitalizing on the knowledge of these interactions. Please see Table 3-1 for actions of the parasympathetic and sympathetic nervous systems.

www.prenhall.com/colbert

Every time you get connected to the Web site, you will get closer to connecting to how the nervous systems connect together. See an animation of parasympathetic and sympathetic innervation of major organs on the Web site and click on the organs to see what the actual parasympathetic and sympathetic responses would be.

STOP & REVIEW

Have you ever heard the saying, "That made the hairs on the back of my neck stand up"? Would you consider this a sympathetic or parasympathetic response, and why?

NERVOUS SYSTEM CONDUCTION

To understand how drugs affect neurotransmission, you must know how messages are transmitted or conducted from one nerve (neuron) to another. When a resting nerve receives stimulation, an electrical impulse carries the signal along the nerve fiber or axon. At the terminal end of each axon is a small junction or synapse that may connect either to another nerve or to a muscle or gland. Regardless of where the connection leads, for the impulse to be carried on, a chemical neurotransmitter substance must now travel across the synapse. These chemicals are manufactured and stored at the terminal end of the axons and released upon stimulation by the electrical impulse. The two main neurochemical substances stored or manufactured at the ends of the nerve fibers are **acetylcholine (ACh)** and **norepinephrine (NE).** See Figure 3-3, which demonstrates the transmission of a nerve impulse.

Types and Location of Neurotransmitters

The somatic nervous system, which controls the skeletal muscles, is a one-junction system where the stimulus travels via a single nerve axon and then travels to one gap or synapse. The neurotransmitter must then pass the signal on to the brain for sensory input such as pain or on to the effected skeletal muscle for motor output to control the muscle (see Figure 3-4). Notice that ACh is the neurotransmitter substance found within the somatic system, and the only kind of synapse in the somatic system is the neuromuscular junction that connects the nerve to the skeletal muscle or the synapse to the CNS, which brings in sensory information.

The autonomic branch of the PNS has two junctions to traverse in order for the signal to reach the intended site of an involuntary muscle or gland. The first neuron is a presynaptic or preganglionic neuron. A **ganglion** (plural, ganglia) can be thought of as simply a nerve that lies outside of the CNS. Therefore, the first part of the journey from the brain is to the first junction (synapse) and ganglia beyond. The second neuron is a postsynaptic or postganglionic neuron, and it travels from the ganglia to the target site of either an involuntary muscle (cardiac or smooth) or a gland.

Both the parasympathetic and the sympathetic system have preganglionic and postganglionic neurons. The neurotransmitter substance at both preganglionic sites is ACh. ACh is also found at the postganglionic site of the parasympathetic system. However, the neurotransmitter substance that carries the impulse to the involuntary muscle or gland at the postganglionic junction of the sympathetic system is norepinephrine (NE). See Figure 3-5, which now adds the autonomic branches of the peripheral nervous system.

LEARNING HINT

Remember that ACh is the neurotransmitter substance everywhere (skeletal, sensory, both preganglionic junctions and the postganglionic junction of the parasympathetic nervous system), but NE is only found at the postganglionic junction of the sympathetic system.

The only neurotransmitter for the somatic system is ACH

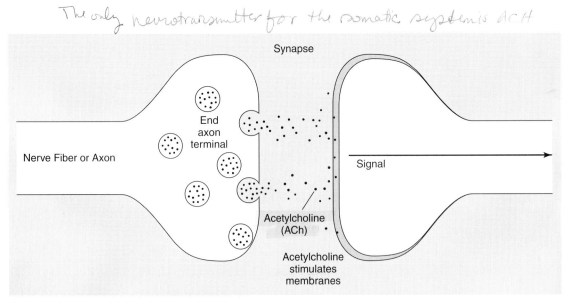

Figure 3-3 Transmission of a Nerve Impulse

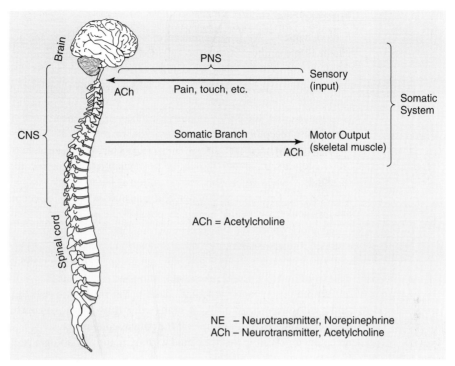

Figure 3-4 Somatic Nervous System Transmission

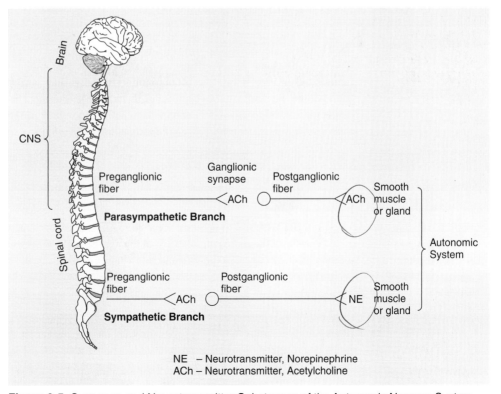

Figure 3-5 Synapses and Neurotransmitter Substances of the Autonomic Nervous System

Receptors

offer a place for tx.

From Chapter 1, we learned that receptor sites are "where the action is." Once the neuro-chemical transmitter substance is released, it will bind to a receptor to elicit a response. If the stimulus begins in the ANS, it must first release ACh across the presynaptic junction and diffuse and bind to postsynaptic receptors found on the postsynaptic nerve to pass the signal on. The receptors that the neurotransmitter ACh binds with as it diffuses across the presynaptic junction in either the parasympathetic or the sympathetic system are called **nicotinic receptors.** These receptors simply pass the signal on to the postsynaptic neuron to then be carried to the target gland, organ, smooth muscle, or cardiac muscle (see Figure 3-6).

Receptors are also found on the postsynaptic junction located on involuntary muscles or glands. This is where the "main" action is, so to speak, and is referred to as the neuro-effector site. Once the neurochemical transmitter binds to receptor sites there, it initiates biochemical triggers that result in physiologic responses depending on what the nerve innervates (connects to). After the chemical transmitter has interacted with the receptor and initiated a response, its job is done and action is terminated. The neurotransmitter must be destroyed or removed after receptor activation. The neurotransmitters that don't bind are destroyed by enzymes or taken back into the synapse, or they diffuse away.

In the postsynaptic junction of the parasympathetic nervous system, the neurotransmitter substance is ACh. ACh binds with **muscarinic receptors** found on involuntary muscles or glands. For example, if the parasympathetic system is stimulated and muscarinic receptors innervating the heart bind with ACh, the physiologic reaction will be the parasympathetic response of slowing heart rate.

Block
parasympathetic = look
Acyty

Stimulate
sympathetic = norephi

STOP & REVIEW

Identify where nicotinic and muscarinic receptors can be found in the parasympathetic and sympathetic nervous systems.

However, if the sympathetic nervous system is stimulated and the impulse reaches the postsynaptic site, norepinephrine will be released and bind with the **adrenergic receptors** found on the glands or smooth or cardiac muscle. For example, if the sympathetic system is stimulated and adrenergic receptors found in the heart bind with NE, the physiologic reaction will be the sympathetic response of increasing heart rate. The adrenergic receptors are further classified as alpha or beta receptors, and these will be further discussed in Chapter 5. See Figure 3-7, which shows the synapses, neurotransmitters, and receptors of the ANS.

www.prenhall.com/colbert

Go to the Web site to actually view animations showing autonomic neurotransmission in both the parasympathetic and the sympathetic nervous systems. View it several times if needed to understand this vital physiologic process.

LEARNING HINT

Remember that the nicotinic receptors are found at preganglionic sites and help to pass the impulse along to the postganglionic neuron. The muscarinic receptors are at the actual effector site of the parasympathetic nervous system.

Receptor Classification

Receptors are classified by the type of neurotransmitter they respond to at the various nerve endings. The receptors that bind with acetyl*choline* are termed cholinergic receptors. Cholinergic receptors can be of two types, termed muscarinic or nicotinic depending upon their location.

The receptors that bind with NE are called **adrenergic receptors.** Sympathomimetics stimulate NE adrenergic receptors of either the **alpha** or **beta** type depending on where they are

(handwritten notes in margin: "Beta heart", "Beta lung", "sympathetic", "blood vessel")

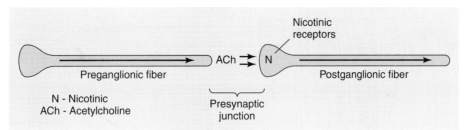

Figure 3-6 Preganglionic Transmission in the ANS
This occurs in both parasympathetic and sympathetic systems, with only the length and location of the nerve fibers being different.

LEARNING HINT

We didn't forget about the somatic branch of the PNS. Remember that this is a one-branch system innervating skeletal muscles, and nicotinic receptors are found at the receptor sites as shown in Figure 3-8. Again, more on this in the chapter on skeletal muscle relaxants.

found in the body. Alpha receptors, found primarily in smooth muscle of blood vessels, can be of two types, either $alpha_1$ or $alpha_2$. Generally, alpha stimulation causes vasoconstriction. Beta receptors are termed either $beta_1$ or $beta_2$. $Beta_1$ receptors are found primarily in the cardiac muscle, where stimulation results in positive chronotropic (increase in rate), dromotropic (increase in conduction), and inotropic (increase in contraction) effects on the cardiac system. They are further discussed in Chapters 9 and 10. $Beta_2$ receptors are found abundantly within the smooth muscle of the airways and in certain blood vessels. $Beta_2$ receptor stimulation results in vasodilation and bronchodilation. $Beta_2$ agonists are the foundation for treatment of bronchospasm and are further discussed in Chapter 5. See Figure 3-8 for the receptors found at nerve endings.

One other type of adrenergic receptor not yet mentioned is the **dopamine receptors** found in renal tissues. Their stimulation causes relaxation of the renal arteries and increases perfusion to the kidneys. These will also be discussed in Chapter 9. See Table 3-2, which shows the various adrenergic receptor types, their location, and their action when stimulated.

(1) Sympathetic Division

(2) Parasympathetic Division

Receptors	
M = Muscarinic receptor	N = Nicotinic receptor
α = alpha receptor	β = Beta receptor
	= Nerve terminal

Figure 3-7 Synapses, Ganglia, Neurotransmitters, and Receptors of the ANS
Note: Adrenergic receptors are classified as alpha (α) or beta (β).

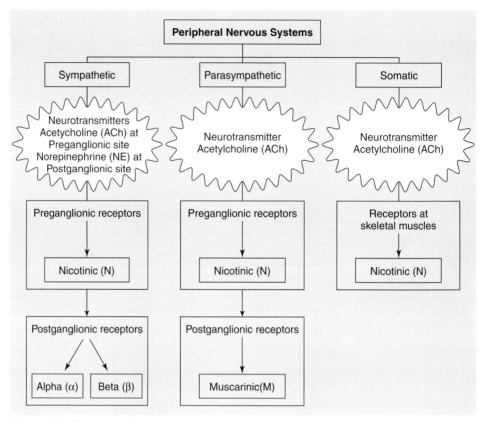

Figure 3-8 Receptors Found at Nerve Endings

Table 3-2 Types of Adrenergic Receptors (Adrenoreceptors)

Type	Tissue	Action
Alpha$_1$	vascular smooth muscle	contracts
	pupil	dilation (mydriasis)
	pilomotor smooth muscle	goosebumps
Beta$_1$	heart	stimulates rate and force
Beta$_2$	respiratory	bronchodilates
	somatic motor (voluntary muscle)	tremors
Dopamine	renal	relaxes arteries

State the effects on the heart, blood vessels, or lungs from stimulating the following receptors: alpha, beta$_1$, beta$_2$, and muscarinic.

ANS DRUG TERMINOLOGY

Physiologically, the ANS acts as two major divisions: the parasympathetic and sympathetic. Again recapping the systems, one can think of the sympathetic system as a response system and the parasympathetic as a homeostatic or maintenance system. They work together to balance each other out. The sympathetic system is not essential for life, but it allows for adjustments to activity and stresses that occur in life. The parasympathetic nervous system controls essential activities and conserves energy for daily body maintenance and metabolic functioning. Each division of the ANS has a direct effect on organ systems such as the heart and lungs, and we will use these two organs as examples in the following classification system. Drugs that affect the function of the ANS are classified in four categories: *neurotransmitter*

1. Drugs that stimulate or mimic the parasympathetic receptors are called **cholinergics** or **parasympathomimetics.** Their responses would be to slow the heart rate and cause bronchoconstriction. Remember from Chapter 1 that these drugs could also be called cholinergic agonists, since agonists stimulate a receptor. In addition, they can be called muscarinic drugs, because they stimulate the muscarinic receptors found in the parasympathetic system.
2. Drugs that block parasympathetic receptors are called **anticholinergics** or **parasympatholytics.** Their response would be to speed the heart and cause bronchodilation in opposition to what the parasympathetic system would do if stimulated. Remember that these drugs could also be called cholinergic antagonists or antimuscarinic agents.
3. Drugs that stimulate or mimic the sympathetic receptors would be termed **adrenergics** or **sympathomimetics.** They would include alpha- and/or beta-adrenergic drugs depending upon the receptor they stimulate. More specifically, beta₁ adrenergics would speed the heart rate, and beta₂ adrenergics would bronchodilate.
4. Drugs that would antagonize the sympathetic response are called **antiadrenergics** or **sympatholytics.** They are also referred to as blockers, and therefore a beta blocker would block the expected effects of bronchodilation and increase in heart rate and thus cause bronchoconstriction and a decrease in heart rate.

LEARNING HINT

Think of the adrenalin rush when you think of the sympathetic nervous system being stimulated to connect adrenergic to sympathetic.

CONTROVERSY

It certainly does get confusing when several terms can mean the same thing. For example, a parasympatholytic can be called an anticholinergic or a parasympathetic antagonist or a vagolytic, after the major nerve (vagus) of the parasympathetic system. We can even throw in the term antimuscarinic. Lung sounds have several different terms that can mean the same thing because of carryover, such as a rale (older term), which is the same thing as a crackle. Attempts have been made to standardize lung sound terminology to be less confusing. Do you think the same could apply to nervous system terminology?

As you can again see, functionally the sympathetic and parasympathetic divisions are opposite. Simulating one autonomic division may increase the activity of an organ, and stimulation of the other division may inhibit the activity. Drug therapy can disrupt the balance in sympathetic and parasympathetic activity. For example, sympathetic influences on the heart cause increased force of contraction and heart rate, and parasympathetic influence results in bradycardia and decrease in contractile force. Smooth muscles in the vessels are relaxed with a decrease in sympathetic activity and vasoconstricted with an increase in sympathetic activity.

STOP
& REVIEW

Which of the four autonomic categories could cause bronchodilation? Which would cause a decrease in heart rate?

Direct- and Indirect-Acting Agents

Drugs can affect different steps in the neurotransmission process. Thus far we have talked about stimulating the receptors (agonists), which is a direct-acting agent. Indirect-acting agents that block the receptor site (antagonists) have also been mentioned. However, other indirect methods, such as increasing or decreasing transmitter substances by enhancing or inhibiting the enzymes that break them down, still need to be discussed. We will take one final look at the four classifications of autonomic drug interactions and further develop the concept of indirect-acting drugs.

Parasympathomimetic

Acetylcholine is the main neurotransmitter in all autonomic preganglionic sites and at parasympathetic postganglionic synapses. Acetylcholine is synthesized from acetyl–coenzyme A (acetyl–CoA) and choline by the enzyme choline acetyltransferase. ACh is a simple molecule, yet it has activity at several different receptors. ACh is not a useful drug therapeutically, because it is not specific enough at receptors and it is rapidly broken down in the body. As previously discussed, drugs that act on acetylcholine receptors are called cholinergic or parasympathomimetics.

Acetylcholine action is terminated when it is metabolized by **acetylcholinesterase (AChE).** Cholinergic drugs are subdivided according to whether they act directly at the receptor by increasing production of ACh or indirectly through inhibition of AChE, the enzyme that breaks down ACh. In either scenario, the action of ACh is enhanced either directly by increasing production or indirectly by preventing its rapid breakdown, thus allowing ACh to remain active longer.

AChE inhibitors are also widely used in agriculture as an insecticide (malathion, parathion). In addition, they have unfortunately been used as nerve gas in chemical warfare; overstimulation of the parasympathetic nervous system results in severe bradycardia, hypotension, and death.

Muscarinic agonists are direct-acting parasympathomimetic agents and therefore stimulate the parasympathetic nervous system by increasing ACh production at the effector site. Methacholine is a drug with muscarinic activity. Chemically it is close to acetylcholine, and it is used clinically as part of a bronchial challenge test to cause bronchoconstriction (parasympathetic response) and thereby diagnose asthma. Asthma, of course, would normally be a contraindication for a parasympathomimetic drug, but here the drug is used in small doses for diagnostic purposes.

Drugs can also act specifically at the nicotinic receptor sites where ACh is the neurotransmitter substance. Remember, ACh transmits both sympathetic and parasympathetic impulses from preganglionic neurons to nicotinic ganglionic receptors on postganglionic neurons. Nicotinic receptors are also found at the skeletal muscles in the somatic nervous system. Nicotinic agonists are classifed by whether they stimulate predominantly at the ganglionic level in the autonomic branch of the PNS or at the skeletal muscles of the somatic branch at the neuromuscular level. See Table 3-3 for sample cholinergic agonists and their indications.

Differentiate ACh and AChE. Now relate these terms to direct- and indirect-acting agents.

Parasympatholytics

Parasympatholytic drugs or anticholinergic drugs are pharmacologic antagonists of the parasympathetic nervous system. Cardiovascular effects from anticholinergics, like atropine, include tachycardia, bronchodilation, and drying of secretions, which are all oppo-

Table 3-3   Sample Cholinergic Agonists and Indications

Drug	Indication
Direct-Acting—increased ACh production	
Bethanechol	urinary retention
Succinylcholine	neuromuscular blockade–intubation
Pilocarpine	glaucoma
Indirect-Acting—decreased AChE activity	
Neostigmine	myasthenia gravis
Pyridostigmine	reversal of neuromuscular blockade
Malathion	insecticide
Nerve gas	chemical warfare

LEARNING HINT

A mnemonic used for atropine toxicity is "dry as a bone, red as a beet, mad as a hatter, and blind as a bat." "Dry as a bone" refers to decreased sweating, salivation, and lacrimation. "Red as a beet" refers to the vasodilation of arms, head, neck, and trunk that occurs with atropine overdoses. "Mad as a hatter" refers to CNS toxicity effects such as delirium. "Blind as a bat" refers to the pupil changes. You can see that excessive blockage of the parasympathetic system may not be tolerated well by patients.

site parasympathetic stimulant responses. Atropine derivatives such as ipratropium bromide, mentioned in Chapter 5, are used for their bronchdilation effects. In addition, atropine is part of the Advanced Cardiac Life Support (ACLS) course for treatment of bradycardia.

Anticholinergic drug subgroups are antimuscarinic, because the drugs block the effect at the postganglionic site where muscarinic receptors are found. They can also block the nicotinic receptors. Nicotinic blockers are further divided according to the two sites where nicotinic receptors are found: the ganglia and the skeletal muscles. Ganglionic blockers are not used clinically, because they block both sympathetic and parasympathetic nerves. Neuromuscular blockers produce skeletal muscle paralysis and can be used for surgery or in critical care when patients need to be totally motionless, or to facilitate mechanical ventilation. The significance of this will be discussed in the chapter on skeletal muscle relaxants. See Table 3-4 for some examples of anticholinergic drugs.

Sympathomimetic

To review: adrenergic drugs stimulate and therefore act like the sympathetic nervous system, which dominates in times of stress. It is a survival response that enables the body to prepare to face or flee from a perceived danger. The autonomic sympathetic nerves kick into high gear automatically, so you don't have to think before you act, and precious life or death time isn't wasted. In danger, the heart rate increases, pupils dilate, blood flow increases in the vital organs where it is needed, and the lungs bronchodilate to take in more oxygen. At the same time, some nonessential areas are shut down so energy can concentrate where it is needed the most.

Drugs that act on norepinephrine receptors are called sympathomimetic or adrenergic agonists and mimic sympathetic responses. In the sympathetic or adrenergic system, NE transmits most of the impulses in the sympathetic postganglionic synapse. NE synthesis is more complex than ACh synthesis. NE is released from the sympathetic nerve endings by

Table 3-4   Anticholinergic Drug Class

Category and Function	Drug
Antimuscarinic	atropine
	ipratropium bromide
Nicotinic blockers	
At ganglionic sites	hexamethonium
At skeletal muscle sites—Neuromuscular	
Nondepolarizing	pancuronium
Depolarizing	succinylcholine

the same mechanism as ACh, but the termination is different. Once released, NE crosses the synaptic cleft and binds to postsynaptic adrenergic receptors. There is not an enzyme that immediately breaks down NE to interfere or inactivate its action at the synaptic cleft. Instead of being metabolized immediately, NE is recycled back into the synaptic knob to be stored for future use. This process is called **reuptake.** Excess norepinephrine that does not participate in the reuptake process can eventually be metabolized by the enzymes monoamine oxidase (MAO) and catechol-*o*-methyl-transferase (COMT). The reuptake and metabolism by COMT and MAO will be important concepts in Chapter 5.

Sympathomimetics can also be either direct or indirect acting. Direct-acting sympathomimetics increase NE production and therefore bind with the adrenergic receptors found on the postsynaptic junction of the sympathetic nervous systems. These receptors can be either alpha or beta receptors depending upon location and action. Indirect sympathomimetics will inhibit the reuptake and enzyme deactivation of NE thereby preventing its breakdown. See Figure 3-9 for sympathomimetic drug subgroups.

Contrast the mechanisms of neurotransmitter inactivation in the parasympathetic and sympathetic nervous systems.

<u>CLINICAL PEARL</u>

What, no cheese, wine, or chocolate? There is a group of drugs called MAO inhibitors that interact with sympathomimetic amines and lead to hypertension. MAO is a digestive enzyme that normally breaks down catecholamines. Any food or cold medication that contains sympathomimetics such as pseudoephedrine shouldn't be used with an MAO inhibitor. Wine, cheese, and chocolate have sympathomimetic components. This is one of the first drug–diet interactions that was ever recognized.

Adrenergic agents may be catecholamines or noncatecholamines. Catecholamines include dobutamine, dopamine, epinephrine, isoproterenol, and norepinephrine. They all have a common basic chemical structure and are destroyed if ingested orally by digestive enzymes. Noncatecholamine adrenergic drugs include the examples of phenylephrine and albuterol. They are used for local or systemic vasoconstriction and bronchodilation, respectively, and will all be discussed in upcoming chapters.

Epinephrine or adrenalin is considered the prototype sympathomimetic, with effects on alpha$_1$, alpha$_2$, beta$_1$, and beta$_2$ receptors, and it is used to treat anaphylactic shock. Norepinephrine, an alpha agonist, causes vasoconstriction and therefore can be used to treat low blood pressure. Alpha adrenergic agents applied locally or taken orally can relieve symptoms of nasal congestion by constricting swollen vessels in the nasal passageways. Phenylephrine topically does the same thing by acting directly on alpha receptors. Alpha, beta, and dopamine drugs are used for applications in cardiovascular and respiratory medicine and will be discussed further in following chapters. See Table 3-5 for representative sympathomimetic drugs.

Sympatholytics

Just like adrenergic agonists, sympatholytics or adrenergic blockers have many cardiovascular indications. However, their general effect is to block or slow the effects of the sympathetic system. These drugs consist of alpha and beta blockers used to treat tachy-

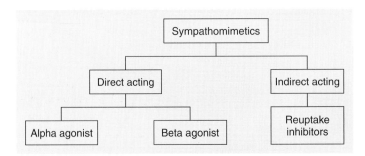

Figure 3-9 Sympathomimetic Drug Subgroups

epinephrine – beta' effects

Table 3-5   Sympathomimetic Drugs

Drug	Indications
Catecholamines *Cardiac situation*	
Epinephrine	anaphylaxis
Norepinephrine	hypotension
Isoproterenol	asthma
Dopamine	shock
Dobutamine	shock, heart failure
Other sympathomimetics	
Phenylephrine	nasal decongestant
Albuterol	asthma

beta —
alpha —

CLINICAL PEARL

Beta blockers can mask the signs and symptoms of hypoglycemia such as tremor and tachycardia, so they are used cautiously in patients with diabetes.

LEARNING HINT

Have you ever experienced the anxiety of stage fright? Performing artists and public speakers have been known to use beta blockers to control tremor, anxiety, and palpitations before appearances.

Stimulate receptor
alpha vasoconstriction
B blocker ↓ BP

arrhythmias and hypertension. In addition to their cardiovascular indications, alpha blockers have direct action on the urethral sphincter to reduce urinary hesitancy in prostate hypertrophy. Adverse effects of beta blockers can include bradycardia, atrioventricular blockade, and exacerbation of asthma. However, there are more selective beta$_1$ blockers, which affect only the heart, with minimal effects on the beta$_2$ receptors found in the lungs. This will be covered in more depth in Chapters 9 and 10. Subgroups of adrenergic blocking drugs or sympatholytics are described in Table 3-6 along with sample drugs and indications.

Table 3-6   Sympatholytic Drug Subgroups

Sympatholytic Subgroup	Drug	Indication
Alpha blocker	Doxazosin	hypertension benign prostate hypertrophy
Beta blocker	Propranolol	hypertension

REVIEW QUESTIONS

beta blocker

1. Which branches comprise the peripheral nervous system?
   I. somatic
   II. parasympathetic
   III. sympathetic
   IV. central nervous system
   (a) I and II
   (b) I, II, III, and IV
   (c) IV only
   (d) I, II, and III
2. Tell whether the following pertain to the sympathetic nervous system (S), parasympathetic nervous system (P), or both (B).
   __S__ fight or flight
   ____ digestion
   ____ ACh at preganglion
   ____ NE
   ____ ACh at postganglion
3. Match synonymous terms in the autonomic nervous system:
   ____ sympathomimetic
   ____ parasympathomimetic
   ____ sympatholytic
   ____ parasympatholytic
   (a) cholinergic
   (b) anticholinergic
   (c) adrenergic
   (d) antiadrenergic
4. Bronchodilation can be achieved using which agent?
   I. parasympatholytic
   II. sympatholytic
   III. sympathomimetic

IV. parasympathomimetic
(a) I and II
(b) II, III, and IV
(c) III only
(d) I and III

5. Skeletal muscles are found in:
(a) blood vessels
(b) airways
(c) heart
(d) diaphragm

6. Contrast the two branches of the autonomic nervous system.

7. Differentiate afferent and efferent nerve impulses.

8. Give the physiologic response to the following:
beta$_2$ stimulation
beta$_1$ stimulation
alpha$_1$ stimulation
beta$_2$ inhibition

9. What would the anticholinergic response be in the eyes, lungs, and heart?

10. What would the adrenergic response be in the eyes, lungs, and heart?

GLOSSARY

acetylcholine   the chemical neurotransmitter of skeletal muscles, the preganglionic sites of both the parasympathetic and the sympathetic nervous system, and the postganglionic sites of the parasympathetic nervous system.

acetylcholinesterase   also known as cholinerestase. The enzyme that deactivates acetylcholine.

adrenergic agents   agents that stimulate the sympathetic nervous system.

adrenergic receptors   receptors of the sympathetic nervous system that include alpha and beta receptors.

afferent nerves   nerves that carry impulses to the brain and spinal cord. Also known as sensory nerves.

alpha receptors   receptors found in the sympathethic nervous system that generally cause vasoconstriction.

antiadrenergics   agents that block the effects of the sympathetic nervous system.

anticholinergic   agents that block the effects of the parasympathetic nervous system.

autonomic nervous system   the nervous system that controls the involuntary responses and is divided into the parasympathetic and sympathetic branches.

beta receptors   receptors found in the sympathethic nervous system that are divided into beta$_1$ and beta$_2$ subcategories. Beta$_1$ receptors are primarily found in the heart and when stimulated cause an increase in rate and force of contraction. Beta$_2$ receptors are primarily found in the lungs and when stimulated cause bronchodilation.

central nervous system   the nervous system comprised of the brain and spinal cord.

cholinergic   referring to the parasympathetic nervous system, where acetylcholine is the neurotransmitter substance at all ganglionic sites.

dopamine receptors   adrenergic receptors found in renal tissue that when stimulated relax the renal arteries and therefore increase renal perfusion.

efferent nerves   nerves that carry impulse away from the brain and spinal cord. Also known as motor nerves.

ganglion   nerve cell body outside of the brain and spinal cord.

muscarinic receptors   receptors found at the postganglionic site of the parasympathetic nervous system.

nicotinic receptors   receptors found at the skeletal muscles in the somatic system and at all preganglionic sites in the parasympathetic and sympathetic nervous systems.

norepinephrine   the chemical neurotransmitter substance found at the postganglionic junction of the sympathetic nervous system.

parasympathetic   branch of the peripheral nervous system that maintains normal body functions and homeostasis.

parasympathomimetic   agent that stimulates the parasympathetic system.

parasympatholytic   agent that blocks or anatagonizes the effects of the parasympathetic system.

peripheral nervous system   part of the nervous system comprised of all nerves outside of the brain and spinal cord; includes the somatic and autonomic nervous systems.

reuptake   process wherein norepinephrine is deactivated at the sympathetic postganglionic sites.

somatic nervous system   the part of the nervous system that controls skeletal muscles and therefore voluntary movement.

sympathetic   branch of the peripheral nervous system that prepares the body for stress and emergencies (a.k.a. the flight or fight system).

sympathomimetic   agent that stimulates the sympathetic system.

sympatholytic   agent that blocks or antagonizes the effects of the sympathetic system.

 www.prenhall.com/colbert

Use the address above to access the free, interactive Companion Web site created specifically for this textbook. Enhance your studying by viewing videos and animations, answering practice quiz questions, and reviewing an audio glossary and much more related to Chapter 3.

CHAPTER 4

Medicated Aerosol Treatments

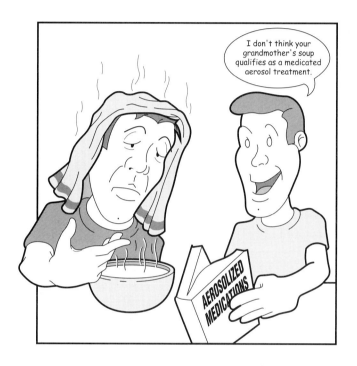

OBJECTIVES

Upon completion of this chapter you will be able to

- Define key terms related to aerosol therapy
- Describe the main goals of aerosol therapy
- State the advantages and disadvantages of the inhalation route of administration
- Describe the factors that affect aerosol depostion
- List advantages and limitations for using a metered dose inhaler (MDI), small volume nebulizer (SVN), and dry powder inhaler (DPI)
- Describe the proper technique for using an MDI, SVN, and DPI

ABBREVIATIONS

propellet MDI

CFCs	Chlorofluorocarbons	HHN	hand-held nebulizer
OTC	over-the-counter	MDIs	metered dose inhalers
DPI	dry powder inhaler	SVN	small volume nebulizer
HFAs	hydrofluoroalkanes		

(openey) MDI

INTRODUCTION

The inhalation route is a very quick-acting and effective route to deliver humidification and/or medications directly to the respiratory system. The delivery of a nonmedicated aerosol such as sterile water is referred to as a bland aerosol. Bland aerosols will be discussed in Chapter 6 under bronchial hygiene and mucokinetic agents. Now, however, we are focusing on aerosolizing a medication that will be inhaled into the respiratory system and then absorbed into the rich capillary network of blood vessels within this system. Administering a drug via the inhalation route is highly advantageous, since it allows you to deliver the medication to the needed site of action directly and thus minimizes the systemic absorption. This in turns minimizes the occurrences or level of severity of side effects that may be associated with the drug.

For example, inhaled steroids are now becoming a mainstay for moderate-to-severe asthma treatment, because they reduce the inflammatory response of the lung. You could administer an oral form of the steroid, but you would have to take a much higher dosage orally to get high enough levels in the entire bloodstream to eventually travel to the lungs to produce the desired effect. Conversely, you can lessen the dosage significantly by inhaling an aerosol of the steroid, because it will be delivered right to the needed site to reduce the inflammation. The side effects of steroids are numerous and dosage dependent, so the inhalation route offers a way to minimize the serious systemic side effects yet maximize the effects on the lungs.

The inhalation route does offer several challenges to the practitioner. One challenge is to teach the patient to self-administer the medicated aerosol effectively. Another is to achieve consistent dosage delivery, considering that there are many variables that affect deposition within the respiratory system. This chapter will give you the needed background to understand the different delivery devices and factors that will maximize optimal medicated aerosol delivery to the respiratory system.

BASIC CONCEPTS OF MEDICATED AEROSOLS

What Is Aerosol Therapy?

An **aerosol** is a suspension of solid or liquid particles within a gas. For example, when we sneeze, we create an aerosol of liquid droplet particles that are suspended in the rapidly exhaled gas from our lungs. A dust storm also creates an aerosol, but now the aerosol particles are solid in nature. **Aerosol therapy** can deliver either solid or liquid aerosol particles into the respiratory tract for therapeutic purposes. The three main goals of aerosol therapy include:

1. To humidify inspired gas, which may be dry or humidity-deficient. An example would be an intubated patient whose natural humidification system (upper airways) is bypassed.
2. To improve the mobilization and elimination of secretions. Examples include patients with thick tenacious secretions who are having difficulty expectorating, or patients who have a dry, nonproductive cough and need a sputum induction to obtain a sample for analysis.
3. To deliver medications to the respiratory tract.

Each of these indications will be discussed in depth in future chapters. The first two indications will be further discussed in Chapter 6, which deals with mucokinetics. The third indication will be discussed in various chapters treating specific categories of drugs that can be administered via aerosol therapy. This chapter will focus on the principles of effective aerosol delivery to the respiratory system.

Advantages and Disadvantages

The advantages to delivering drugs via the aerosol route center around two major facts. First, the lungs have a large surface area and rich corresponding vasculature for drug absorption. As you remember from Chapter 1, blood flow influences the extent and rate of absorption. Therefore, medications delivered via the inhalation route act very quickly. Secondly, the aerosol route is delivering the medication locally to the site of need and is not systemically diluted in the entire bloodstream or affected by the GI tract or the first-pass effect mentioned in Chapter 1. This allows for smaller effective dosages of the drug, thereby reducing potential side effects. From a patient perspective, the inhalation route is effective and convenient if proper instruction and education are given.

There are also disadvantages to the inhalation route. First, because several factors influence the exact amount that actually gets to the lungs, it is difficult to get precise dosages each time. Often the patient will self-administer aerosol medications, and therefore this route also requires good patient education and compliance for safe and effective use. In addition, specialized equipment is utilized to deliver the aerosol and must be properly maintained for function and infection control.

If the healthcare practitioner understands the principles of aerosol medication delivery, knows the proper use of the various aerosol delivery devices, and can effectively instruct and educate the patient, then the disadvantages are minimized.

Why does the inhalation route have a quick onset of action?

Technical Background

Let's return to the sneeze as an example of an aerosol. The liquid particles (the very small water droplets from the lungs) are suspended in a gas (the air expelled from the lungs). The aerosol particles can travel and settle out on inanimate objects such as the floor, or they can be breathed in by another individual and settle in that person's lungs. This is why the sneeze (or cough) represents a likely transmission for certain pulmonary diseases. We certainly don't want the possibly contaminated aerosol particles of a sneeze to travel into someone else's lungs, and hopefully the aerosol droplets will all impact upon a tissue (the Kleenex type, or a similar brand) and be properly discarded. However, it is beneficial to deliver certain types of medication into the lungs in an aerosol form.

A **medicated aerosol** simply means a suspension of a liquid or solid drug in a carrier gas. However, what determines how this medicine gets delivered into the lungs? Let's start with four technical terms that are used in reference to medicated aerosols. These are all factors that influence drug delivery within the lungs. First, **stability** refers to the tendency of an aerosol to remain in suspension. The current delivery devices that create aerosols all produce stable aerosols that will not destabilize (rainout) before they reach the lungs. However, because of this stability, it is important for the patient to hold their breath so that the

Table 4-1 Advantages and Disadvantages of Medicated Aerosols

Advantages	*Disadvantages*
Smaller required doses	Difficult to deliver consistent precise dose
Quick drug response	Requires patient compliance and education
Fewer, less severe side effects	Equipment maintenance
Painless and convenient	

particles will rainout into the lungs and not be quickly breathed right back out into the room, where they have no pharmacological effect.

Secondly, **penetration** refers to how far into the lungs the aerosol particles travel. This is related to several factors, such as the size of the aerosol particle, the patient's breathing pattern, and their disease state. Optimally, you want the aerosol to penetrate to the desired level of action. How you accomplish this mainly depends on the breathing pattern, which will be discussed shortly.

The third term is **deposition,** which refers to the aerosol particles falling out of suspension. Ideally, we want them to fall out into the desired area of the lungs. Deposition, like penetration, is a factor of how the patient breathes and their disease state.

The final term is **inertial impaction.** Even though these particles are very small, they nevertheless have weight and must obey the laws of physics. They will develop inertial energy depending on the speed of the delivery device and/or the rate of breathing. If something gets in their way, such as a bifurcation of the lung, and their inertial energy is such that they cannot negotiate the turn, they will impact upon the airway wall.

What factors influence drug delivery within the lungs?

Aerosol Size Matters

One final technical aspect of aerosol particles is size. Size is one of the most important factors in determining whether the aerosol will get to the lung. Aerosol particle sizes are in **microns,** which equal one millionth of a meter. Critically small variances in size will determine how far the aerosol can penetrate.

For example, 10- to 15-micron particles will get stuck in the upper airways (nose and mouth). Many nasal sprays produce particles in this range, because this is where you want deposition to occur. Slightly smaller particles, within the 5- to 10-micron range, penetrate to large bronchi. Particles of 1 to 5 microns penetrate to the lower airways, where most bronchoactive drugs are needed. Most aerosol-generating devices will therefore produce aerosol particles within this range. Particles of less than .5 microns have so much stability that while they may penetrate to the alveoli, they may also be breathed right back out (see Figure 4-1, which shows where various particle sizes will deposit).

Breathing Pattern

If the particles are within the proper range, how much aerosol actually gets to the lung depends greatly on the patient's breathing pattern. Remember that one of the disadvantages of the inhalation route was an imprecise dosage. Even if the aerosol-generating device is used properly, studies estimate that only around 10% to 50% may actually get into the lungs under optimal conditions. If poor technique is used, only 1% to 2% may actually deposit in the lungs.

If you visualize the tracheal bronchial tree, it is a maze of sharp turns that present a great potential for inertial impaction that would interfere with even distribution of the aerosol within the lungs. Rapid inspiratory flows can cause turbulence that favors inertial impaction and deposition higher in the respiratory tract. Slow inspiration produces more laminar flow and results in deeper penetration of the aerosol particles.

Looking at all factors, one can see why the optimal breathing pattern for effective aerosol delivery to the lungs is a slow, deep breath with a hold. Slow breathing minimizes the inertial impaction that can cause the medication to rainout in the upper airways. Deep breathing allows for maximum penetration within the lungs. A breath hold allows for these

Margin notes

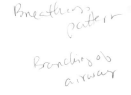
Breathing pattern

Branching of airway

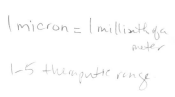
1 micron = 1 millionth of a meter

1-5 therapeutic range

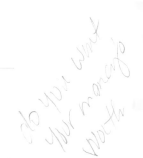
do you want your money worth

LEARNING HINT
If you were an aerosol particle and tried to reach the bottom of the tracheal bronchial tree, would it be better to travel very fast or very slow? Well, picture a fork in the road (not the kind you eat with); you need to take one of the roads to get deeper into the lungs. You must slow down in order to negotiate the curve of your choice.

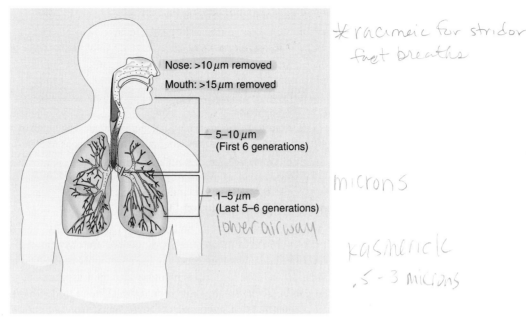

[handwritten: # racmeic for stridor fast breaths]

[handwritten: microns]

[handwritten: kasmenick .5 - 3 microns]

[handwritten: lower airway]

Figure 4-1 Deposition of Variously Sized Aerosol Particles Within Respiratory System

very small, stable particles to deposit out of the aerosol and onto the lung tissue. Therefore, a slow deep breath through the mouth with an *inspiratory hold* is the optimal breathing pattern for maximal penetration and deposition within the lungs.

[handwritten: other target areas:]

There are, however, indications for medicated aerosol delivery to just the upper airway. The upper airway includes the oropharynx, larynx, trachea, and supraglottic area. Topical anesthetics can be delivered to the supraglottic regions prior to intubation or bronchoscopy procedures. Glottic edema can cause upper airway swelling, which could asphyxiate a patient, and vasoconstrictors can be given to shrink the swelling and maintain a patent airway.

[handwritten: for stridor]

If your target for aerosol deposition is the upper airway, larger particles, of a size between 5 and 10 microns, should be used and delivered by fast inspiratory flow rates, which will increase deposition in the larynx and supraglottic area. In other words, taking a fast breath in will cause all the particles to crash (impact) on the walls of the upper airways, because they cannot negotiate the curves.

< CONTROVERSY >

Although it may be clinically beneficial to have a nebulizer that produces larger particle sizes (5 to 10 microns) to target the upper airway, small volume nebulizers generally produce most of their particle sizes less than this range to achieve peripheral distribution and deposition.

CLINICAL PEARL

Disease states can even influence aerosol distribution in the lungs. COPD patients may have aerosol particles distributed more centrally than non-COPD patients, who have more particles in the peripheral portions of the lungs.

In summary, in most situations you are striving for deposition in the peripheral regions of the lung, so a *slow, deep* breath through the mouth with an *inspiratory hold* is best. If upper airway deposition is desired, a fast inspiratory flow rate is required. Table 4-2 quantifies general guidelines on aerosol deposition.

Table 4-2   Optimal Breathing Pattern

Peripheral Distribution	*Oropharynx, Larynx, Trachea, and First Six Airway Generations*
Slow (inspiratory flow of less than 30 L/min) deep breath, with a 10-second breath hold. Aerosol particle size range should be 1–5 microns.	Fast inspiratory flow (above 30 L/min) to increase deposition in the larynx and supraglottic area. Normal flow at 30 L/min would increase deposition in the trachea and the first six generations of airways (larger airways) with aerosol particles in the range of 5–10 microns.

Types of Aerosolized Drugs

So what types of drugs can be aerosolized and delivered into the respiratory system? The list may surprise you, because many people are only familiar with the over- the-counter (OTC) nasal decongestant sprays or the commonly prescribed bronchodilators used to treat asthma. In addition to steroids mentioned in the Introduction, several other drug classifications can be given via the inhalation route. A more in-depth discussion will be included in each chapter that deals with each of these specific classifications. The following represents a *brief* description of these drug classifications:

Nasal Decongestants. Found primarily as OTC squeeze bottles that you spray into your nostrils. These produce larger particles, which settle in the nasal region. Basically they are fairly powerful vasoconstrictors and thereby decrease the blood flow to the stuffy nose. This in turn allows the nasal passageway to become clearer, because the vessels shrink and open up the passageways. Since this is a vasoconstrictor, it can increase blood pressure, which should be monitored. A representative drug would be Neo-Synephrine.

Bronchodilators. Bronchodilators enlarge the diameter of the airway through a number of different mechanisms, most of which include relaxing the smooth muscle that surrounds the airways. Some representaitve drugs include Proventil, Atrovent, Maxair, and Serevent. These and others are discussed in Chapter 5.

Antiasthmatics. This is a relatively new category of drugs, ones that desensitize the allergic response and therefore prevent or decrease the incidence of asthma. Representative drugs would be cromolyn sodium and nedocromil sodium, which are discussed in Chapter 7.

Corticosteroids. These drugs are being used increasingly in moderate and severe asthma attacks to reduce the inflammatory response within the lung. It is speculated that they help prevent or lessen what is called late-phase asthma, which can be very severe and occur hours after the initial attack. Representative drugs include Vanceril, Flovent, and Azmacort. These and others will be discussed in Chapter 7.

Mucolytics. This category of drugs breaks down the secretions within the lungs to make it easier to expectorate and clear the lungs. In addition to nebulization, sometimes these medications are directly instilled into the lungs in liquid form via an endotracheal tube or bronchoscope. A representative drug is Mucomyst. This drug and others will be discussed in Chapter 6.

Antimicrobials. Much promise lies in this new area where aerosolized antibiotics and antiviral agents have been and continue to be developed to fight both bacterial and viral infections involving the respiratory system. Representative drugs include gentamicin, amphotericin B, ribavirin, and pentamidine. These and others will be covered in Chapter 8.

Surface-Acting Agents. These drugs have been dramatic in the replacement of surfactant in premature infants and reducing the need for oxygen and mechanical ventilation. Representative drugs are Survanta and Exosurf and will be discussed in Chapter 6.

AEROSOL DELIVERY DEVICES

Metered Dose Inhalers (MDIs)

The most common type of aerosol treatment is the **metered dose inhaler (MDI).** MDIs are small portable aerosol delivery devices that can effectively deliver medication to the respiratory system. They basically consist of a propellant contained in the canister filled with medication. Since they are usually self-administered, they require patient education and cooperation.

CONTROVERSY

The propellants used in MDIs are blends of liquefied gas **chlorofluorocarbons** (CFCs, freon), which are bad for the environment because they enlarge the hole in the ozone layer. In addition, some patients are sensitive to these propellants and may experience bronchospasm. Therefore (primarily because of the damage to the ozone layer), the United Nations Environment Program has called for phasing out the production of CFCs. Pharmaceutical companies went to work and developed **hydrofluoroalkanes** (HFAs), which do not hurt the ozone layer and are not dangerous to some patients. The current studies are conflicting as to which of the types of propellents give better lung deposition. Further studies are indicated, and we will keep you updated on the Web site.

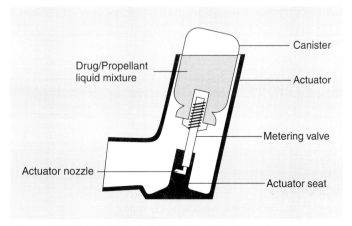

Figure 4-2 Schematic of MDI Delivery Systems

Spacers and Special Considerations

The particles that are exiting the MDI have a very high flow rate because of the pressurized delivery system. Therefore, inertial impaction in the oropharynx is a likely occurrence. To minimize this, reservoir or **spacer devices** have been developed (see Figure 4-3). These devices allow for three major advantages.

CLINICAL PEARL

There are some inexpensive alternatives that patients can use temporarily as a spacer. Examples include a six-inch piece of corrugated aerosol tubing and even cardboard toilet paper rolls for one-time emergency use. However, these are temporary, and we recommend a proper spacer, which can be reused and cleaned properly.

1. They form the aerosol in a holding chamber or reservoir, which then allows the particles to slow down and gives the patient time to coordinate their inspiration. In addition, many of the initial particles are larger than 5 microns, and the reservoir allows enough time to vaporize them to the point of 1 to 5 microns, so lung deposition is better.
2. Many patients, as they depress the canister, move the MDI and end up spraying their nose or eyes. The spacer device allows you to have something stable in your mouth as you depress the canister that will direct the flow of aerosol into the oral cavity and eventually into the lungs.
3. Patients often have difficulty coordinating the activation of the device and taking a slow deep breath. The spacer makes this a more forgiving process, because the aerosol is formed in a holding chamber. If the patient lags behind in breathing in, it is of little consequence with a spacer. If they lag behind without a spacer, the aerosol is already impacted in the mouth, or if they moved, on the nose or eyes.

www.prenhall.com/colbert

Spacers and valved holding chambers are technically different. Go to the Web site for an explanation of these differences.

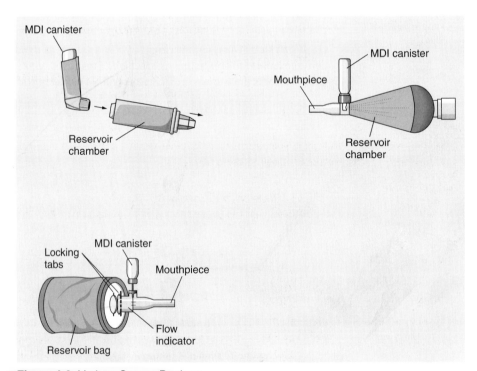

Figure 4-3 Various Spacer Devices

Administering an MDI Treatment

Some studies have shown that up to 60% to 70% of patients do not use their MDIs correctly. Therefore, we will present a narrative on the steps and factors in administering an MDI treatment and follow with a simplified and streamlined set of specific steps.

If the MDI hasn't been used for days or weeks, the propellant may be lost or the first dose not properly charged. Therefore, shake the MDI first and discharge one waste dose to prime the valve with drug and propellant if you have not used it for 24 hours.

The next step is to exhale and place the spacer device within your mouth. If you don't have a spacer device, hold the MDI 2 to 3 centimeters away from your open mouth. Depress the canister and take a slow, deep breath in through your mouth, continuing until your lungs are filled, to allow for maximum distribution throughout the lungs. Hold this breath for 8 to 10 seconds to allow for deposition of the medicated aerosol, and then breathe out normally.

Often a second dose is needed or prescribed, and it is important to wait a few minutes to allow the first dose to work. Most of the short-acting bronchodilators work very rapidly and waiting a minimum of one to two minutes will allow the airways to open and the next dose to deposit in lower generations.

MDI Instructions

1. Assemble the inhaler and hold inhaler upright. (Don't forget to take off the cap! If you're wearing a cap of your own, you can leave it on.)
2. Shake the MDI well. (Remember to discharge a waste dose if it has been more than 24 hours since you last used the inhaler.) *if needed*
3. Exhale normally.
4. Place the spacer device in your mouth, keeping your tongue down so it doesn't obstruct flow. If no spacer device is available, use the open-mouth technique, and position the inhaler about 2 to 3 cm away from mouth.
5. Begin to take a *slow deep* breath through your mouth, pressing down on the canister as you continue to inhale.
6. Breathe in until your lungs are full; then *hold* your breath for 10 seconds, or as long as you can.
7. Breathe out normally.
8. Wait 1 to 2 minutes before taking the next puff in the same manner. If a third puff is prescribed, wait another 1 to 2 minutes again.
9. Reassemble and store (put the cap back on).

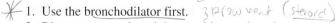

NOTE: If you are using an <u>inhaled steroid</u>, use the same procedure as for a bronchodilator, with the following considerations. *1 Albuterol / 2 Atrovent / 3 Pulmovent (steroid)*

1. Use the bronchodilator first.
2. Rinse your mouth and throat with mouthwash or water after finishing.

CLINICAL PEARL

If you are administering a short-acting bronchodilator and any other inhaled medication, there are additional considerations. The bronchodilator should be given first to open the airways so that the additional medications can be widely distributed in the lungs. In addition, inhaled steroids can deplete or wipe out the normal bacteria in the mouth, and therefore it is critical to rinse the mouth after steroids to prevent an opportunistic oral infection.

CLINICAL PEARL

Having the patient tip their head backward slightly as if sniffing produces maximal opening of the airway and can improve drug delivery to the lungs.

Instruct a classmate on the proper use of an MDI. If possible, obtain a placebo (contains no drug) MDI for optimal practice.

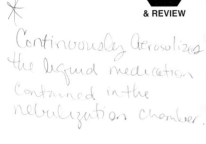

Continuously aerosolizes the liquid medication contained in the nebulization chamber

Small Volume Nebulizer

Whereas the MDI only forms an aerosol when activated, the **small volume nebulizer (SVN)** continuously aerosolizes the liquid medication contained in the nebulization chamber (see Figure 4-4). The aerosol is formed by a continuous flow of gas that is either compressed air or oxygen. The treatments usually last between 8 and 12 minutes and allow for numerous breaths to administer the medication versus the 1 or 2 puffs of an MDI. Although the device may be creating the aerosol, it is not assisting the patient in the breathing process.

Again, the ideal breathing pattern is a slow deep breath with an inspiratory hold for maximum deposition to the periphery. However, someone in acute respiratory distress will have a difficult time holding each breath over this extended time. In that case, the practitioner can encourage the patient to periodically (as often as possible for the patient) take slow deep breaths and hold and allow for treatment breaks.

CLINICAL PEARL

Shakespeare asks the question, "What's in a name?" The answer may be plenty when you have various names to describe the same thing. Some hospitals call SVNs hand held nebulizers (HHNs), or spontaneous nebulizer treatment, or jet nebulizer treatment. Others use the brand name of the nebulizer device.

CONTROVERSY

Since the SVN forms an aerosol on both inspiration and exhalation, a large portion is lost to the atmosphere. Therefore, some devices have a thumb control port so that the patient can create nebulization on inspiration only. However, these are often difficult for the patient to control with each breath and are not widely used.

The spontaneous aerosol treatment can be given with a mouthpiece or a mask. A mask is not preferred, since it reduces deposition in the lung. Much of the medication gets deposited on the face, or, in the case of one of the authors, the beard. However, situations that involve, for example, obtunded or comatose patients or children who cannot maintain a good seal around a mouthpiece may necessitate the use of a mask to deliver the aerosol. The

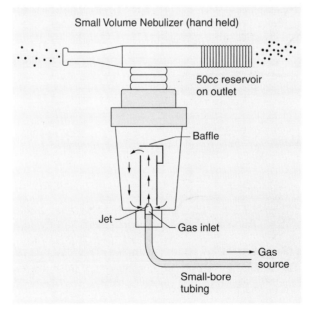

Small Volume Nebulizer (hand held)

50cc reservoir on outlet

Baffle

Jet

Gas inlet

Gas source

Small-bore tubing

Figure 4-4 Schematic of SVN Device

SVN is bulkier to use, since you need an external pneumatic (gas) power source. Care and cleaning of the SVN is also more involved than for the MDI.

---

www.prenhall.com/colbert

Go to the Web site to see a video of an SVN treatment and to learn how to clean and care for the equipment.

Continuous Nebulization

There are certain instances such as status asthmaticus for which aerosolized bronchodilators need to be administered continuously. SVNs can be adapted with an infusion pump for this purpose. In addition, specialized nebulizers created for this purpose such as the Mini-Heart can be used. Studies have shown this to be safe, and it may be more effective in patients with severe pulmonary dysfunction.

Dry Powder Inhaler

> **CLINICAL PEARL**
>
> Patients should be instructed not to exhale into the DPI, as this may blow out the powder and therefore reduce the dosage. In addition, the added humidity from the breath may wet the powder and reduce delivery.

From the definition of an aerosol, we can also see that an aerosol can contain solid particles suspended in a gas. **Dry powder inhalers (DPI)** are devices that actually deliver the drug in powder form to be delivered into the lungs for absorption (see Figure 4-5). DPIs have no propellant or external power sources and are small self-generating devices. In other words, the patient must generate sufficient inspiratory flow rates (equal to or greater than 60 liters per minute) for the device to properly aerosolize the dry powder. This may be difficult in acute respiratory distress or for small children, especially during an asthmatic attack (see Table 4-3).

Table 4-3 Advantages and Disadvantages of DPI

Advantages	*Disadvantages*
Relatively small and easy to use	Few drugs available in powder form
Contains no harmful propellants	Some patients might react to the carrier substance
Easy to tell how much drug is left	Inspiratory flow of more than or equal to 60 L/min is required
Eliminates timing and technique problems with MDIs	
Can be used in cold environments (e.g., ski slopes) where propellants won't work	

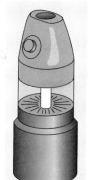

Figure 4-5 DPI Device

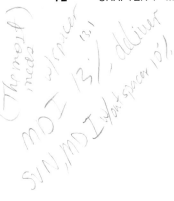

www.prenhall.com/colbert

Go to the Web site to see a video of a of DPI treatment and to learn about the drugs that currently can be given via this method.

Choosing the Proper Treatment

How do you choose among the MDI, SVN, or DPI? This choice depends on several factors. Generally, if a patient is able to follow instructions and demonstrates correct use of an MDI, it is the preferred way to go. However, the patient must have an adequate inspiratory capacity and be able to hold their breath. This is very important, since they are only getting two or three chances for good aerosol deposition. MDIs work well with patients in mild distress or who are taking a drug for prophylactic treatment. An unstable breathing pattern or respiratory distress would limit the effectiveness of an MDI.

The SVN is indicated if the patient is unable to follow the instructions to complete an effective MDI treatment or if the respiratory pattern is unstable. For example, the patient may be in distress, tachypneic and unable to take a slow deep breath with a hold. The SVN now allows for numerous breaths over time, which provides more deposition in cases of acute respiratory distress. SVNs may make more sense in an acute asthmatic attack, although the research hasn't been conclusive. The SVN with a mask is an option available for disoriented or comatose patients who are spontaneously breathing.

DPIs are less frequently used, because only a few drugs are available in this form. However, because of their portability (they are easy to place in pockets) and ease of use, they may be prescribed to children who have adequate inspiratory flow rates to properly use the device. However, only two drugs are currently available, and high inspiratory flow rates are needed. They also work well in cold weather conditions, where the MDI propellants may be hampered.

In summation, if you have a patient who can follow instructions and has a stable breathing pattern, and if the prescribed drug is available in that form, the MDI is the best way to go. We strongly recommend using a spacer with an MDI (even in these cost-containment days), because spacers help coordinate a better and more effective dose into the lungs and minimize the amount that gets deposited in the mouth. However, for disoriented patients, patients unable to use an MDI for whatever reason, or patients with an unstable breathing pattern (fast rate, unable to hold breath or to deep breathe), an SVN would be more effective. Remember, SVNs are bulkier and require an outside gas source and more meticulous cleaning, but if a patient can't use a MDI, this now becomes a way to deliver medication into the lungs.

www.prenhall.com/colbert

MDIs and SVN treatments are also delivered while a patient is on a mechanical ventilator. This requires special considerations, which are discussed on the Web site.

CLINICAL PEARL

SVNs may require unit dose drug packaging if patients are unable to prepare the correct dosage using a dropper.

STOP

& REVIEW

Give at least one patient situation for each form of medicated aerosol treatment—MDI, SVN, and DPI—where that form would be preferred.

The Future

The aerosol route holds much promise for the future. Research is currently being done on inhaled insulin for diabetics. Gene replacement therapy, where a defective gene is replaced to treat certain genetic diseases such as cystic fibrosis, is showing some promise via the aerosol route. Morphine has been aerosolized in intubated patients to decrease anxiety and pain; however, this is still being studied. The Web site that corresponds to this book will allow us to keep you up to date on all these developments. You can find updates on specific new aerosolized drugs in the chapter that pertains to their respective drug category.

SUMMARY

Aerosol drug delivery is used for a wide range of drug classifications. Like any pharmacological route of therapy, aerosol therapy has many advantages and disadvantages. To make clinical decisions about different methods of aerosol delivery, apply general pharmacological principles introduced previously and reinforced in this chapter. You will achieve effective therapy only with careful attention to technical factors such as stability, penetration, deposition, inertial impaction, and breathing pattern. No other route of therapy is so dependent on the patient and the delivery technique.

REVIEW QUESTIONS

1. To deliver a topical anesthetic to the supraglottic tissues prior to bronchoscopy, which of the following techniques would be best?
   (a) Use of an MDI that delivers particles in the range of 1 to 5 microns and slow mouth breathing with breath hold
   (b) Giving an oral medication and waiting for the systemic effects
   (c) Use of a nebulizer that delivers particles in the range of 5 to 10 microns, high inspiratory flow rates, and mouth breathing
   (d) Use of a nebulizer that delivers particles of 10 to 15 microns, high inspiratory flow rates, and nose breathing

2. Slow inspiratory flow rates would
   (a) decrease penetration
   (b) enhance deposition in the upper airways
   (c) increase inertial impaction
   (d) maximize delivery to the lung periphery

3. The ideal particle size for aerosol delivery to the small airways is
   (a) 10 to 15 microns

   (b) 1 to 5 microns
   (c) .5 microns
   (d) 100 microns

4. What is the ideal pattern for DPI administration?
   (a) fast and deep
   (b) slow and deep
   (c) fast and shallow
   (d) slow and shallow

5. Chlorofluorocarbons are being phased out as MDI propellants because they
   (a) have problems with stability
   (b) are expensive
   (c) have an unpleasant smell
   (d) damage the ozone layer

6. List and describe the three main goals of aerosol therapy.

7. Contrast the advantages and disadvantages of aerosol therapy.

8. You are asked to evaluate patients for aerosolized bronchodilator therapy. Which delivery device would you recommend for the following patients?
   (a) a 16-year-old cooperative and alert male with exercise-induced asthma
   (b) an 88-year-old female with dementia
   (c) an 18-month-old infant

(d) a 58-year-old with COPD who is in the emergency department in acute respiratory distress

9. Describe the steps in the proper technique of administering a bronchodilator MDI treatment. What additional steps would be taken if an MDI corticosteroid was also ordered?

10. Describe the role of continuous nebulization aerosol therapy.

CASE STUDY

Chief Complaint

Mr. Blue is an anxious-appearing 60-year-old male diagnosed with COPD 6 months ago. He was discharged from the hospital a week ago and now complains that the new inhaled medications are "not working." He also complains of a white tongue and throat and a strange taste in his mouth.

Past Medical History

His last hospitalization was for pneumonia; he was diagnosed at that time with congestive heart failure and prescribed home oxygen. Family history revealed positive for lung cancer in his mother. Social history: he is a 50-pack/year smoker.

Medications

(bronchodilator) albuterol MDI 2 puffs qid and prn
(corticosteroid) beclomethasone MDI 2 puffs qid

What supports the statement that Mr. Blue is not correctly using his MDIs? What specific instructions would you emphasize during your patient education session? Are there any other suggestions you would make at this time to improve his health?

GLOSSARY

aerosol   suspension of liquid or solid particles in a gas.

aerosol therapy   delivery of aerosol particles into the respiratory system for therapeutic purposes.

chlorofluorocarbons (CFCs)   older propellant for MDIs; damaged the ozone layer and were reactive in some patients, so are therefore currently banned.

deposition   aerosol particles falling out or raining out of suspension.

dry powder inhaler (DPI)   medicated aerosol delivery device that delivers a powered (solid) aerosol to the respiratory system.

hydrofluoroalkanes (HFAs)   replacing CFCs as MDI propellant, because they do not damage the ozone layer and are not as reactive in patients.

inertial impaction   the impacting of aerosol particles upon airway walls because of inertial energy.

medicated aerosol   medicine that has been made into an aerosol to be delivered into the respiratory system.

metered dose inhaler (MDI)   a medicated aerosol delivery device that delivers measured doses (metered puffs) of aerosol from a small gas-powered canister.

micron   one millionth of a meter; the order of magnitude of how small these aerosol particles are.

penetration   how deep the aerosol particles travel into the respiratory system.

pneumatically powered   another name for gas-powered.

small volume nebulizer (SVN)   a medicated aerosol delivery device that uses a gas-powered source to form and deliver the aerosol continuously over a period of usually 8 to 12 minutes.

spacer   reservoir device used with aerosol delivery devices such as MDIs to optimize aerosol drug delivery.

stability   tendency of an aerosol to remain in suspension.

    www.prenhall.com/colbert

Use the address above to access the free, interactive Companion Web site created specifically for this textbook. Enhance your studying by viewing videos and animations, answering practice quiz questions, and reviewing an audio glossary and much more related to Chapter 4.

CHAPTER 5

Bronchodilators

Medical Daffy Definition #101

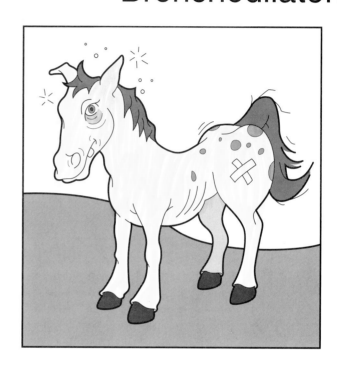

Broncho-di-lator—a bucking rodeo horse who has a very poor prognosis.

OBJECTIVES

Upon completion of this chapter you will be able to

- Define key terms relative to bronchodilator pharmacotherapy
- Describe the neurological control of bronchial smooth muscle, including the sympathetic and parasympathetic nerves, their chemical mediators, and how bronchodilation is achieved
- Differentiate bronchospasm and bronchoconstriction
- Describe three pharmacologic methods for bronchodilation (sympathomimetic, anticholinergic and xanthine) and the mode of action of each
- State the indications, contraindications, adverse reactions, onset of action and dosage range for each bronchodilator
- Recommend appropriate bronchodilator therapy for various patient situations, including drug, dosage, frequency and route of delivery
- Describe appropriate techniques for monitoring the patient's response to bronchodilator therapy

Main contributing author Terri Price

ABBREVIATIONS

AMP	adenosine monophosphate	FEV_1	forced expiratory volume in one second
α	alpha receptor		
β_1	beta$_1$ receptor	β_2	beta$_2$ receptor
cAMP	cyclic AMP	PVC	premature ventricular contraction
PEFR	peak expiratory flow rate		

INTRODUCTION

Imagine yourself being called to the emergency department to treat an asthmatic who is struggling to breathe. The treatment needs to work quickly and be safe. The administration of inhaled bronchodilators is the most important aspect of treating such emergencies. With the prevalence of asthma, COPD, and respiratory disease in general, bronchodilators are one of the most commonly prescribed drug classifications. The practitioner must be thoroughly knowledgeable in the actions, adverse reactions, dosages, onset of action, and duration of action of the various agents. In addition, the practitioner must be knowledgeable about the mechanisms of **bronchoconstriction** in various disease states to be able to select the most beneficial agent for individual patients. The practitioner must also be able to select the best delivery system, instruct patients to develop techniques that assure optimal delivery of the medication, and assess the patient's response to the treatment.

AIRWAY ANATOMY AND PHYSIOLOGY

Before discussing the specific agents, a brief review of airway anatomy and physiology is needed. The conducting airways of the lung are made up of three layers, the *mucosa*, the *submucosa*, and the *adventitia*. The mucosa layer contains the ciliated cells that move the mucus toward the pharynx to keep the lumen of the airway cleared of debris. The submucosal layer contains bronchial glands, smooth muscle, capillary network, and elastic tissue. The smooth muscle of this layer plays a very important role in bronchospasm. Much of this chapter concerns the mechanisms by which various drugs relax the bronchial smooth muscle. Finally, the adventitia is a sheath of connective tissue that surrounds and supports the airways.

The large airways begin with the trachea, which divides to form bronchi. Between the submucosa and the adventitia of the large airways are plates or incomplete rings of cartilage that provide support to prevent the airways from collapsing. Somewhere between the 5th and the 14th generation below the subsegmental bronchi, the bronchi become bronchioles. The term bronchiole means small bronchi or small airways. They are 1 to 2 mm in diameter and lack the supporting cartilage of the large airways. The smooth muscle of the submucosa changes from sheets of muscle surrounding the bronchi to long strands that spiral and crisscross around the bronchioles. This configuration of muscle fibers reduces the diameter and length of the airway when the smooth muscle contracts. See Figure 5-1.

Bronchoconstriction versus Bronchospasm

The term bronchoconstriction refers to a decrease in the diameter of the airway. This may be the result of three distinct mechanisms: **bronchospasm,** airway edema, or secretions. Sometimes all three may be contributing factors in a patient's bronchoconstriction.

- *Bronchospasm* is the actual spasm of the smooth muscle in the bronchial wall. The airway diameter is reduced, which causes a reduction in airflow and increased work of breathing. Bronchodilating drugs are indicated for treatment of this problem.

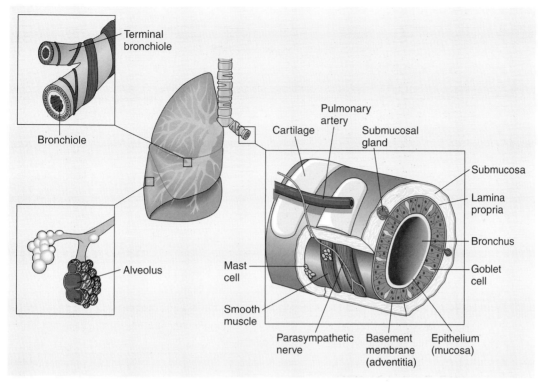

Figure 5-1 The Cross-Sectional Anatomy of a Bronchus, Bronchiole, and Alveolus

- *Edema* occurs when insult or injury to the mucus membranes causes dilation of the blood vessels and accumulation of fluid in the tissues. The swollen tissue reduces the diameter of the lumen of the airway, and breathing becomes more difficult. In this case, treatment should be aimed toward constricting the blood vessels to reduce swelling or toward administration of steroids to block the inflammatory response. These agents will be discussed in Chapter 7.
- *Secretions* contained within the airway reduce the airway diameter. This is often the result of impairment of the normal mucocilliary clearance mechanism of the lungs. Effective bronchial hygiene techniques coupled with wetting agents and mucolytics may be indicated for this process, and they are discussed in Chapter 6. See Figure 5-2 which illustrates these three types of bronchoconstriction.

LEARNING HINT

To get a feel for a reduced airway diameter, while seated and with noseclips on, breathe through a straw and note the difficulties you experience in breathing. You can remove the noseclips and straw and easily return to normal; the bronchoconstricted patient must rely on appropriate medical treatment to return to normal breathing.

Regardless of the cause of the reduction in airway diameter, a bronchoconstricted patient will experience increased airway resistance, increased work of breathing, and dyspnea. To select the best bronchodilator, the practitioner must understand the pathophysiology of the disease and the mechanism of the bronchoconstriction. This chapter will focus on treating bronchoconstriction due to bronchospasm.

STOP & REVIEW

Explain the statement "Bronchospasm always results in bronchoconstriction, but not all bronchoconstriction is caused by bronchospasm."

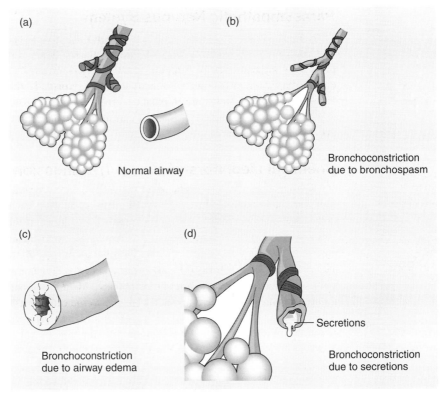

Figure 5-2 Normal Bronchi, Bronchospasm, Mucosal Edema, and Mucus Narrowing the Airway

NEUROLOGICAL CONTROL OF BRONCHIAL SMOOTH MUSCLE

The bronchi are innervated by the autonomic branch of the PNS, as discussed in Chapter 3. Since the nervous system plays such an important role in maintaining airway diameter, it will be reviewed again briefly. These concepts are central to understanding the pharmacologic treatment of bronchoconstriction.

The autonomic nervous system is comprised of two divisions, the sympathetic nervous system and the parasympathetic nervous system.

Sympathetic Nervous System

The sympathetic nervous system dominates the body's reaction to stressful circumstances. This so-called fight or flight response to sympathetic activation stimulates the heart, increases cardiac output and blood pressure, dilates the pupils, increases metabolism, and enhances alertness. The response mediated by the sympathetic nervous system also relaxes the bronchial smooth muscle to dilate the airways and lower airway resistance, facilitating increased ventilation. The increased rate and depth of breathing increases ventilation. Ultimately, this results in increased oxygen to the lungs and, in turn, to the blood. Heart rate and blood pressure increase to supply more blood to carry oxygen from the lungs to the tissues. These physiologic changes provide the body with the energy to mount a maximum physical effort.

Parasympathetic Nervous System

maintance

The parasympathetic nervous system dominates the body's maintenance functions such as increased salivation and mucus secretion, increased blood flow to the gut, and increased peristalsis, defecation, and urination. It also decreases heart rate and blood pressure and increases bronchoconstriction and mucus secretion. Normally, the sympathetic and parasympathetic nervous systems are in balance, creating normal airway smooth muscle tone, but circumstances and certain medications can shift the balance in favor of one system over the other (see Figure 5-3).

Chemical Mediators of Neural Transmission

Reviewing from Chapter 3: The impulses of the nervous system are transmitted from nerve to nerve and to the muscles or organs by chemical substances such as norepinephrine (NE) and acetylcholine (ACh). Both systems use ACh to transmit impulses from neuron to neuron. But at the synapse where the neuron meets the muscle, the chemical transmitter for the sympathetic nervous system is NE, and for the parasympathetic nervous system it is ACh. The action of ACh is limited by an enzyme called acetylcholinesterase (or cholinesterase, abbreviated AChE), which quickly metabolizes ACh. The synaptic junctions of the sympathetic nervous system have no such enzyme, so the effects of NE take longer to dissipate. The receptors for the parasympathetic nervous system are referred to as muscarinic and nicotinic. The receptors that are important in the lung are called muscarinic. When stimulated, they cause constriction of bronchial smooth muscle and increased mucus secretion. See Figure 5-4.

Because the parasympathetic system uses ACh at the transmitter between the nerve and the muscle, it is also called the cholinergic system. The sympathetic system's action is based

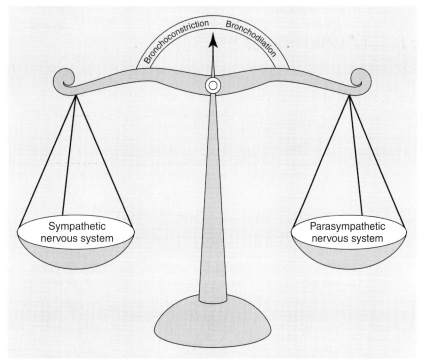

Figure 5-3 Balance Between the Sympathetic and Parasympathetic Nervous System to Maintain Normal Bronchial Smooth Muscle Tone

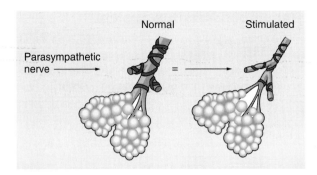

Figure 5-4 Stimulated Parasympathetic Nerve Causing Bronchospasm

on NE as the transmitter. **Epinephrine,** also called adrenaline, is a drug that is very similar to NE, so the sympathetic nervous system is sometimes referred to as the adrenergic system. Figure 5-5 contrasts a parasympathetic neuron with a sympathetic neuron.

Sympathetic Nervous System Receptors

The sympathetic nervous system has essentially three types of receptors. They are referred to as alpha (α), beta$_1$ (β_1), and beta$_2$ (β_2) receptors. (Actually, there are alpha$_1$ and alpha$_2$ receptors as well, but they will not be differentiated for the purposes of this discussion.) Each of the three receptor types is distributed to different parts of the body and when stimulated produces different effects. The α receptors are found mainly in arteries and veins throughout the body, including the vessels within the lungs. They are distributed evenly in the large and small airways, and their stimulation results in vasoconstriction.

The β_1 receptors are found mainly in the heart, where they increase both the rate and the force of contraction of the heart when stimulated. The β_2 receptors are found in the bronchiolar smooth muscle of the lung, the uterus, and skeletal muscle blood vessels. β_2 recep-

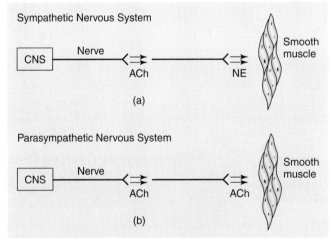

Figure 5-5 Impulse Transmission in the Sympathetic and Parasympathetic Nervous Systems

tors are found throughout the tracheal bronchial tree, but they are particularly concentrated in the small airways. When stimulated, β_2 receptors relax the smooth muscle in the lungs to cause bronchodilation. This action of the β_2 receptors on bronchial smooth muscle is the basis for many of the bronchoactive drugs. In addition, stimulation of the β_2 receptors within the blood vessels of the skeletal muscle causes them to dilate, increasing blood supply and sometimes causing tremor, a common side effect listed for many of the bronchodilators. In the uterus, stimulation of the β_2 receptors can stop contractions due to premature labor. A summary of the sympathetic receptors and their effects can be found in Table 5-1.

The Sympathetic Nervous System in the Lung

The sympathetic nervous system exerts its effects by both direct and indirect means. The presence of nerve fibers results in direct stimulation of the receptor site. These receptors are referred to as neuronal receptors. However, some receptors are not directly wired to the nervous system by nerve fibers. These receptors are indirectly stimulated by circulating catecholamines (NE and epinephrine) within the bloodstream. They are referred to as hormonal receptors, because they respond to chemical mediators that are released into the bloodstream from the adrenal medulla. As the chemical mediators or hormones circulate through the blood stream, they stimulate receptors throughout the body, not just the receptors associated with nerve fibers. Their stimulation results in the same action as if they were transmitted to the receptor by nerve fibers.

The arteries and submucosal glands of the lung are well innervated by sympathetic nerve fibers, while the bronchiolar smooth muscle essentially lacks these fibers and therefore responds to circulating hormones or medications. For example, the α and β_2 receptors of the bronchial smooth muscle are stimulated by the *circulating* hormones epinephrine and NE, which are produced within our bodies. Similarly, when we administer inhaled bronchodilators, the drug combines with the β_2 receptors in the lung, causing indirect or hormonal stimulation of the receptor rather than neuronal stimulation.

Epinephrine stimulates both α and β receptors equally, while norepinephrine acts mainly on the α receptors. But recall that in Chapter 1, we learned that "pure" reactions do not occur with any drug. Even though some drugs are *highly selective* for a particular receptor, there is always some potential for stimulation of other receptors as well.

See Table 5-2 which summarizes these effects.

STOP & REVIEW

Note the similar actions of the sympathomimetic and parasympatholytic agents. The same effect results from very different actions on the ANS. This is the reason for using more than one drug to treat bronchoconstriction. It is a concept that will be reinforced throughout this chapter. What do you think the relationship between sympatholytic and parasympathomimetic agents would be?

Table 5-1   Summary of the Sympathetic Nervous System Receptors, Their Locations, and Their Actions

Receptor	Location	Action
Alpha	arteries and veins	vasoconstriction
Beta 1	heart	increase in rate and force of contraction
Beta 2	lungs, skeletal muscle, and uterus	smooth muscle relaxation

Table 5-2 Summary of the Major Effects of Sympathomimetics, Parasympatholytics, Sympatholytics, and Parasympathomimetics

Effects	*Sympathomimetic*	*Parasympatholytic*	*Sympatholytic*	*Parasympathomimetic*
Bronchial smooth muscle	relaxes	relaxes	constricts	constricts
Mucus secretion		decreases		increases
Heart rate	increases	increases	decreases	decreases
Blood pressure	increases	increases	decreases	decreases
Pupils	dilate	dilate	constrict	constrict
Blood flow to skeletal muscles	increases	increases	decreases	decreases
Salivation	decreases	decreases	increases	increases
Digestion	decreases	decreases	increases	increases
Blood glucose	increases	increases	decreases	decreases
Insulin	decreases	decreases	increases	increases

BRONCHODILATORS

Bronchodilators can be divided into three categories based on the mechanism of their action. These categories are as follows:

- sympathomimetics (beta-adrenergics)
- anticholinergics (parasympatholytics)
- xanthines

The sympathomimetics directly cause bronchodilation by increasing **cyclic AMP (cAMP)**, a substance that causes bronchial smooth muscle relaxation. Anticholinergics block the bronchoconstricting effects of the parasympathetic system by decreasing **cyclic GMP** (cGMP), a substance that causes bronchial smooth muscle constriction. Several mechanisms have been proposed for the bronchodilation action of xanthines, but none have been definitively established. Sympathomimetics and anticholinergics are most commonly administered as inhaled aerosols. Xanthines are taken orally or intravenously. Their different modes of action may lead to the use of combination drug therapy for optimal management of bronchospasm in some patients. See Figure 5-6, showing the change in balance leading to sympathomimetic bronchodilation.

< CONTROVERSY >

For quite some time, xanthines were thought to bronchodilate by increasing levels of cAMP through inhibiting phosphodiesterase, the enzyme that deactivates cAMP. Currently, there are several other theories to explain its mechanism of action. Furthermore, xanthines may not actually produce bronchodilation at all at therapeutic doses, but they are weak bronchodilators at very high doses.

---

www.prenhall.com/colbert

For information on current research on methylxanthine mechanism of action and pharmacologic properties, go to the Web site for this chapter.

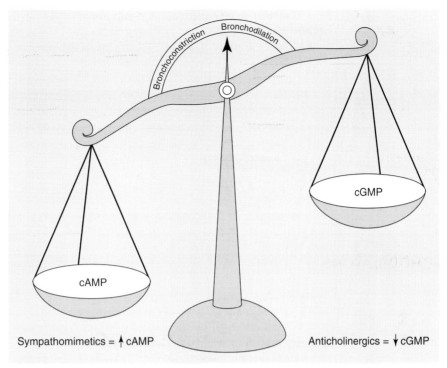

Figure 5-6 Sympathetic Stimulation Favoring Bronchodilation

Sympathomimetic (Adrenergic) Bronchodilators

Stimulation of the sympathetic nervous system causes bronchodilation (β_2) and vasoconstriction (α effect) in the pulmonary system. Drugs that mimic these effects are called sympathomimetic or adrenergic agonists. Sympathomimetics have three potential effects, depending upon the receptor or receptors that are stimulated:

racemic epinephrine

- Alpha (α) stimulation results in vasoconstriction, which reduces blood flow and thereby decreases swelling. In the upper airway, this can result in decongestion. For example, the active ingredient in many OTC nasal decongestants is phenylephrine, a potent α receptor stimulant that temporarily relieves swelling in the nasal passages. α-stimulating drugs can also be administered to the supraglottic region, where soft-tissue swelling can cause airway obstruction.
- β_1 stimulation results in increased heart rate and force of contraction. These drugs will be discussed in later cardiac chapters.
- β_2 stimulation results in bronchial smooth muscle relaxation, inhibition of inflammatory response, and increased mucocilliary clearance. *Dilation of airway*

Mechanism of Action

When a β_2 agonist binds to the $\beta_2$receptor, it activates special stimulatory proteins (G proteins) that activate the membrane-bound enzyme adenyl cyclase. Adenyl cyclase in turn increases synthesis of cyclic adenosine 3'-5'-monophosphate (cAMP). cAMP causes relaxation of smooth muscle by inactivating an enzyme that initiates the interaction of actin and myosin. You may recall that actin and myosin are the proteins that work together to shorten or contract smooth muscle fibers. cAMP also decreases the amount of intracellular calcium, thus causing relaxation since calcium is needed for contraction.

cAMP also has anti-inflammatory properties related to its ability to inhibit mast cell chemical mediator release. This will be discussed in depth in Chapter 7, but it is therorized that the prevention of the influx of calcium not only relaxes smooth muscle but prevents the influx of calcium into mast cells. Calcium influx is believed to cause a powerful contraction and expulsion of the mast cells' chemical mediators, which leads to an inflammatory response.

cAMP is constantly broken down by another enzyme, phosphodiesterase. The cAMP becomes AMP, which is inactive, so does not produce bronchodilation. In fact, when AMP is present in large quantities it actually *interferes* with bronchodilation.

DEVELOPMENT OF THE β AGONISTS

Although natural substances have been used for their bronchodilating effects since ancient times, it wasn't until the 1900s that epinephrine was administered subcutaneously and later by aerosol for the treatment of bronchospasm. Since then, various agents have been developed by altering the structure of the molecule. This has resulted in medications that are more potent, are longer acting, and have fewer side effects. A perfect bronchodilator has yet to be developed, but a better understanding of pharmacokinetics has allowed for many improvements. The basic catecholamine molecule consists of a catechol nucleus and an amine side chain. The nucleus is made up of a benzene ring and two hydroxyl groups. See Figure 5-7.

Drug researchers discovered that by making some changes to the structure of the benzene ring, they could make drugs that are much more resistant to degradation by enzymes, which enables them to stay active longer. β-agonists also needed to be more β_2-specific so that the patients would have fewer cardiac side effects. Increasing the length of the side chain portion of the molecule has in fact resulted in agents that are β_2-specific and therefore safer. (This is sometimes referred to as the "Keyhole Theory of Specificity.")

Changes to the benzene ring have resulted in three chemical classes of sympathomimetic **β-agonists.** They are catecholamines, resorcinols, and saligenins. For example, catecholamines have hydroxyl molecules (OH) attached to their benzene ring at positions 3 and 4, while resorcinols have hydroxyl groups at 3 and 5. Please refer to the diagrams in Figure 5-8. You will also see some pretty dramatic differences when you compare the side chain of epinephrine, a catecholamine, to that of salmeterol, a saligenin. The specific actions and examples of each class will be given.

www.prenhall.com/colbert

To see the chemistry of how β_2 selectivity was enhanced and catecholamines, resorcinols, and saligenins modified, go to the Web site to view an animation.

Figure 5-7 Basic Catecholamine Molecule

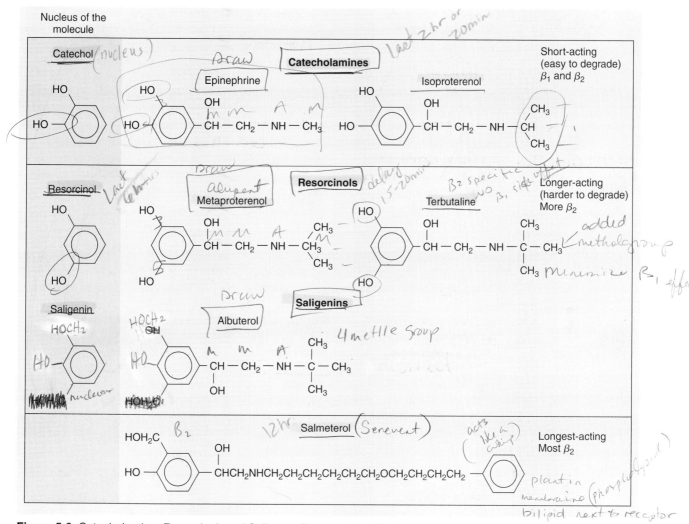

Figure 5-8 Catecholamine, Resorcinol, and Saligenin Chemical Modifications

Note: Increasing length of amine side chain results in more β_2 specificity.

Catecholamines

Catecholamines are the oldest group of inhaled bronchodilators. All sympathetic broncho-dilators are catecholamines or derivatives of catecholamines. Their basic molecular structure consists of a benzene ring and an amine side chain.

Catecholamines are effective and potent dilators. They have a rapid onset and reach their peak effect quickly. But their duration of action is rather short (only about .5 to 3 hours), so they require frequent dosing. This does limit their usefulness in respiratory care, because patients don't like having to take medication so frequently. The catecholamines are rapidly *deactivated* by the enzymes COMT (catechol-*o*-methyltransferase) and MAO (monoamine oxidase). COMT is found in the liver, kidneys, and throughout the body. None of the catecholamines can be given orally, because they are degraded in the GI tract where MAO is found.

Despite their limitations, drugs from this class may be useful when very rapid onset is needed, as in pulmonary function testing or for prevention of bronchospasm that may be caused by other agents such as Mucomyst, which is explained in the next chapter. Examples of catecholamines include epinephrine, norepinephrine, racemic epinephrine, dopamine, isoproterenol, isoetharine, and bitolterol. Only isoetharine and bitolterol are used as inhaled bronchodilators, because they produce fewer cardiac side effects than other drugs in this class. Epinephrine may be used as a bronchodilator when administered by subcutaneous injection, but this is rarely practiced, since it has no proven benefits when compared to the safer inhaled medications. The catecholamine racemic epinephrine is used to treat upper airway swelling, because its primary effect is vasoconstriction, but it also acts as a relatively weak bronchodilator. The other catecholamines (including epinephrine) are used primarily for their effects on heart rate and blood pressure.

℞ ***isoetharine (Bronkosol, Bronkometer).*** Isoetharine is similar to isoproterenol, but its bronchodilator activity is reduced 10-fold, while its cardiac stimulation is reduced 300-fold. Isoetharine, like all catecholamines, is inactivated by heat, light, and air, and turns pink. Unaerosolized medication may become deactivated in the nebulizer or cause the patient's sputum to be tinged with pink. Of course, if this occurs, the medication must be discarded, because it is ineffective.

℞ ***racemic epinephrine (Vaponefrin, MicroNefrin).*** Racemic epinephrine is a synthetic form of epinephrine that has both α and β effects. It is used as a topical vasoconstrictor (α effect) for treatment of airway edema associated with croup and laryngeal edema.

℞ ***bitolterol (Tornalate).*** Bitolterol is called a pro-drug, which means that it differs from the other catecholamines because it is administered in an *inactive* form and must be converted in the body to its *active* form. The process of activation begins upon administration and continues over time. This results in a sustained release that lasts up to 8 hours. Bitolterol is similar to albuterol in effectiveness; however, muscle tremor occurs more frequently (in about 15% of patients). Bitolterol can be given by aerosol solution or MDI.

STOP & REVIEW *Why are catecholamines stored in dark containers?*

Resorcinols

The catecholamines were not suitable for maintenance therapy of bronchospastic airways because of their short duration of action. Drug reasearchers sought to modify the catechol nucleus so that it would be resistant to breakdown by COMT and therefore be longer acting. The result was the development of metaproterenol (Alupent) and terbutaline (Brethine, Brethaire). Another advantage of the resorcinols is that they can be taken orally, because they also resist the action of enzymes in the GI tract and liver. Because of their longer duration, they were the first true maintenance drugs for treatment of reactive airway disease, although they could still be used for rescue therapy because of their rapid onset.

℞ ***metaproterenol (Alupent, Metaprel).*** Metaproterenol (Alupent) is available as a solution for aerosol, MDI, tablets, and syrup for children. From administration to the onset of action is 5 to 15 minutes. The drug is slower to reach its peak effect (30–60 min), but its duration is 4 to 6 hours. Metaproterenol has a more bulky side chain, which makes it more β_2-specific than the catecholamines. It is considered to be β_2-selective, but metaproterenol has substantial cardiac side effects because of its structural similarity to isoproterenol.

℞ ***terbutaline (Brethine, Bricanyl).*** Terbutaline is both β_2-specific and longer acting than catecholamines. Like metaproterenol, terbutaline is β_2-selective, but it has very few cardiac side effects. The onset of action is also 5 to 15 minutes from administration. It reaches its peak effect in about 30 to 60 minutes, and the duration is 4 to 6 hours. Terbutaline is available as an MDI.

STOP & REVIEW

What advantages did the resorcinols provide over the catecholamines?

Saligenins

These are the most recently developed and widely prescribed of all bronchodilators. Owing to another modification of the catechol nucleus, they are also the most β_2-specific. Like the resorcinols, they have the same rapid onset of action and a duration of 4–6 hours. Salmeterol (Serevent) is one of the longest-acting β-agonists available, and levalbuterol is the newest drug available as of the writing of this textbook. Both are examples of saligenins. pirbuterol (Maxair) is structurally very similar so it is also included with this group.

R̶ *an additional side effect is hypokalemia*

albuterol (Proventil, Ventolin). Albuterol is a frequently administered bronchodilator. It is very β_2-specific and therefore has very few side effects, because of its long side chain. The onset of action is 15 minutes. It reaches its peak effect in 30–60 minutes and has a duration of 4 to 6 hours. Albuterol is available in a syrup for children, oral tablets, extended-release tablets, nebulizer solution, MDI, and dry powder inhaler (DPI). Most MDIs use a chlorofluorcarbon-based propellant (CFC). There is a question as to the safety of this propellant; it has been associated with toxicity when patients overuse their MDIs, and there are also environmental safety issues. The CFC propellants are being phased out, and Proventil HFA is now available. DPIs are another safe alternative for patients who have problems with CFC propellants. Please refer to Chapter 4.

pirbuterol (Maxair). Pirbuterol (Maxair) is the result of a very slight modification to the nucleus, but it has the same side chain as albuterol. It is available orally, as a syrup for pediatric patients, and as an MDI with a breath-actuated inhaler device. Pirbuterol is said to be less potent by weight than albuterol and is similar to metaproterenol in both efficacy and toxicity. The side effects are the same as with other β_2-agonists.

non protic

salmeterol (Serevent). ~~(maintance purpose only)~~ Salmeterol is very *lipophilic,* unlike most β-agonists, which are *hydrophilic.* This means that while other β agonists approach the β receptor directly from the extracellular space, salmeterol diffuses into the cell's bilayer phosolipid membrane and enters the receptor from a lateral approach. The long side-chain tail anchors itself into a hydrophobic region of the receptor, and the active saligenin head is left free to continually stimulate the active part of the β_2 receptor by engaging and disengaging itself. This action provides prolonged (12-hour) duration of action. Salmeterol's long action makes it *ideal for maintenance* (prevention of bronchospasm), but it *cannot be used as a rescue treatment* for acute bronchospasm because of its very slow onset. Rescue medication such as albuterol should be given *in addition to* the patient's regularly scheduled dose of salmeterol (Serevent) for treatment of acute episodes.

onset 20min
peak effect 3–5hr
Duration 12hr

levalbuterol (Xopenex). Levalbuterol (Xopenex) is the first drug in a new subclass of inhaled β-agonists. It is an R-isomer saligenin, which seems to be a more potent dilator than albuterol, with fewer side effects. It is also metabolized more slowly. Onset of action is about 15 minutes after administration. It takes 30–60 minutes for the drug to reach its peak effect, and it lasts for 3 to 8 hours.

3rd dose .31mg
MDI = Xop

Summary of Therapeutic Effects of β-Agonists

Pulmonary		*Cardiovascular*
bronchodilation	vasodilation	inotropism/increased cardiac output
anti-inflammatory	increased mucociliary clearance	decreased peripheral vascular resistance

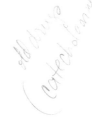

Side Effects of β-Agonists

Most of the side effects of β-agonists are associated with the older drugs such as epineph-rine and isoproterenol. Each new drug developed was made more β_2-selective by altering the chemical structure of the catecholamine molecule. But even the newer β_2-selective agents can cause some side effects.

Tachyphylaxis and tolerance are terms used to describe the desensitization of the β_2 re-ceptor to β-adrenergic drugs. More specifically, tachyphylaxis refers to the decreased re-sponse to a drug that occurs shortly after administration. In the case of β-agonists, this may occur within seconds of administration. This effect is transient, meaning that if the drug is stopped, the receptors rapidly return to their responsive state.

Tolerance is a decreased response to a drug that occurs with long-term use. After hours of exposure to β-agonists, there is an actual decrease in the number of β_2 receptors. This process is called **downregulation.** These receptors are not so easily restored, and new re-ceptors must actually be synthesized. Infection and inflammatory mediators also decrease responsiveness to the medication. Administration of systemic corticosteroids can reverse desensitization of the β_2 receptors due to both tachyphylaxis and downregulation. However, inhaled corticosteroids do not appear to reverse these processes.

> ## CONTROVERSY
>
> The **Asthma Paradox** is the term that describes the unexpected increase in asthma deaths despite better understanding and treatment of the disease. The question of whether the use of β-agonists somehow increases the severity or risk of death from asthma has yet to be answered. Numerous studies have appeared on the effects of various adrenergic agonists in asthma, but they show conflicting results. There are several theories that attempt to explain the Asthma Paradox. Some of them implicate β-agonist usage, while others suggest that delays in seeking proper medical attention, increased exposure to allergens, or underusage of anti-inflammatory agents are the possible causes.

In general, β-agonists are considered to be safe and effective, especially when deliv-ered by inhalation. The guidelines based on Expert Panel Report 2 by the National Heart, Lung, and Blood Institute of the National Institutes of Health recognize that β-agonist ther-apy plays an important role in the management of asthma.

Summary of Side Effects of β-Agonists

tachycardia	nervousness
arrhythmias/palpitations	insomnia
increased pulse and blood pressure	dizziness
hyperglycemia	headache
hypokalemia	nausea
tremor	

Please refer to Table 5-3, which lists and compares the sympathomimetic bronchodilators, including their brand names, routes and dosages, times of onset and peak action, durations, and receptor selectivities.

Classification by Duration of Action

In the clinical setting, it is often more practical to classify sympathomimetics by the duration of their action rather than by their chemical classification. Traditionally bronchodilators have been classified as either short-acting or long-acting. With the introduction of agents such as salmeterol that last up to 12 hours, it may be necessary to reconsider this traditional classification. Recent publications suggest placing bronchodilators into four time-duration categories: ultrashort-acting, short-acting, intermediate-acting, and long-acting. The catecholamines, **epinephrine, isoproterenol,** and isoetherine, with a duration of 2–3 hours, would be ultrashort-acting. The resorcinols, metaproterenol, terbutaline, and bitolterol, lasting up to 6 hours, would be short-acting. Albuterol and bitolterol, once considered long-acting, would be reclassified as intermediate-acting, with a duration of 8 hours. Because of their relatively rapid onset of action, these all can be used as **rescue therapy.** They can provide

Table 5-3 Comparison of Some Typical Inhaled Sympathomimetics

Drug	Route	Dose	(maintenance) Frequency	Onset (min)	Peak (min)	Duration (hrs)	Receptor
CATECHOLAMINES							
epinephrine							
Adrenalin	Neb	.25–.5 ml	Q4–Q6 Hr	3 to 5	5 to 20	1 to 3	α, β
Primatene Mist	MDI						
racemic epinephrine							
Vaponefrin	Neb	.25–.5 ml	QID	3 to 5	5 to 20	.5 to 2	α, β
Micronefrin	Neb	.25–.5 ml	QID	3 to 5	5 to 20	.5 to 2	α, β
AsthmaNefrin	Neb	.25–.5 ml	QID	3 to 5	5 to 20	.5 to 2	α, β
isoproterenol							
Isuprel	Neb	.25–.5 ml	QID	2 to 5	5 to 30	.5 to 2	β_1 and β_2
Isuprel Mistometer	MDI	1–2 puffs	QID	2 to 5	5 to 30	.5 to 2	
isoetharine							
Bronkosol	Neb	.25–.5 ml	QID	1 to 6	15 to 60	1 to 3	$\beta_2 > \beta_1$
RESORCINOLS							
bitolterol							
Tornalate	MDI	2 puffs	BID–QID	3 to 4	30 to 60	5 to 8	$\beta_2 > \beta_1$
metaproterenol							
Metaprel	MDI	2 puffs	TID–QID	1 to 5	60	6	$\beta_2 > \beta_1$
Alupent	Neb	.2–.3 ml	TID–QID	1 to 5	60	6	$\beta_2 > \beta_1$
terbutaline							
Brethaire	MDI	2 puffs	Q4–Q6 Hr	5 to 30	30 to 60	3 to 6	$\beta_2 > \beta_1$
SALIGENINS							
albuterol							
Ventolin	MDI, DPI, Neb	2 puffs	TID–QID	15	30 to 60	5 to 8	$\beta_2 > \beta_1$
Proventil	MDI, DPI, Neb	.25–.5 ml	TID–QID	15	30 to 60	5 to 8	$\beta_2 > \beta_1$
levalbuterol							
Xopenex	Neb	.63–1.25 mg	TID	15	30 to 60	3 to 8	$\beta_2 > \beta_1$
pirbuterol							
Maxair	MDI	2 puffs	Q4–Q6 Hr	5	30	5	$\beta_2 > \beta_1$
salmeterol							
Serevent	MDI, DPI	2 puffs	Q12 hr	20	3 to 5 Hr	12	β_2

Table 5-4   Classification of Sympathomimetics by Duration of Action

Ultrashort-Acting (2–3 hrs)	Short-Acting (5–6 hrs)	Intermediate-Acting (8 hrs)	Long-Acting (12 hrs)
Catecholamines	*Resorcinols*	*Saligenins*	
isoproterenol	metaproterenol	albuterol	salmeterol
Isuprel	Alupent	Ventolin	Serevent
isoetharine	terbutaline	Proventil	
Bronkosol	Brethaire	levalbuterol	
epinephrine	pirbuterol	Xopenex	
	Maxair	bitolterol	
		Tornalate	

for the rapid relief of symptoms; however, they may need to be readministered rather frequently. A drug such as salmeterol, of course, is a true long-acting bronchodilator, with a duration of 12 hours. It is most beneficial as a **maintenance therapy,** because is it takes too long to work, but it does last a long time. See Table 5-4 for a comparison of these drugs in table form.

STOP & REVIEW

Contrast rescue versus maintenance bronchodilator therapy.

As indicated in Table 5-3, all of the β-agonists are available for inhalation either by aerosol, MDI, or DPI. All but the catecholamines can be given orally (tablets or syrups). Remember, catecholamines are deactivated in the stomach.

Delivering the drug directly to the target organ (the lung) is obviously desirable in order to reduce side effects, but the efficacy of the inhalation route during acute attacks of airway obstruction has been questioned. Maximum aerosol deposition depends on the patient's ability to take a slow deep breath followed by a breath hold. Shortness of breath may certainly compromise the patient's technique. Furthermore, the reduction in diameter of the spastic airways may decrease deposition of aerosol particles in the bronchioles. In spite of this, there are several studies that have failed to show any significant difference between inhaled and parenteral (intravenous or subcutaneous) administration of β-agonists. There has been no reason found to avoid the inhalation route during severe acute episodes of bronchospasm. In fact, the *Guidelines for the Diagnosis and Management of Asthma* by the National Heart, Lung, and Blood Institute recognize the benefit of frequent (every 20 minutes) and continuous nebulization of selective β_2-agonists such as terbutaline and albuterol during severe acute asthma attacks.

Though recognized as sometimes necessary, this aggressive dosing is not standard therapy. There is a risk of serious arrhythmias (PVCs, or **premature ventricular contractions**), hypokalemia, hyperglycemia, and significant tremor. Patients must be closely supervised and monitored with a cardiac monitor. In most instances, this would require the patient to be in an ICU or emergency department. In spite of this, frequent and continuous nebulization with terbutaline or albuterol can be both safe and effective.

ANTICHOLINERGIC (PARASYMPATHOLYTIC) BRONCHODILATORS

Another class of bronchodilators is called anticholinergic. Their mechanism of action is entirely different from that of the sympathomimetics. Remember that the parasympathetic nervous system plays an opposing role to that of the sympathetic system. Stimulation of the parasympathetic nervous system increases bronchoconstriction and mucus production. Administration of an anticholinergic can block the effects of the parasympathetic system and therefore cause bronchodilation.

The prototypical anticholinergic agent is atropine. It is an alkaloid found in several plants, including *Atropa belladonna* (the nightshade plant) and *Datura.* There is evidence to suggest that the ingredients from these plants have been used for thousands of years for their effects on the CNS. As early as the seventeenth century, the fumes from burning *Datura* were inhaled for cough and shortness of breath. In the 1980s, interest in anticholinergic agents as adjuncts to β-adrenergics was renewed. The renewed interest was largely due to a better understanding of the role that the parasympathetic nervous system plays in bronchospasm and also due to the introduction of ipratropium bromide, an atropine derivative with fewer side effects. Ipratropium bromide (Atrovent) is the most commonly used anticholinergic bronchodilator.

Mechanism of Action

In contrast to the structure of the sympathetic nervous system, the lungs are directly innervated by the vagus nerve, which is a major nerve of the parasympathetic nervous system. Nerve fibers reach the airway epithelium, submucosal glands, smooth muscle, and probably mast cells. The muscarinic receptors are present in the airways from the trachea to the bronchioles; however, they are concentrated in the large airways.

When a parasympathetic nerve fiber is stimulated, ACh is the neurotransmitter that stimulates a muscarinic receptor in the bronchial smooth muscle. Once stimulated, the inactive enzyme GTP is converted to its active form, cGMP. However, cGMP causes constriction of the bronchial smooth muscle. See Figure 5-9. Stimulation of parasympathetic nerves in the lung also causes other parasympathetic responses, such as slowing of the heart rate and increased secretions.

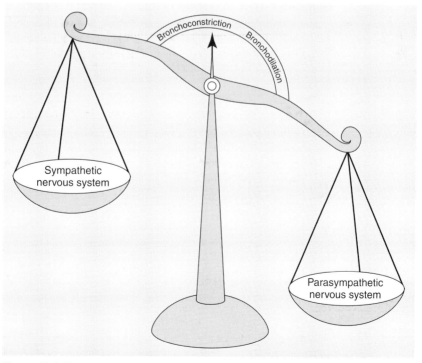

Figure 5-9 Parasympathetic Stimulation Favoring Bronchoconstriction

Parasympatholytic (anticholinergic) agents block ACh at the muscarinic receptor site in the airways (see Figure 5-10). Effects of parasympatholytics include drying of pulmonary secretions, increased heart rate, and bronchodilation. Notice that these are opposite (-lytic) effects to those of parasympathetic stimulation. The degree of bronchodilation that can be achieved with an anticholinergic bronchodilator is dependant upon the degree of bronchial tone already present due to the parasympathetic system. In healthy individuals, there will be minimal airway dilation following the administration of an anticholinergic agent, because there is only a basal level of parasympathetic tone to be blocked. However, in certain disease states, the parasympathetic activity is increased, and significant bronchodilation can be achieved with administration of an anticholinergic agent.

For example, a portion of the bronchospasm seen in COPD patients is caused by vagally mediated innervation of airway smooth muscle. In other words, the bronchospasm is due to overstimulation of the parasympathetic nervous system, and this problem should respond to an anticholinergic agent. Inhalation of irritants such as cigarette smoke, cold air, high inspiratory flow rates, noxious fumes, and histamine release cause a nerve impulse to be sent from the airway to the CNS, then from the CNS back to the airways by way of the parasympathetic nervous system, which constricts the airway smooth muscle and increases mucus secretion and cough. This parasympathetic reflex bronchoconstriction can be blocked very effectively by an anticholinergic agent such as ipratropium bromide.

CLINICAL PEARL

Anticholinergics are also indicated for allergic and nonallergic rhinitis, because they block muscarinic receptors in the mucus-producing glands in the nose.

℞ atropine sulfate

Atropine sulfate is the prototypical parasympatholytic and does relax airway smooth muscle. However, it is not commonly used as a bronchodilator because of its many side effects. It inhibits mucus production and reduces mucociliary clearance. CNS effects can occur even at small doses. Restlessness, irritability, drowsiness, fatigue, and mild excitement have been reported. At higher doses, disorientation, hallucinations, coma, and acute psychotic reactions can occur. Relaxation of the muscles that control the lens of the eye causes blurred vision. Vagal blockade increases heart rate. The GI effects of atropine include dryness of the mouth (due to blockade of salivary gland secretion) and decreased motility in the gut. Clinically, atropine is primarily a cardiac drug and will be discussed in Chapter 9.

CLINICAL PEARL

The inhibition of mucus production and impaired mucociliary clearance can cause thick retained airway secretions, which obstruct the airways and can lead to collapse of the lung.

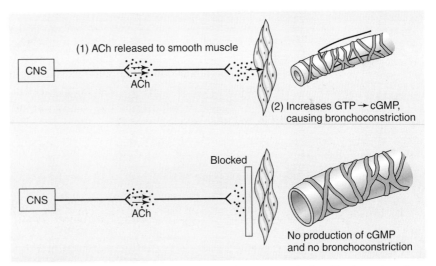

Figure 5-10 Diagram of Parasympathetic Neurotransmission Blockage Leading to Bronchodilation

℞ **ipratropium bromide (Atrovent)**

℞

Ipratropium bromide (Atrovent) is available as a solution for nebulization, MDI, and as a nasal spray pump. It is also available with albuterol (a sympathomimetic) in a single MDI canister **(Combivent)** for patients that have demonstrated a response to both classes of drugs. The onset of bronchodilation begins within minutes, but then increases more gradually to its peak effect in 1–2 hours. The duration of bronchodilation is about the same as that of a β-agonist in asthmatics, but it acts for 1–2 hours longer than a β-agonist in COPD patients. It has little or no effect on mucociliary clearance from the lung, even though it does decrease hypersecretion of mucus in the nose. This is one of the main reasons why it is preferred over atropine. It has little or no effect on heart rate, blood pressure, or the GI tract, but there are rare cases of dry mouth, headache, blurred vision, cough, nausea, and nervousness (see Table 5-5).

STOP

& REVIEW

Why would atropine be contraindicated in cystic fibrosis patients who have thick tenacious secretions?

MONITORING OUTCOMES OF INHALED BRONCHODILATOR THERAPY

Patients should be assessed before, during, and after treatment in order to get an accurate assessment of the effectivness of the medication(s). The practitioner should obtain baseline data such as heart rate, respiratory rate, auscultatory breath sounds, and oxygen saturation by pulse oximeter. Measuring arterial blood gases may also be indicated if acid base status is in question. The practitioner should inquire about the patient's perceived level of **dyspnea** (subjective), observe the patient's breathing pattern and use of accessory muscles. Measurement of **peak expiratory flow rate** (PEFR) or **forced expiratory volume in 1 second** (FEV_1) can be measured before and after the treatment. They can be sensitive indicators of airway obstruction and actually *quantify* airway obstruction and post-treatment improvement. However, both PEFR and FEV_1 are effort dependent. They are only valuable if the patient gives a maximum effort. Patients in acute bronchospasm may be unable to perform the forced exhalation required, because it can cause coughing and increase bronchspasm.

Signs of a positive bronchodilator response include improved appearance, less dyspnea, decreased use of accessory muscles, improved vital signs, increased sputum production, decreased wheezing coupled with increased intensity of breath sounds, increase in FEV_1 or PEFR, and improved oxygenation.

Table 5-5 Common Parasympatholytics

Drug and Trade Names	Dosage	Frequency	Onset (min)	Peak (hrs)	Duration (hrs)
ipratropium bromide					
Atrovent Solution for Nebulization	500 μg/unit dose	TID, QID	1 to 5	.25	4 to 8
Atrovent MDI	2 puffs	QID	15	1 to 2	4 to 6
ipratropium bromide and albuterol					
Combivent MDI	2 puffs	QID	15	2	6 to 8

> **www.prenhall.com/colbert**
>
> Get connected to the Web to view the correct technique for performing a peak flow maneuver (PEFR).

Side effects are relatively uncommon with the newer β_2-selective sympathomimetics. They are even less common when the drug is given by inhalation, compared with oral and intravenous administration. But though adverse reactions may be uncommon, some patients are more sensitive than others, and problems are possible. The most common side effect is muscle tremor due to stimulation of β_2 receptors in the skeletal muscles. There are also some β_2 receptors in the heart and blood vessels, so increased heart rate and vasodilation are possible. It is generally accepted that an increase in heart rate of greater than 20% of the baseline heart rate or 20 beats per minute is significant. If either tremor or increase in heart rate develops, the treatment should be stopped, the patient monitored until the effects subside, and the physician notified. The entire event should be documented in the patient's medical record. Often, when the practitioner changes the route of administration (from oral to inhaled), the selection of a more β_2-selective agent or a smaller dose may alleviate any unwanted effects from bronchodilator therapy.

STOP & REVIEW

List the positive clinical responses to bronchodilator therapy.

XANTHINES

℞ **Theophylline** and its salt, **aminophylline** are the primary xanthines used clinically. However, there are also a few other well-recognized members of the xanthine group (or methylxanthines, as they are sometimes called). These include theobromine and caffeine. All of these substances can be found naturally in certain plants. For example, caffeine is found in coffee beans and cola. Tea leaves contain both caffeine and theophylline. Caffeine and theobromine are found in cocoa. Various parts of these plants have been used for their stimulant effects on the CNS for centuries. Xanthines are administered orally or intravenously, and there are many different brand names. Even though they are not administered by aerosol, it is importatat for the practitioner to understand the role they may play in bronchodilation.

Mechanism of Action

The traditional explanation of the xanthines' mode of action is that they produce bronchodilation by inhibiting phosphodiesterase, which is the enzyme that deactivates cAMP. This indirectly increases bronchodilation by increasing cAMP. Though this is true, at the dosages commonly used in humans, theophylline is a relatively poor inhibitor of phosphodiesterase, and therefore a weak bronchodilator. Several other theories of how xanthines work have been investigated, but at this time, there is no definite explanation for how they work. In fact, it is possible that there are multiple mechanisms behind their actions.

Nonbronchodilating Effects of Theophylline

Even though theophylline is a weak bronchodilator, it has several other effects that produce clinical improvement. For example, theophylline has been shown to increase the *strength and endurance of muscle contraction,* including that of the diaphragm. This may help prevent respiratory failure by increasing the patient's ventilatory drive. The diuretic effect of xanthines is well known to those who drink caffeinated beverages such as coffee, tea, and cola.

CLINICAL PEARL

Xanthines may be prescribed as maintenance therapy for COPD and this will be discussed in the "putting it all together" section of this book. Caffeine is used in the treatment of apnea of prematurity because of its stimulation of the CNS.

Table 5-6 Common Xanthines

Elixophyllin	Theo-Dur
Slo-Phyllin	Theobid
Slo-Bid	Respbid
Theolair	Sustaire

Xanthines have a slow onset and long duration and are well tolerated by many patients. However, patients should be monitored closely, because there is wide variability in its therapeutic effect. This variability in response is most likely due to its being metabolized at different rates by different people. In addition, a variety of other medications react with xanthines, increasing side effects and serum drug levels. Toxicity can result, and patients with liver disease and congestive heart failure (CHF) must also be carefully monitored. The therapeutic range for theophylline is narrow (5–15 μcg/ml). Side effects increase when blood concentrations are close to 20 μg/ml, and toxic levels can exist (>20 μg/ml). Serum levels should be monitored as appropriate. Side effects involve the CNS, cardiovascular effects, and the GI tract. CNS side effects include dizziness, headache, restlessness, irritability, insomnia, and seizures. Cardiovascular side effects include diuresis, palpitations, tachycardia, arrhythmias, and hypertension. GI side effects include nausea, vomiting, diarrhea, epigastric pain, and anorexia. See Table 5-6 for a listing of common xanthines.

SUMMARY

To obtain the best possible results from inhaled bronchodilators, the healthcare practitioner responsible for administering these medications must be familiar with the three mechanisms of bronchoconstriction (bronchospasm, airway edema, and mucus plugging) as well as the numerous agents for treatment, their doses, route of administration, and potential for side effects.

Bronchodilation can be achieved via three classes of medications. These include β-adrenergic agents, anticholinergic agents, and xanthines. The β-adrenergic agents work by stimulating the sympathetic effects of bronchodilation in the lungs. Ideal agents are β_2-specific, to avoid unwanted cardiac (β_1) side effets. Anticholinergic agents work by blocking the parasympathetic response of bronchoconstriction and thus cause bronchodilation.

Although the xanthines theophylline and aminophylline are traditionally classed as bronchodilators, they are actually poor bronchodilators at therapeutic levels. Their real benefit as a maintenance drug in COPD may be due to increased ventilatory drive or by strengthening the contraction of the diaphragm, thereby increasing airflow and improving ventilation. Since they have a long duration of action, they may be used to control symptoms through the night. However, their benefits should always be weighed against their numerous side effects, especially since there are now long-acting sympathomimetics available.

REVIEW QUESTIONS

1. You are called to the emergency department to assess a 14-year-old girl. She became short of breath after receiving a kitten for her birthday. Upon assessment, you note that her respirations are 31/min and her heart rate is 110. On auscultation, you note a prolonged expiratory wheeze. Which of the following medications would you recommend?
   (a) ipratropium bromide
   (b) albuterol
   (c) salmeterol
   (d) caffeine
   Why?

2. Which of the following are advantages of ipratropium bromide over atropine for treatment of bronchospasm?
   (a) fewer cardiac side effects
   (b) no effect on mucus clearance from the lung
   (c) more rapid onset of action
   (d) all of the above
3. Which of the following would you recommend for an asthmatic patient who complains of waking up in the early morning hours with shortness of breath?
   (a) albuterol
   (b) epinephrine
   (c) ipratropium bromide
   (d) salmeterol
4. How should a patient who is receiving a xanthine be monitored to determine the appropriate dose?
   (a) Measure peak expiratory flow rate (PEFR) before and after administration of the medication
   (b) Measure the FEV_1 before and after the administration of the medication
   (c) Serum blood levels of the medication should be measured
   (d) Auscultate breath sounds after administration of the medication
5. A patient with asthma has failed to improve after treatment with nebulized albuterol. Which of the following would be most appropriate?
   (a) ipratropium bromide (Atrovent)
   (b) salmeterol (Serevent)
   (c) isoproterenol (Isuprel)
   (d) levalbuterol (Xopenex)
6. Explain the reason you chose the drug you did for the patient in Question 5.
7. What is the typical nebulizer dose for albuterol and for metaproterenol?
8. Which route of administration for a β-adrenergic bronchodilator would be least likely to produce side effects: oral, intravenous, or inhaled?
9. A patient with COPD experiences increased bronchospasm after using his albuterol inhaler. His doctor feels that it may be due to the CFC propellant in his MDI. What do you suggest?
10. Explain why a bronchodilator may not be helpful in treating a child with croup.

CASE STUDY 1

A 66-year-old male with a history of COPD is admitted to the emergency department with shortness of breath. He is not currently taking any medication for his breathing. The patient states that he usually only gets short of breath on exertion, but he developed a "cold" several days ago that made his breathing worse. He has been placed on oxygen. The doctor wants him to have breathing treatments. What medication, dose, and route of administration would you suggest?

How should the effectiveness of the treatments be monitored?

After several days of breathing treatments and antibiotics, the patient is ready for discharge, but he still becomes short of breath during the night. What maintenance medication(s) do you suggest?

CASE STUDY 2

A 9-year-old boy has just been diagnosed with mild asthma. He frequently wheezes while playing soccer, but has no other symptoms. What medication, dose, and route of administration would you suggest?

How should he monitor his asthma and his response to his medication?

GLOSSARY

β-agonist   see **beta agonist**

Asthma Paradox   the phenomenon of increasing incidence of and mortality from asthma despite a better understanding of the pathophysiology and improved drugs for treatment of asthma. The reasons for the Asthma Paradox are still open to debate.

beta agonist (β-agonist)   a drug that combines with a β receptor and stimulates the activity of that receptor.

bronchoconstriction   narrowing of the bronchioles due to swelling, mucus obstruction, or spasm of the smooth muscle of the airway.

bronchospasm   narrowing of the bronchioles due to contraction of the smooth muscle surrounding the airways.

cyclic AMP   enzyme produced when β_2 receptors are stimulated; it affects the activities of a variety of cells, including the relaxation of bronchial muscle.

cyclic GMP   enzyme that has the opposite effect of cyclic AMP; it causes bronchoconstriction.

downregulation   the long-term process of decreasing the sensitivity of β-receptors to β-agonists because of a reduction in the number of receptors.

dyspnea   air hunger resulting in difficult or labored breathing.

epinephrine   also called adrenaline, a hormone produced by the adrenal medulla. It acts as the circulating neurotransmitter for the sympathetic nervous system, stimulating both α and β receptors; it is also a potent catecholamine administered for its effects on the sympathetic nervous system.

maintenance therapy   medications that provide long-term control of symptoms, such as shortness of breath and wheezing; usually taken daily.

peak expiratory flow rate   measurement of maximum flow rate generated during a forced exhalation. Used to indicate the degree of airflow obstruction.

premature ventricular contraction   potentially serious abnormal heartbeats that originate in the ventricles.

rescue therapy   rapid-acting medications used to provide prompt relief of symptoms such as shortness of breath and wheezing in asthma.

ventilatory drive   the strength of the stimulus to breath, controlled by the CNS; influences the rate and depth of breathing.

www.prenhall.com/colbert

Use the address above to access the free, interactive Companion Web site created specifically for this textbook. Enhance your studying by viewing videos and animations, answering practice quiz questions, and reviewing an audio glossary and much more related to Chapter 5.

CHAPTER 6

Mucokinetics and Surfactants

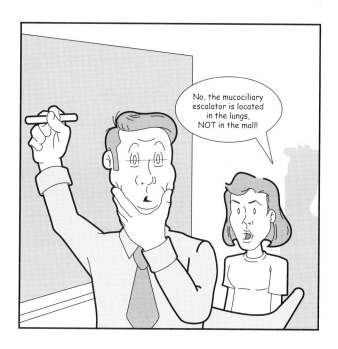

OBJECTIVES

Upon completion of this chapter you will be able to

- Define key terms related to mucokinetic and surfactant agents
- Describe the production, function, and clearance of mucus in the healthy lung
- State the indications for bland aerosols and mucolytic agents
- Compare and contrast the mechanisms of action of bland aerosol and mucolytic agents
- Describe how surface tension relates to oxygenation and work of breathing
- Describe the role of surfactant in the lungs and surfactant replacement agents
- Describe the mechanisms of action of expectorants and antitussive agents

ABBREVIATIONS

DNase	deoxyribonuclease	IRDS	Infant Respiratory Distress Syndrome
SP	Surface Proteins		
RDS	Respiratory Distress Syndrome	ml/kg	milliliters per kilogram
		NaCl	sodium chloride, or salt

Main contributing author Terri Price

INTRODUCTION

This chapter encompasses a rather diverse group of drugs with widely varying effects. We will need to review the physiology of mucus production, mucus function, and the impact that various disease states have on them. We will look at the role of bland (unmedicated) aerosols and mucolytics and the importance of bronchial hygiene techniques in the management of retained secretions. The consequences of retained secretions can be very serious and include infections, airway obstruction, and collapse (atelectasis). It is therefore important to understand the pharmacologic aids available to you to assist in good bronchial hygiene.

Finally, we will take a closer look at the lower respiratory tract, where surfactant plays a critical role in maintaining the integrity of the alveolar surface. This integrity is vital to the role of adequate gas exchange and therefore must be maintained. This chapter will provide the reader with a basis for understanding current and future roles for surfactant replacement therapy.

THE MUCOCILIARY SYSTEM

Anatomy and Physiology

Remember the mucosa, submucosa, and adventitia that were discussed in Chapter 5 (see Figure 6-1)? The mucosa (inner layer) is made up of different types of specialized epithelial cells, which rest on a basement membrane. Most numerous are the pseudostratified ciliated columnar epithelia, but there are also secretory cells such as goblet cells, serous cells, and clara cells. The goblet cells produce a relatively small amount of mucus, which is secreted into the airway. The serous cells produce less viscous mucus, which makes up the sol layer of the mucus. We'll get to that in a minute. The role of the clara cells is not com-

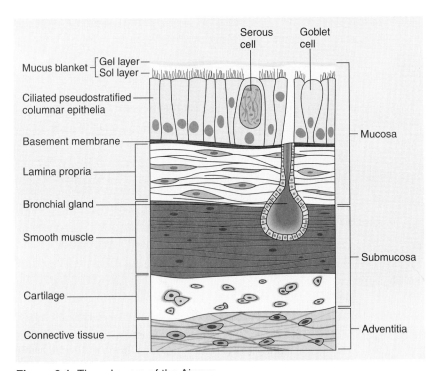

Figure 6-1 Three Layers of the Airway

pletely clear, but they are known to have a high degree of metabolic activity and contain a lot of enzymes. The bronchial glands are found in the submucosal layer. They produce most of the mucus found in the airways. Together, the **goblet cells** and **bronchial glands** produce about 100 ml of mucus each day. Most of the mucus is reabsorbed, but about 10 ml reaches the pharynx each day, where it is usually swallowed.

The mucociliary system, or mucociliary escalator as it is sometimes called, consists of the mucosal blanket that lines the airways from the naso and oropharynx to the terminal bronchi. It also includes the cilia, which propel the mucus up the airway. Cilia are tiny hairlike projections that arise from the surface of the mucosal cells. There are about 200 cilia per cell, and they are about 6 μm in length. The cilia beat about 1,000 times per minute in a coordinated fashion in order to propel the mucus toward the upper airway. In healthy lungs, the mucus moves forward at a speed of about 2 cm/min.

The mucociliary system is an important part of the pulmonary defense system. It protects the lungs from inhaled debris, and it contains enzymes that give it antimicrobial properties that help prevent infection. Mucus helps to warm and humidify inspired gases, and it prevents excessive loss of heat and moisture from the airways. It is important to note that no cilia or mucus are found in the lower airways from the respiratory bronchioles to the alveoli.

Structure and Composition of Mucus

The layer of mucus (or mucosal blanket) that covers the surface of the airways is about 5 to 10 μm thick and is made up of two distinct layers, the gel layer and the sol layer. The gel layer floats on top of the sol layer. It is about 1–2 μm thick and, as its name implies, it is rather gelatinous. It is sticky and works a lot like flypaper to trap inhaled particles and bacteria. The sol layer is deeper (about 4–8 μm thick) and has a more watery consistency, which enables the cilia to beat freely. The beating of the cilia within the sol layer helps propel the gel layer toward the larynx.

The mucus molecule itself is very large and complex. It is about 95% water, so it is imperative that there is a sufficient amount of water available in the body to produce normal mucus. Once formed, mucus does not absorb water readily. The remaining 5% of mucus composition comprises the long, flexible strands of protein and lipid molecules that form polypeptide chains, with many carbohydrate side chains attached. The side chains are crossconnected with disulfide, physical, ionic, and hydrogen bonds (see Figure 6-2).

See Table 6-1 for a summary of the functions of mucus in the healthy lung.

Proper function of the mucociliary system is critical to the maintenance of a healthy pulmonary system. The volume, consistency, and structure of mucus produced can be altered in various disease states, including primary pulmonary disease and systemic dehydration. Mucus production increases when the respiratory tract is irritated and during increased parasympathetic stimulation. In certain disease states (such as cystic fibrosis, pneumonia, and chronic bronchitis), mucus production increases significantly. The airways can produce more than twice the normal amount of mucus. Simultaneously, mucus clearance can also be impaired, resulting in an overwhelming accumulation of mucus in the

Table 6-1   Mucus Function in the Healthy Lung

Function
prevention of water from moving into and out of the epithelia
shielding epithelia from direct contact with toxic materials, irritants, and microorganisms
prevention of infection due to the action of antimicrobial enzymes
lubrication of the airway

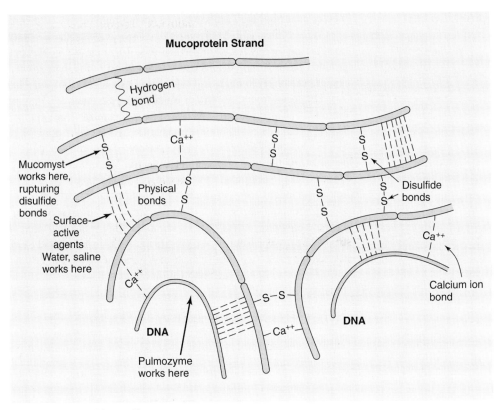

Figure 6-2 The Mucus Structure

lungs. See Table 6-2 for a more complete listing of disease states that increase the volume and/or thickness of mucus.

The frequency with which the cilia beat is also adversely affected by disease state, environmental conditions, and chemicals. Many factors can slow or stop the beating action of the cilia, which decreases the rate of mucus clearance from the lung. Thick mucus, dry gas, smoke (including cigarette smoke), noxious gases, infection, positive pressure ventilation, foreign bodies (including endotracheal tubes), high concentrations of oxygen, and certain drugs such as atropine are all known to slow the beating of the cilia. Table 6-3 identifies factors that impair the function of the cilia.

The result of either increased mucus production or impaired mucus clearance can be a pulmonary system that is completely overwhelmed with thick, retained secretions that ob-

Table 6-2   Diseases That Increase the Volume or Thickness of Mucus

Disease
chronic bronchitis
asthma
cystic fibrosis
acute bronchitis
pneumonia

Table 6-3   Factors That Impair
Ciliary Activity

Factor
endotracheal tubes
extremes of temperature
high concentrations of oxygen
dust, fumes, and smoke
dehydration
thick mucus
infections

struct the airways. Though the mechanisms controlling mucus composition and production are not completely understood, the pharmacologic approach to secretion management generally falls into one of the following broad categories:

- those that increase the depth of the sol layer (water or saline solution and expectorants)
- those that alter the consistency of the gel layer (mucolytics)
- those that improve ciliary activity (sympathomimetic bronchodilators and corticosteroids)

There are a variety of pharmacologic agents and bland aerosols that alter the structure of mucus. Mechanical techniques such as deep breathing, assisted coughing, and suctioning can be applied to aid in the removal of secretions. Respiratory care practitioners are frequently called upon to assist with mobilization of retained secretions by applying various combinations of humidity, bland and medicated aerosols, and mechanical techniques.

Of course, the purpose of this chapter is to focus on the pharmacologic approaches for the control of mucus. This includes bland aerosols, which increase mucus clearance, mucus production, and productive coughing. Mucus-controlling drugs (mucolytics) achieve their effect by changing the molecular structure of the mucus gel so that the cilia can work more efficiently. The pharmacologic basis for mucus-controlling agents that are currently available will be reviewed in this chapter. Since mucus is composed largely of water, the importance of maintaining adequate systemic hydration is also a very important aspect of maintaining proper consistency and clearance of mucus. See Table 6-4 for factors that lead to dehydration and thereby thicken mucus.

LEARNING HINT

Pharmacologic agents and bland aerosols alter the structure of mucus, while mechanical techniques such as deep breathing, assisted coughing, and suctioning can be applied to aid in the removal of secretions.

Table 6-4   Factors That
Lead to
Dehydration and
Thick Mucus

Factor
increased respiratory rate
increased depth of breathing
systemic fluid loss
infections

BLAND AEROSOLS

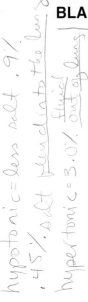

(handwritten margin notes:) hypotonic = less salt .9% / .45% salt pulled into the lungs / hypertonic = 3.0% fluid out of lungs

Definitions

Bland aerosols do not affect the mucus molecule directly; they dilute the mucus by altering its water content. They are also referred to as wetting agents. Bland aerosols include the following agents:

- water
- normal saline *.9% Normal body concentration 9mg/ml*
- hypotonic saline *less salt*
- hypertonic saline *more salt*

Historically, treatment of thick, retained secretions has been aimed at thinning thick mucus by adding water or saline to the respiratory tract by inhalation. Once formed, the gel layer of the mucus is somewhat resistant to the addition and removal of water. However, it is critical to have an adequate amount of water available as mucus is being formed so that the mucus will have normal **viscoelastic** properties.

Bland aerosols may not be as effective as once thought at thinning thick mucus by topical hydration or mixing, but instead their benefit may be due to a different mechanism. All bland aerosols are somewhat irritating to the airway (although they are not all equally irritating). Irritation tends to increase the production of thinner mucus, possibly by stimulating the goblet cells' and bronchial glands' production of mucus. Mucus clearance is increased by restoring the sol layer and stimulating cough, and this effect can be clinically useful.

Delivery Methods

There are several methods available for delivering water and saline to the lung. One method is through the use of humidification devices, which work by bringing dry gas into contact with water, where the gas passes over or bubbles through the water. The water molecules evaporate and therefore increase the humidity of the gas. Another method of delivering water to the airway is by the use of nebulizers. Nebulizers produce aerosols, which are small droplets of solution suspended in a gas. When the aerosol is inhaled, water particles are deposited in the airway. The final method is to instill the liquid directly into the respiratory tract. We will discuss each of these techniques briefly below.

Humidifiers. Simple humidifiers are mainly used for oxygen delivery (see Figure 6-3). The amount of humidity that they add to the gas is highly variable depending on how long the gas is in contact with the water, the surface area available between the gas and the water, and the temperature of the gas. The type of humidifier commonly used in conjunction with oxygen therapy is intended to minimize the drying effects of oxygen, not to serve as therapy for thick secretions. Heating inspired gas greatly increases the amount of water vapor that the gas can carry. Systems that deliver heated, humidified gas are most often used with mechanical ventilators. In-depth knowledge of how to deliver and monitor gas that is heated to body temperature and 100% relative humidity is an important aspect of ventilator management.

Aerosols. The most common method for administering water and saline solutions to the respiratory tract is by aerosol. Small-volume (hand-held) nebulizers, large-volume nebulizers, and ultrasonic nebulizers have all been used. Small-volume nebulizers typically contain 3–5 ml of which only about 1 ml is actually deposited in the lung. For this reason, the use of small-volume nebulizers is medication delivery, as discussed in Chapter 4, and sputum induction, when stimulating the cough is the goal of the therapy.

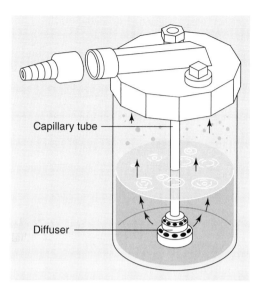

Figure 6-3 A Simple
Humidifier

Large-volume and ultrasonic nebulizers are capable of delivering significant volumes of aerosol to the lungs (see Figure 6-4). Although they are clinically very useful, ultrasonic nebulizers have been shown to cause runny, watery secretions in infants. Secretions of this consistency also impair the function of the mucociliary system. This condition has been, again, compared to trying to rake water.

Direct Instillation. Direct instillation of fluid (usually normal saline) into the respiratory tract is sometimes performed on patients with artificial airways, during bronchoscopy,

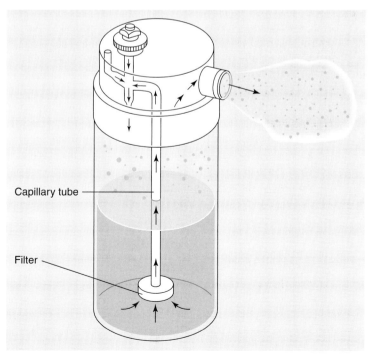

Figure 6-4 A Nebulizer

and on rare occasions through a transtracheal catheter. Fluid injected into the upper airway is very irritating and causes a strong cough.

The once common practice of *routinely* instilling saline into the airway during suctioning is now discouraged. It was once thought to improve mucus clearance by thinning thick secretions, but it is now understood that the saline does very little to thin thick secretions, and only about 20% of the instilled fluid is recovered during suctioning. The main benefit appears to be that it does stimulate a vigorous cough. Current evidence suggests that this practice should be reserved for situations where patients do not cough adequately during suctioning and during bronchoscopy. During bronchoscopy, the patient's airway is anesthetized, so that coughing is minimal. More of the instilled solution can be recovered by suctioning through the bronchoscope.

www.prenhall.com/colbert

Get connected to the Web to see examples of humidifiers and nebulizers.

Bland Solutions

Sterile and Distilled Water. Sterile water is free of microorganisms, but it may also contain additives to make it bacteriostatic. Distilled water is both sterile and pure (no additives, and all other constituents [such as naturally occurring minerals] are removed). Although any solution intended for inhalation must be sterile, water does not need to be distilled. In fact, distilled water tends to be a bit more irritating than sterile water. Sterile water is commonly used as the diluent for other aerosolized medications, in humidifiers, in large-volume nebulizers, and in croup tents.

A cool mist of sterile water may have a soothing (humectant) effect on inflamed upper airways, as in croup, but there is little evidence that a significant amount of water deposits in the lower airways. It is also theorized that because sterile water is hypotonic, it is more readily absorbed by mucus and that it may thin mucus more effectively than saline, but again, there is little objective evidence that either water or saline mix well with mucus.

Devices that produce very dense aerosols tend to be more irritating to the airways. Dense aerosols are more likely to cause cough, and even bronchospasm in susceptible individuals (such as asthmatics). However, the irritation and cough make these aerosols useful for sputum induction. It is a good idea to monitor the breath sounds of patients receiving aerosol treatments for sputum induction, because wheezing may indicate bronchospasm.

Normal Saline. Normal saline (0.9% sodium chloride) is physiologically normal. Since it is **isotonic** with body fluids (meaning that it has the same concentration of sodium and chloride as what is found in the body), it is less irritating and not as likely to cause bronchospasm as water. It is frequently used as a diluent for other aerosolized medications, such as bronchodilators.

Hypertonic Saline. **Hypertonic** saline is any solution that contains more than .9% sodium chloride. The most commonly available solutions contain 5% and 10% NaCl. These solutions are very irritating and are only used for sputum induction, particularly when the patient has a dry, nonproductive cough (remember, the airway responds to irritation by producing more mucus.) Because of the higher salt concentration, the aerosolized particles are hygroscopic, meaning that they attract water. Therefore, more water tends to move from the mucosal membranes to the airway in order to dilute the salt.

Table 6-5 Common Concentrations of Saline

.45%	(half normal)
.9%	(normal)
5%	(hypertonic)
10%	(hypertonic)

Hypertonic saline solutions are more likely to cause bronchospasm than any of the other bland aerosols. Therefore, it may be necessary to pretreat some patients with a bronchodilator. It is certainly advisable to monitor the patient throughout the treatment and be prepared to stop the treatment or administer a bronchodilator if necessary.

Hypotonic Saline. Saline is also available in a solution of .45%, or half normal saline. Commercially available solution for ultrasonic nebulizers is usually the .45% strength. **Hypotonic** saline is less irritating than either sterile water or hypertonic saline, and it is less likely to cause problems with sodium retention than normal saline (.9%). In addition to ultrasonic nebulizers, it can be used in any large-volume nebulizer or as the diluent for nebulized medications.

Why might hypertonic saline be better than sterile water or normal saline for sputum induction for a patient who has a dry, nonproductive cough?

MUCOLYTICS

Definition

When there is infection and/or dehydration of the pulmonary system, the gel layer of the mucus becomes thickened. Waste products of inflammation such as white blood cells (leukocytes), DNA, and other cellular debris add to the thickening of the mucus. Thick mucus cannot be mobilized by the action of the cilia, and when the cilia cannot keep the gel and sol layers in motion, the layers *combine* and a vicious cycle of thickening mucus ensues. In this situation, humidity, mucolytic agents, and expectorants, or combinations of these agents, may be needed.

Mucolytics are drugs that control mucus by their direct action of altering the structure of the mucus molecule. In essence, they facilitate expectoration of mucus by liquefying it. Mucolytics break down the complex molecular strands to thin the thick mucus. There are currently two mucolytic agents that are approved by the FDA for administration by aerosol to treat abnormal pulmonary secretions. They are Mucomyst and Pulmozyme. Investigation continues in this area, and new agents may be forthcoming. Check the Web site for updated information.

Generic   Trade mark

℞ **n-acetylcysteine (Mucomyst, Mucosol).** Acetylcysteine is used to treat thick, viscous secretions, such as may be seen in cystic fibrosis, chronic bronchitis, tuberculosis, and acute tracheobronchitis. It acts by disrupting the disulfide bonds in the mucus. The long mucopolysaccharide strands are cross-connected with numerous bridges, including disulfide bonds. The long strands become a matted network of complex molecules. Breaking the disulfide bonds releases the mucopolysaccharide strands. The structure of the gel layer is broken down, and the viscosity and elasticity of the mucus therefore is reduced (see Figure 6-5).

Dose and Administration. Mucomyst can be given by aerosol or by direct instillation to the tracheobronchial tree. It is supplied in 10% and 20% solution strengths, and the dosages are as follows:

　　20% Solution: 3–5 ml TID or QID
　　10% Solution: 6–10 ml TID or QID

For instillation, 1 to 2 ml of either strength can be used.

Adverse Reactions. The most serious side effect of Mucomyst is bronchospasm, which may occur when the drug is administered by nebulization. Mucomyst is most likely to cause bronchospasm in patients with reactive airway disease, but it can also occur in patients without any primary pulmonary disease. The 10% strength Mucomyst is less likely to cause bronchospasm than the 20% solution.

When Mucomyst is to be nebulized, most clinicians opt to use the 20% solution in combination with a short-acting bronchodilator to prevent bronchospasm. Bronkosol is ideal because, as you may recall from Chapter 5, it has a very rapid onset of action (1–6 min) and may reach its peak effect in as little as 15 min.

Other complications of Mucomyst include nausea, **rhinorrhea, bronchorrhea,** and **stomatitis.** Rhinorrhea and stomatitis are secondary consequences of irritation of mucus membranes. Excessive thin and watery secretions result. Bronchorrhea is the term used to describe excess thin watery secretions in the airways. Rhinorrhea is what you would commonly call a runny nose.

Once a larger mucus molecule is broken down, it must be cleared, or mucus plugging can result. Deep breathing and coughing are essential for clearing the mucus from the airways. Mucus plugging can occur in patients with ineffective cough or artificial airways. It is advisable to monitor patients carefully for changes in breath sounds or signs of respiratory distress. Suction equipment should be available for patients who cannot cough effectively.

Although it is tasteless, some patients object to the disagreeable odor caused by the release of hydrogen sulfide. Nausea and vomiting have been attributed to the smell. Muco-

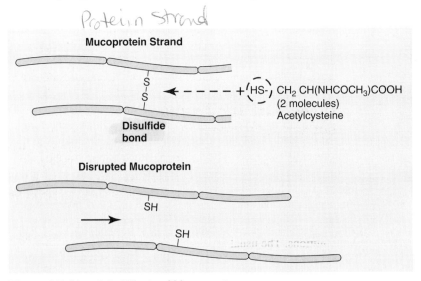

Figure 6-5 Mucolytic Effects of Mucomyst

CLINICAL PEARL

The hydrogen sulfide smell of Mucomyst has been compared to rotten eggs, but it is actually tasteless. If the patient is to drink it, mixing it with cola makes it more palatable and reduces the risk of making the patient vomit.

myst is corrosive to metal and irritating to mucus membranes, so patients should rinse their mouths and nebulizers (if they have metal parts) after treatments.

Other Uses. N-Acetylcysteine (Mucomyst) is also used as an antidote to protect the liver from damage in acetaminophen (Tylenol) overdose. In this situation, Mucomyst is given orally. It may be mixed in cola or given by nasogastric tube. The package insert is a good reference for complete information on dosing, but we recommend calling the poison control center.

CF

℞ **dornase alfa (Pulmozyme).** Dornase alfa or Pulmozyme is a clone of the natural human enzyme that digests extracellular DNA. Dornase alfa is a solution of recombinent human deoxyribonuclease (DNase). It received FDA approval in 1994.

Pulmonary secretions in cystic fibrosis are extremely thick and sticky because of abnormal chloride exchange mechanisms, which increase sodium and water absorption from the airway. This thickens airway mucus, impairs mucus clearance, and leads to infection. Because of their chronic pulmonary infections, cystic fibrosis patients have large numbers of neutrophils that congregate in the airways. As the neutrophils break down, a lot of their DNA is also left in the airways. This results in further thickening of the mucus.

Pulmozyme is indicated as **maintenance therapy** in the management of the viscous pulmonary secretions seen in cystic fibrosis. It is a proteolytic enzyme that breaks down the DNA material, decreasing the viscosity of the mucus and restoring its ability to flow. The change in sputum viscosity is dose dependent, higher doses producing thinner mucus.

Dose and Administration. Pulmozyme is available in single-dose ampules containing 2.5 mg of drug in 2.5 ml of solution, administered once a day. Further analysis has suggested that patients older than 21 years of age with a forced vital capacity (FVC) greater than 85% of predicted may benefit from twice-a-day treatment. Pulmozyme should not be diluted or mixed with other medications. The solution should be refrigerated and protected from light. Medication that has been at room temperature for more than 24 hours or appears discolored should be discarded. The manufacturer recommends that Pulmozyme should be nebulized only with the Hudson T Up-draft II disposable nebulizer, Marquest Acorn II and Pulmo-Aide compressor, or PARI LC (reusable) Jet Plus with PARI PRO NEB compressor, because these are the only ones that it has been tested with.

Adverse Effects. Pulmozyme has been shown to be safe and well tolerated. Side effects are minimal but include voice alteration, pharyngitis, laryngitis, rash, chest pain, and conjunctivitis. It is contraindicated in patients with hypersensitivity to dornase alfa or to Chinese Hamster Ovary cell products (from which it is derived).

Other Mucolytic Agents

sodium bicarbonate. Sodium bicarbonate is a weak base, and mucus becomes less adhesive in an alkaline environment. The sodium bicarbonate increases the pH of the mucus, weakening the bonds of the polysaccharide chains. The hypertonicity of sodium bicarbonate also causes an increase in respiratory tract secretions by osmosis. Alkalinization also activates proteases that are found in purulent sputum to help digest the excess protein molecules.

Dose and Administration. Sodium bicarbonate is usually available in 1.4%, 5%, and 7.5% solutions. The usual dose is 2–5 ml of 2.5% solution, given by small-volume nebulizer or instilled down the endotracheal tube (2–10 ml) Q4–Q8 hours. The 1.4% solution is nearly isotonic, which makes it less effective. The 7.5% can be irritating to the airways. The 5% concentration is well tolerated but is often diluted with an equal volume of sterile water, which brings it down to 2.5%. Sodium bicarbonate is compatible with other mucolytics, and there is some evidence that it potentiates the effects of Mucomyst. It can be mixed with β-adrenergic bronchodilators only if it is nebulized immediately, or the alkalinity will deactivate the bronchodilator drug.

Adverse Reactions. The only adverse reactions are that 5% and 7.5% solution can be irritating to the mucosa, and instilling very large amounts could result in systemic absorption and increased pH.

CLINICAL PEARL

Pioneer folk medicine recommended dissolving baking soda (sodium bicarbonate) in boiling water and breathing in the vapors for colds. How did they know?

Expectorants

Expectorants increase the production and expectoration of mucus by increasing the amount of fluid in the respiratory tract and stimulating cough. They are one of the main ingredients in many OTC cough and cold medications. Expectorants are thought to work either by increasing vagal gastric reflex stimulation (parasympathomimetic) or by absorption into the respiratory glands to directly stimulate mucus production. Hypertonic saline, which was discussed earlier in this chapter, is also considered to be an expectorant. **Guaifenesin** is one of the most commonly used expectorants. Other examples include **terpin hydrate, ammonium chloride,** and **potassium iodide.**

> ⬡ CONTROVERSY ⬡
>
> There is some controversy over the effectiveness and use of expectorants. One problem is the difficulty in obtaining objective data to assess their effectiveness. The simplest and most frequently recommended method for preserving mucus clearance is still to drink plenty of water and other liquids that do not cause diuresis. Tea and alcohol should be avoided because of their diuretic effects.

Antitussives/Cough Suppressants

Stimulation of vagal sensory endings in the larynx, bronchi, or even the stomach can cause a cough. The cough that results from irritation of these nerve endings may not be contributing to clearance of the airways, as it may be dry and nonproductive. More coughing leads to more irritation of the nerve endings, and so on. It may be necessary to suppress this type of dry, hacking, nonproductive cough. Cough suppressants depress the cough center, which is thought to be located in the medulla. There are both narcotic and nonnarcotic preparations to choose from. **Codeine** is one of the common narcotic cough suppressants, and **dextromethorphan** is a nonnarcotic cough suppressant.

Cough suppressants should never be given to patients with thick retained secretions. They need to cough to clear them. You can also find combinations of drugs in OTC cold preparations, such as an antitussive and an expectorant. The rationale is that a frequent, dry hacking cough is better replaced by a less frequent but more productive cough. However, the practice of combining an expectorant to stimulate mucus production with an antihistamine to dry secretions in OTC medications is questionable.

Ethanol (Ethyl Alcohol)

Ethyl alcohol is a surface-active agent that decreases the **surface tension** of respiratory secretions. Historically, it was used to treat fulminant alveolar pulmonary edema. This is a condition of very severe and rapid onset of alveolar edema. It is most commonly associated with severe acute congestive heart failure. Fulminant pulmonary edema has a very rapid onset and tends to be much more severe than the interstitial edema frequently associated with chronic congestive heart failure. The signs and symptoms include life-threatening hypoxemia, cyanosis, diffuse wet crackles, and foamy secretions that may be tinged with pink. The surfactant in the lung mixes with the alveolar fluid and results in the formation of foamy secretions. The foamy bubbles are a significant barrier to oxygen diffusion from the lungs to the blood. This leads to profound hypoxemia and can be life threatening. Alcohol decreases the surface tension of the bubbles, causing them to become unstable and dissipate, relieving the airways of the obstructive foam and allowing for better diffusion of oxygen.

However, ethanol is an irritant and an astringent, which can be harmful to delicate pulmonary tissue. It can increase the leakage of fluid into the airway and depress pulmonary defense mechanisms against infection. It can cause mild intoxication, depress ciliary function, or cause bronchospasm. It is also very important to note that isopropyl alcohol or denatured alcohol is highly toxic and cannot be used. There is no data to indicate that alcohol provides any benefit over traditional medical treatment of pulmonary edema, and it has a real potential for hazards; it is no longer part of the standard treatment for pulmonary edema.

Conclusion

The mucociliary system preserves and protects the lungs from disease and dehydration. The normal structure and function of the mucociliary system should be maintained. When possible, avoid factors that contribute to excess mucus production, such as smoking, pollution, and allergens. When the integrity of the mucociliary system is compromised, therapy should be geared toward increasing mucus clearance and restoring adequate hydration. This may be achieved through a variety of mechanisms, including the following:

- administration of bronchodilators
- adequate systemic hydration
- deep breathing and coughing
- postural drainage
- mucolytics
- expectorants

SURFACE-ACTIVE AGENTS

Alveolar Physiology and Surfactant Synthesis

Throughout Chapter 5 and so far in Chapter 6, we have been discussing the anatomy and physiology of the conducting airways. We have also explored many of the pharmacologic agents that act on the airways themselves and the mucus they contain. Now we will turn our attention to the area of the lungs beyond the terminal bronchioles, where gas exchange takes place. This is known as the respiratory zone of the lungs, and it includes the respiratory bronchioles, alveolar ducts, alveoli, and pulmonary capillaries (see Figure 6-6).

The walls of the respiratory bronchioles are made up of very thin, flattened squamous cells and a thin layer of connective tissue. They lack the smooth muscle and mucus-producing cells of the conducting airways. Alveolar ducts branch from the respiratory bronchioles, and the walls of the alveolar ducts are made up entirely of alveoli. Each alveolar duct ends in a cluster of alveoli, which together are called an alveolar sac. Each alveolar sac opens into about 10 to 16 alveoli.

About 8% of the alveolar cells are Type I pneumocyte cells. They are very large, thin, and flat. They cover about 93% of the alveolar surface and allow for the diffusion of gases. Interspersed on the alveolar surface are the Type II pneumocytes. Even though there are twice as many of them, they are very small, comprising only 7% of the alveolar surface (see Figure 6-7).

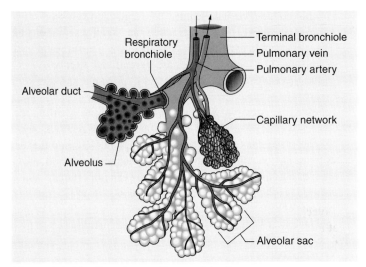

Figure 6-6 The Respiratory Zones of the Lung

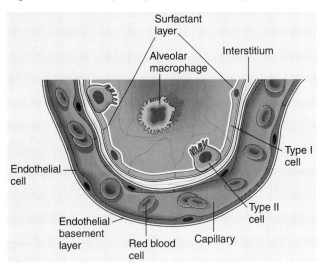

Figure 6-7 The Alveolar Surface

The Type II pneumocytes play a very important role in the lung. The Type II cells manufacture a complex substance called **surfactant.** Surfactant consists mainly of phospholipids (dipalmitoyl lecithin), neutral lipids, and the surface proteins (SP), SP-A, SP-B, SP-C, and SP-D. The theorized role of each of these proteins is listed in Table 6-6. Surface proteins B and C (SP-B and SP-C) appear critical to maintain normal surfactant function, while SP-A and SP-D are not (see Table 6-6).

Table 6-6 Surfactant Proteins

Protein	Function
SP-A	has host defense properties activates macrophage function facilitates phagocytosis of pathogens
SP-B	critical to surface tension–lowering property of surfactant
SP-C	facilitates surfactant spreadability
SP-D	functions as host defense mechanism by binding to pathogens

Surfactant Function

Surfactant is critical in maintaining the condition of the alveolar surface so that gas exchange can occur. Clinically, surfactant performs the following three critical functions:

- prevents alveolar collapse
- enables the lung to expand easily
- prevents leakage of fluid from the alveolar capillary membranes

To understand the importance of surfactant, we must first understand surface tension. The surface of a liquid acts as if there were an elastic skin constantly pulling in, attempting to contract the liquid into the smallest surface area. This force is called surface tension. It is created by uneven forces of attraction on the molecules at the surface of the liquid. The molecules under the surface have equal forces of attraction all around them. The molecules at the surface are in contact with air (this is called the gas–liquid interface); there is no attraction between the surface molecules and air, so the surface molecules are pulled inward and down, creating the force called surface tension (see Figure 6-8). It is this surface tension that makes liquid contract into a small sphere, such as, for example, the water drops that "bead" on a freshly waxed car. Without surface tension, the water drop would spread out into a large puddle.

The surface of alveoli also has a layer of fluid, comprised largely of water. The greater the surface tension of the fluid, the smaller the sphere becomes, and in turn, the smaller the sphere becomes, the greater the surface tension gets. By the law of LaPlace, the alveoli will eventually decrease to their critical volume. Below this volume, the force of the surface tension will cause the alveoli to collapse, resulting in atelectasis. Once alveoli collapse, the pressure required to reopen them is much greater than the pressure required to inflate an alveolus that is just above its critical volume. This pressure is called the critical pressure.

Surfactant is secreted by the Type II pneumocytes and stored in vesicles called lamellar bodies. The lamellar bodies unravel in the alveoli, and the surfactant forms a thin film called a monolayer on the inner surface of the alveoli. The air–liquid interface is replaced with an air–lipid interface, which has a much lower surface tension. In this way, the alveoli are stabilized above their critical volumes and do not collapse. Lower surface tension allows the alveoli to expand into a larger sphere, which provides a larger surface area, for

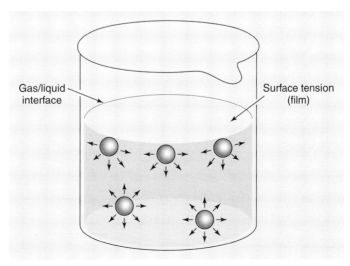

Figure 6-8 Surface Tension

greater gas diffusion. The lower surface tension also makes it easier to inflate the alveoli, which results in a lower work of breathing.

How can the law of LaPlace be used to explain why a balloon can be very difficult to blow air into initially but once started, becomes easier?

The action of surfactant and its effect on surface tension is a very dynamic process. Surface tension varies with alveolar volume. On inspiration, the alveolar volume increases, spreading the surfactant molecules further apart, and surface tension increases. This helps to prevent alveolar overdistension. On exhalation, the surfactant molecules are tightly packed, decreasing surface tension and preventing collapse (see Figure 6-9).

Surfactant has a relatively short half-life and must be continuously replaced at the alveolar surface. During exhalation, old surfactant is squeezed out of the monolayer, and new surfactant is added on inspiration. Under normal circumstances, most of the surfactant (90% to 95%) is taken back up and recycled by the Type II pneumocytes.

Since inflation and deflation are important in maintaining a healthy monolayer and low surface tension in the alveoli, you can see that lung collapse or atelectasis disrupts surfactant production. Hypoxia can also damage the Type II pneumocytes and interrupt surfactant production, and repeated collapse and reopening of alveoli cause a lot of lung damage, inflammation, and leaking of protein-rich fluid into the alveoli. This also disrupts surfactant function.

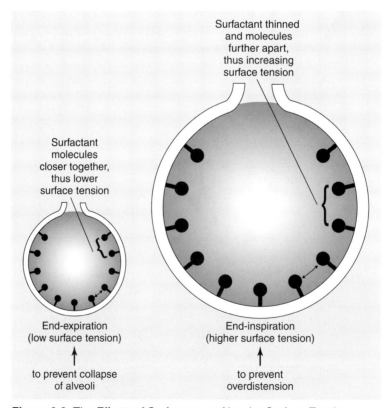

Figure 6-9 The Effects of Surfactant on Alveolar Surface Tension

Infants born prematurely may not have mature Type II pneumocytes. What complications might evolve?

Indications for Surfactant Replacement Therapy

The surfactant that is produced naturally in lung tissue is called **endogeneous surfactant. Exogeneous** surfactants are those that are produced outside of the body and administered as a therapy. The major indication for surfactant replacement therapy is to prevent or treat infants with Respiratory Distress Syndrome (RDS). RDS is a disease associated mainly with prematurity and low birth weight. The Type II pneumocytes in these infants are not mature enough to produce surfactant. In other cases, the Type II pneumocytes can be damaged from the hypoxemia that results from perinatal asphyxia. In either case, an inadequate amount of surfactant leads to alveolar collapse, hypoxemia, and increased work of breathing for the infant.

General Techniques of Surfactant Administration

Surfactant is administered intratracheally. This requires placement of an endotracheal tube. The tube must be positioned properly above the carina to ensure even distribution to both lungs. The baby should be suctioned to remove any secretions that would interfere with medication delivery. The techniques for delivering Survanta and Exosurf differ somewhat, so the technique for each drug will be reviewed briefly.

Surfactant can be given immediately after birth, as close to the first breath as possible, to premature infants with very low birth weight. This early administration is called prophylactic (preventative for RDS). Rescue therapy is administered 6 to 8 hours after birth to treat RDS once signs and symptoms have already developed.

Types of Exogenous Surfactants

There are two types of exogenous surfactants that are currently available, natural/modified and synthetic. We will discuss the advantages and limitations of each type and review an example of each type.

℞ *colfosceril palmitate (Exosurf).* Exosurf is a synthetic surfactant. Synthetic surfactants are mixtures of synthetic components that are produced in the laboratory. This means that the drug is free of infection and foreign proteins, which is an advantage, but it may not perform as well as natural surfactant because of the organic chemicals that are substituted for the natural proteins.

Dose and Administration. The dose is 5 ml/kg of Exosurf administered intratracheally. Multiple doses can be given 4–6 hours apart if there has not been a good response to a single dose. Two or three doses are usually given if the clinical response of the baby indicates the need for further treatment. This is just a guideline; clinical assessment and judgment are required.

Exosurf is supplied in a powder form and must be reconstituted with the liquid supplied by the manufacturer. It needs to be mixed thoroughly but gently so that it does not form bubbles. The reconstituted solution is instilled down the baby's endotracheal tube through the sideport of a special adaptor provided by the manufacturer. The medication can be instilled through the sideport while the infant is attached to the ventilator. After instillation of half of the dose, the baby is turned 45 degrees to the right side for 30 seconds, while ventilation continues. He or she is then returned to the supine position while the second half is instilled. He or she is turned 45 degrees to the left for 30 seconds, then returned to supine, and the catheter is removed. This procedure is to distribute the surfactant as widely as possible throughout the lung.

beractant (Survanta).

Survanta is a natural/modified surfactant comprised of natural bovine (cow) lung extract modified with three other additives. Natural surfactant is obtained from animals or humans by means of alveolar wash or amniotic fluid. The surfactant is then extracted from the liquid by centrifugation or simple filtration. The surfactant is modified by adding and removing certain components to improve its function in the lung, reduce protein contamination, and ensure sterility. This preparation consumes a lot of time, which adds to the cost of the drug. There is also a concern over the possibility of viral infection and immunologic reaction to foreign proteins. However, the advantage of natural surfactants is that they contain the phospholipids and proteins (SP-B and SP-C) necessary for absorption and spreading.

Dose and Administration. The dose is 4 ml/kg administered by direct tracheal instillation. The dose can be repeated in 6 hours for up to 4 doses if required on the basis of clinical judgment. An endotracheal tube with a sideport can be used, or the baby can be briefly disconnected from the ventilator while a 5 French catheter is placed directly in the endotracheal tube to instill the Survanta. The manufacturer recommends that the baby be placed in four positions: inclined 5–10 degrees, head turned to the right, then head turned to the left, then reclined 5–10 degrees with the head to the right, and finally with head turned to the left. If the catheter is being placed directly into the endotracheal tube, the catheter is withdrawn and the infant returned to the ventilator after each instillation.

Adverse Reactions. A steady improvement in oxygenation is usually seen following surfactant administration, but one must keep in mind that these drugs often produce rapid changes in lung compliance. It is critical to make appropriate adjustments in the ventilator settings. There are several hazards one must be aware of. They can be divided into those that occur during administration and those that occur after administration.

During administration:

- reflux of solution
- transient decrease in oxygenation
- bradycardia and/or hypotension

After administration:

- hyperoxygenation
- hyperventilation (decrease in $PaCO_2$)

Uncommon side effects include:

- apnea
- pulmonary hemorrhage
- bronchospasm

The patient should be monitored closely and appropriate ventilator changes made following surfactant administration. As the baby's lung compliance improves, tidal volumes

CLINICAL PEARL

The transient decrease in oxygen is due to the initial diffusion barrier of the drug. This is very transient and should not be significant, especially with proper preoxygenation. The bradycardia and/or hypotension can be secondary to hypoxemia or could be a result of vagal stimulation.

may increase significantly. Ventilator pressure may need to be decreased to prevent alveolar damage or rupture. Oxygen levels in the baby's blood may also increase, allowing for the baby's oxygen concentration to be decreased. Monitoring may include chest X-ray, chest movement or tidal volume changes, arterial blood gases, and oxygen saturation measurements.

Surfactant Replacement Therapy Indications

Surfactants have been used anecdotally and successfully to treat several other conditions, including the following:

- meconium aspiration syndrome
- full-term infants with RDS
- pulmonary hemorrhage
- congenital diaphragmatic hernia
- severe pneumonia
- pulmonary infections
- any condition where there is loss of surfactant and low lung volume

Surfactant Administration in Adult Patients

So far, surfactant has not been proven to be successful in treatment of adults and children with ARDS. Only a few studies of adults with ARDS have been done, and the results have been conflicting. One large trial where Exosurf was nebulized continuously for 5 days showed little improvement and no difference in outcome. The actual dose that was delivered to the lungs in this study is not known. It has been suggested that the delivered dose may not have been sufficient.

A smaller study, where Survanta was instilled directly into the lungs of adults, showed a decrease in mortality from 43.8% in the control group to 17.8% in the group who received Survanta. These results suggest that there may be some benefit, but more research is needed. The dose and delivery technique may need to be modified for adults. This could make treatment extremely costly (one estimate was $5,000 per dose for adults). Finally, there are differences in the pathophysiology of ARDS. In IRDS, the problem is a primary surfactant production deficiency, while in ARDS, the surfactant deficiency is secondary to lung injury and inflammatory response. This may account for the different response to surfactant replacement therapy.

 Exosurf, Survanta, **Infasurf,** and **Curosurf** are available in the United States, and there are several other surfactants that are available throughout the world. See Table 6-7 for the commercially available surfactants.

Table 6-7 Commercially Available Surfactants

Generic Name	Trade Name	Type
colfosceril	Exosurf	synthetic
beractant	Survanta	natural/modified
poractant alfa	Curosurf	natural/modified
calfactant	Infasurf	natural/modified
bovactant	Alveofact	natural/modified

www.prenhall.com/colbert

Get connected to the Web for updates on the latest developments in surfactant replacement therapy.

REVIEW QUESTIONS

1. What layer(s) comprise the mucosal blanket that covers the airways?
   (a) sol
   (b) gel
   (c) (a) & (b)
   (d) none of the above

2. Bland aerosols are aerosols that:
   (a) have no taste
   (b) are boring
   (c) are colored
   (d) are nonmedicated

3. A patient with a dry nonproductive cough that requires a sputum induction for TB (tuberculosis) testing may benefit most from what solution?
   (a) hypertonic
   (b) hypotonic
   (c) sterile water
   (d) isotonic

4. Concerning the drug dornase alfa (Pulmozyme):
   I. indicated for maintenance therapy for secretions in cystic fibrosis patients
   II. ruptures disulfide bonds in sputum
   III. should not be mixed with other medications
   IV. should be refrigerated and protected from light
   (a) I, II, and III

   (b) I, III, and IV
   (c) I and IV
   (d) IV only

5. During surfactant replacement administration, the patient should be monitored for what hazards or conditions?
   I. improved lung compliance
   II. transient decrease in oxygenation
   III. reflux of solution
   IV. bradycardia
   (a) I, II, III, and IV
   (b) I and II
   (c) I and III
   (d) II, III, and IV

6. State four functions of mucus in maintaining a healthy pulmonary system.

7. What is the typical dose range for Mucomyst, and how can it be delivered?

8. What precaution can be taken to prevent the bronchospasm that is sometimes associated with Mucomyst?

9. State one advantage of natural (endogenous) surfactant over artificial surfactants.

10. State three critical functions of surfactant in the lung.

11. What is the primary indication for surfactant replacement therapy?

12. How is surfactant administered?

CASE STUDY 1

A COPD patient is admitted with pneumonia. He has a frequent strong nonproductive cough. The patient states that when he does cough up sputum, it is very thick and yellow. Upon auscultation, you note that he has expiratory rhonchi bilaterally and crackles over the right middle and lower lobes. He is already receiving aerosol treatments with al-buterol and ipratropium bromide. He is also on antibiotics.

(a) What other medication may help to reduce the viscosity of this patient's sputum?

(b) What other therapies and recommendations do you have for this patient?

CASE STUDY 2

A baby boy is born at 33 weeks' gestation. He is admitted to the neonatal intensive care unit with respiratory distress, nasal flaring, and grunting. His oxygen requirement is also increasing dramatically.

(a) What pathological process should be suspected?

(b) What medication is indicated, and when and how should it be given?

(c) What patient parameters should be monitored before and after medication administration?

GLOSSARY

bronchial gland   mucus-producing exocrine glands found in the submucosa. They are stimulated by parasympathetic nerves and secrete a relatively watery fluid.

bronchorrhea   excessive discharge of respiratory tract secretions.

endogeneous surfactant   complex mixture of phospholipids and proteins produced in the lung by the Type II pneumocytes. It plays a crucial role in reducing alveolar surface tension and preventing alveolar collapse.

expectorant   substance that improves expectoration of respiratory secretions by increasing the output from the bronchial glands.

exogenous surfactant   surfactant drugs that are produced outside of the patient's own body. They may be obtained from humans or animals, or synthesized in the laboratory.

goblet cell   found in the mucosal epithelium, these secretory cells produce gelatinous mucus. Topical irritation and exposure to irritants increase their size and number.

hydrophilic   molecules or substance that is attracted to water.

hypertonic   a solution containing a greater concentration of salt than is normally found in the body.

hypotonic   a solution containing a lower concentration of salt than is normally found in the body.

isotonic   a solution containing the same concentration of salt as that found in the body.

maintenance therapy   agent used to treat a chronic disease state rather than the acute phase.

rhinorrhea   excessive secretion from the nose.

stomatitis   inflammation of the mucous lining in the mouth.

surface tension   force of contraction at the surface of a liquid that pulls the molecules at the surface inward and down.

surfactant   complex mixture of phospholipids and proteins produced in the lung by the Type II pneumocytes. It plays a crucial role in reducing alveolar surface tension and preventing alveolar collapse.

viscoelastic   used to describe the ability of mucus to change shape (spread or flow) when a force is applied to it and then return to its normal shape.

www.prenhall.com/colbert

Use the address above to access the free, interactive Companion Web site created specifically for this textbook. Enhance your studying by viewing videos and animations, answering practice quiz questions, and reviewing an audio glossary and much more related to Chapter 6.

CHAPTER 7

Anti-Inflammatory and Antiasthmatic Agents

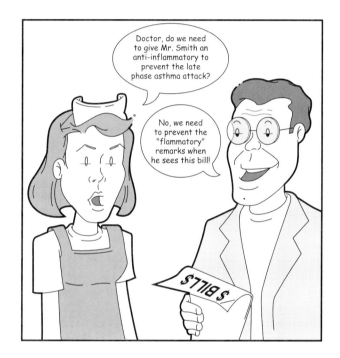

OBJECTIVES

Upon completion of this chapter you will be able to

- Describe the inflammatory process as it relates to airway disease
- List the chemical mediators involved in allergic reactions
- Discuss physiology of corticosteroids
- Define hypothalamic pituitary adrenal axis, suppression, and steroid dependency
- Be able to describe the pharmacotherapy of oral, parenteral, and inhalational corticosteroids
- Be able to differentiate the anti-inflammatory and antiasthmatic classes of medications available to treat asthma according to their mechanism of action and clinical usage

ABBREVIATIONS

HPA	hypothalamic pituitary axis	FEV_1	forced expiratory volume in
PDE	phosphodiesterase		1 second
ACTH	adrenocorticotropic hormone	EIB	exercise-induced bronchospasm
CAM	cellular adhesion molecule	BHR	bronchial hyperresponsiveness
PGE	prostaglandin	CRF	corticotropin-releasing factor
PGF_{2_a}	prostaglandin F_{2_a}	PEFs	peak expiratory flows
PGE_1	prostaglandin E_1	CRH	corticotropin-releasing hormone
PGE_2	prostaglandin E_2	H_2	histamine 2
IgE	immunoglobulin E	CBC	complete blood count
MRI	mediator release inhibitor		

INTRODUCTION

In Chapter 5, we learned about the role of bronchodilators to treat bronchospasm within the smooth muscle layer of the airway. Bronchospasm can be the result of an immediate reaction to an airway irritant, but the story doesn't end there. What about the subsequent airway inflammation that can result from bronchospasm or from disease processes such as asthma or chronic bronchitis or from mechanical lung trauma? In this chapter we will focus on the anti-inflammatory and antiasthmatic classes of medications frequently used in association with bronchodilators to treat and/or lessen the subsequent pulmonary inflammation. To distinguish the roles of these classifications of drugs, it is first important to review how the airway can be affected by inflammation and what the various pathways are that lead to the inflammatory response.

Lung inflammation can be due to diseases, infections, inhalation of toxic substances, or trauma. The resulting mucosal edema, bronchoconstriction, and increased mucus production can be life threatening because of increases in airway resistance from swelling and decreasing ventilation leading to poor gas exchange.

Inflammation occurs in response to a stimulus that causes release of chemical mediators that travel to the site of injury. There are several different pathways containing chemical mediators that lead to the inflammatory process within the lungs. Different drugs discussed in this chapter will work on different mediator pathways. This is the rationale for combination drug use to attempt to attack the specific pathway(s) leading to the inflammatory response in each particular situation.

THE INFLAMMATORY PROCESS

The Immune Response

The major function of the body's natural defense mechanism—the immune system—is to neutralize, destroy, and eliminate foreign materials called antigens. It accomplishes this by the ability of white blood cells (leukocytes) to produce specific antibodies to combat foreign invasion. **Antigens** stimulate both the immune and inflammatory processes. Table 7-1 lists some of these common antigens.

The **immune** system has two functional units: **humoral** (circulating) immunity and **cell-mediated** immunity. Either or both units can respond to an antigen and activate the

Table 7-1 Common Antigens

dust mites	smoke
animal dander	sulfites
mold	viruses
pollen	bacteria

white blood cells known as lymphocytes, as well as macrophages. Humoral immune response involves activation of **B lymphocytes,** while cell-mediated immunity involves production of **T lymphocytes.**

B lymphocytes produce antigen-specific antibodies called **immunoglobulins** that act to remove or destroy the antigen. We currently know of five major classes of immunoglobulins that are found naturally in the body or are produced by B lymphocytes in response to foreign objects (see Table 7-2 for a list of the classes of immunoglobulins). T lymphocytes remove or destroy antigens directly or may act indirectly, with help from macrophages and neutrophils.

Mast Cell Chemical Mediator Release

The most common immune system–produced antibody involved in allergic asthma and rhinitis (runny stuffy nose) is immunoglobulin E (IgE). Once IgE becomes exposed to an antigen, it fixes itself to the surface of a mast cell membrane. Mast cells can be found throughout the body, but for our discussion we are focusing on those found in the respiratory tract. In essence, once the antigen attaches to the mast cell, the mast cell becomes "sensitized" and awaits reexposure of the antigen much like a police officer waiting to leap out and grab a known perpetrator, one he's seen before. Upon reexposure, an antigen–antibody reaction then occurs, which consists of a cascade of **chemical mediators** spilling out from the ruptured mast cell (degranulation). Mediators released are histamine and chemotactic factors. Others are products of arachidonic acid metabolism such as leukotrienes, prostaglandins, and thromboxanes.

Within the airway, these chemicals can immediately lead to bronchospasms. Eventually these chemicals and others produced as a result of the mast cell rupture cause **inflammation** and the inflammatory reaction, which causes further airway smooth muscle contraction, mucosal edema, cellular infiltration, and mucus secretions with plugging. See Figure 7-1, which represents the mechanism that leads to mast cell rupture or degranulation.

Table 7-2 Immunoglobulins

Type	Characteristics
IgG	most common, 80% of total immunoglobulins in plasma protects against childhood diseases
IgM	10% of total immunoglobulins, numbers increase in chronic infections
IgE	hypersensivitiy reactions, allergic rhinitis, allergic asthma bound to mast cells
IgA	mucous membranes in respiratory tract, salivary and bronchial secretions transfers immunity to the child
IgD	unknown role, maybe B cell maturation

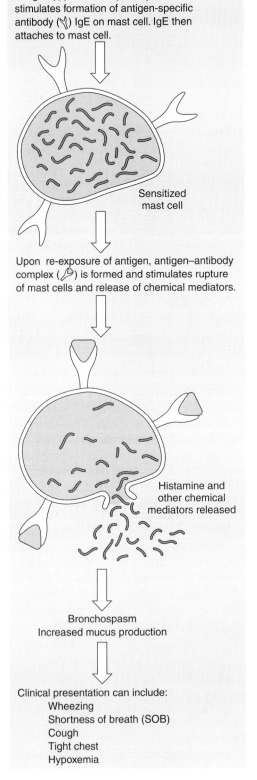

Antigen (▽) enters respiratory tract and stimulates formation of antigen-specific antibody (Ψ) IgE on mast cell. IgE then attaches to mast cell.

Sensitized mast cell

Upon re-exposure of antigen, antigen–antibody complex (🔑) is formed and stimulates rupture of mast cells and release of chemical mediators.

Histamine and other chemical mediators released

Bronchospasm
Increased mucus production

Clinical presentation can include:
    Wheezing
    Shortness of breath (SOB)
    Cough
    Tight chest
    Hypoxemia

Figure 7-1 Mast-Cell Rupture or Degranulation in the Airways

www.prenhall.com/colbert

This is a very simple explanation of an immune system so complex that a thorough treatment of it could comprise a whole separate textbook. For more details of mediators and how they relate to pathophysiology and pharmacology, go to the Web site.

Types of Asthma

Because asthma represents a disease of chronic inflammation, it can be used to illustrate the inflammatory response. Keep in mind that the inflammatory response is a needed body response; it is only hyper-activation of this response that can cause serious consequences.

Asthma has two primary types: allergic asthma and nonallergic asthma. Most people have the allergic kind, caused by an external antigen such as pollen, dust, smoke, or pets. This is the kind that can lend itself to treatment with **immunotherapy,** commonly known as allergy shots, because you know the exact antigen triggering the immune and inflammatory response. Allergy shots work because an allergic individual exposed to small doses of an antigen or allergen produces antibodies specific to the antigen. The antibodies are then sensitized and can recognize and fight the antigen when it returns. While allergy shots may sound like the most logical treatment possible, they are usually used only if drug therapy isn't effective for allergies. This is because immunotherapy treatment can be lengthy, with symptom relief not present until after at least six months of therapy. There is always the risk of anaphylaxis in patients with severe asthma when allergy injections are used, and some believe this is because too many mast cells become sensitized and the subsequent chemical mediator release can then be too great.

Nonallergic asthma is precipitated by infection, cold air, exercise, or stress, with no specific antigen being identified. No immune response is involved, but mast cells still degranulate, which then can result in an acute asthma attack. Lessening the frequency and severity of the attacks from either nonallergic or allergic asthma is accomplished by prophylactic antiasthmatic agents, which stabilize or desensitize mast cells, thus preventing their rupture and chemical mediator release. These agents will be discussed later in this chapter.

CLINICAL PEARL

Allergic asthma can also be called atopic or extrinsic asthma, because it is known to be stimulated from a specific antigen source. Nonallergic asthma can also be referred to as intrinsic or nonatopic asthma.

Phases of the Inflammatory Response

Regardless of the type of asthma, the inflammatory response related to an asthmatic attack and mast cell degranulation can have two distinct phases: early and late. The **early-phase response** of any inflammatory reaction consists of local vasodilation and increased vascular permeability, redness, and wheal (local, usually itchy swelling, or welt) formation. The immediate inflammatory response in asthma results in bronchial contraction, with wheezing, cough, dyspnea, and hypoxemia caused as a result of mast cell degranulation and subsequent histamine and other chemical mediator substances' release. Please see Figure 7-1 again, which illustrates the early phase of the inflammatory response.

Bronchodilators almost always reverse the bronchospasm in the early phase; however, in more difficult cases of asthma, the episode launches a series of steps leading to a slow inflammatory process that develops 6 to 8 hours later. This is termed the **late-phase response** and is very difficult to resolve. The late-phase reaction can be serious, and treatment is aimed at stopping inflammatory progression before it occurs at this stage. White blood cells, including lymphocytes, and other chemical mediators contribute to the late-phase inflammation. White cells infiltrate the asthmatic airways, as evidenced by an increase in eosinophils and neutrophils. Sloughing of airway cells and growth of goblet cells results in hypersecretion of mucus and mucosal swelling. Increased vascular permeability then occurs, causing further mucus secretion and mucosal swelling, which results in mucus plugging. In essence, a "traffic jam" of cellular debris and secretions piles up.

In addition, the destruction of the phospholipid mast cell membrane and its subsequent breakdown by phospholipase produces the fatty acid arachidonic acid. Arachidonic acid then produces two pathways that contribute to the late-phase response. The lipoxygenase pathways consist mainly of **leukotriene** release, and the cyclooxygenase pathway primarily releases **prostaglandins,** all adding to the late-phase responses of submucosal edema, mucus production, and hyperreactive airways. See Figure 7-2, which shows the early and late-phase inflammatory response.

STOP
& REVIEW

Contrast early- and late-phase responses; why do you think this will be important to drug therapy?

LEARNING HINT

On the complete blood count (CBC), the presence of eosinophils hints at the presence an active allergic response.

When we look at Figure 7-2, logic tells us that the optimal blockage of the inflammatory response would be to stabilize the mast cell membrane and not allow it to begin the cascade of mediator release leading to both the early- and late-phase responses. This will be the mechanism of action behind the prophylactic antiasthmatics discussed later in this chapter. In addition, this chapter will discuss other categories of drugs that block specific inflammatory pathways, such as the leukotriene inhibitors, antihistamines, and prostaglandin inhibitors. For now, we will focus on the drug category **corticosteroids,** which have a broad

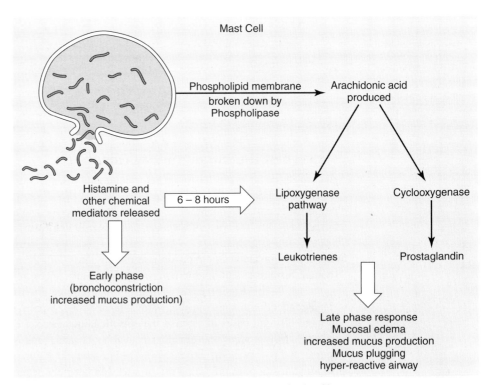

Figure 7-2 The Late-Phase Inflammatory Response in the Airways

Note: Increased neutrophils, monocytes, and eosinophils migrating to inflamed airways also contribute to late-phase response.

spectrum of activity and work on several of the different mediator pathways in both the early- and late-phase inflammatory responses.

www.prenhall.com/colbert

Other drugs currently being researched for their ability to inhibit airway inflammatory response include monoclonal antibodies to specific cytokines as well as cellular adhesion molecules (CAM-1). Go to the Web site for more information on these types of drugs.

CORTICOSTEROIDS

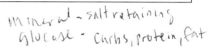

Mineral - salt retaining
Glucose - carbs, protein, fat

Corticosteroid Physiology

Corticosteroids can block both the initial immune response and the subsequent inflammatory process and are therefore a mainstay of treatment for allergic asthma. Before we can talk about corticosteroids and how they work, though, we must review corticosteroid physiology.

Body functions are controlled by the nervous system and the endocrine system working together in an integrated fashion. The endocrine system produces hormones, which are chemical substances secreted into the bloodstream that then circulate and exert physiologic effects on body cells and tissues. The adrenal glands contain two endocrine organs: the adrenal medulla and the adrenal cortex. The adrenal medulla secretes the hormone catecholamines norepinephine (NE) and epinephrine and is functionally related to the sympathetic component (fight-or-flight) of the autonomic nervous system (ANS), as discussed in Chapter 3. In this chapter, though, we will focus on the adrenal cortex. Its role is secretion of steroid substances called adrenocortical hormones or corticosteroids.

Corticosteroids are classified into **mineralcorticoids** and **glucocorticoids.** Depending on the chemical structure of the corticosteroid hormone, drugs differ in their mineralcorticoid and glucocorticoid activity. Mineralcorticoids are corticosteroids with salt-retaining activity that are important for electrolyte balance and fluid volume. Aldosterone is an example of a mineralcorticoid. Aldosterone causes increased sodium and water reabsorption into the bloodstream, which decreases urine production and thereby causes volume expansion within the bloodstream.

Glucocorticoids affect carbohydrate, protein, and fat metabolism and are useful pharmacologically for anti-inflammatory activity and their ability to suppress immunologic activity. Synthetic corticosteroids have been developed to optimize anti-inflammatory activity and minimize mineralcorticoid activity. Although the two classifications seem distinct, glucocorticoids also tend to have some mineralcorticoid activity (see Table 7-3).

CLINICAL PEARL

Spironolactone (Aldactone) is a diuretic that works as an aldosterone antagonist.

Table 7-3   Oral Corticosteroids' Glucocorticoid and Mineralcorticoid Activity

Corticosteroid	*Glucocorticoid Strength*	*Mineralcorticoid Strength*
hydrocortisone	1	1
cortisone	0.8	0.8
prednisone	2.5–3.5	0.8
prednisolone	3–4	0.8
methylprednisolone	4–5	0–0.8
dexamethasone	20–40	0

While immunosupression by high doses of corticosteroids may be beneficial after organ transplantation, this will have implications for precautions you should take while treating transplant patients. Can you think of what precautions you should take and why?

Other corticosteroids that are not as pertinent to cardiorespiratory pharmacotherapy, and therefore will not be discussed here, are sex hormones, which have androgenic, estrogenic, or progestenic activity. Some of these types of corticosteroids have been used by weightlifters or in sexual hormone replacement therapy. The term **steroid** is frequently used instead of corticosteroid in these contexts. All steroids except the sex hormones are essential for survival, and death would result without their presence. (One could of course argue that the sex hormones are needed for the survival of the species.)

Corticosteroids are used to treat many diseases, such as rheumatoid arthritis, cancers, and pulmonary diseases. In respiratory disease, they treat acute and chronic asthma, with a controversial role in COPD, as discussed in Chapter 13. Administration routes used are inhalational, oral, and parenteral.

While treatment with corticosteroids is usually short term and adjunctive, it can also be long term. Corticosteroids can make some patients feel euphoric, and patients frequently want to be on steroids. Unfortunately, therapeutic pharmacological use can alter the balance of natural steroid production. This will be discussed shortly, as it relates to steroid dependence and adrenal suppression.

> **CONTROVERSY**
>
> There must be the appropriate balance of risk and benefit in terms of side effects and gain from corticosteroids. Because corticosteroids are very effective therapeutically yet have several side effects, implications of their clinical use must be understood and jointly agreed on by the patient and healthcare provider alike.

The main internally produced or endogenous glucocorticoid is hydrocortisone. It's important to understand the production and control of the body's endogenous corticosteroids and the hypothalamic pituitary adrenal axis (HPA). Only then can the concept of adrenal suppression and steroid dependence be understood.

Hypothalamic Pituitary Adrenal Axis

The HPA controls corticosteroid release in the body. It is responsible for the normal diurnal variation in steroid blood levels. For example, when we rise in the morning, the body must now ready itself to face the day, and hormone production begins and peaks and troughs throughout the day according to our metabolic needs. One of the factors that influences corticosteroid release in the body is stress. In stressful situations, corticosteroids work to decrease the effects of stress. They do this by raising blood glucose levels so that vital tissues, such as the brain and heart, get the glucose needed in stressful situations. When the hypothalamus is stimulated, it sends impulses that cause corticotropin-releasing factor (CRF) to be released in the anterior pituitary gland. The anterior pituitary gland, under the influence of CRF, then causes adrenocorticotropic hormone (ACTH) to be released into the bloodstream. ACTH then circulates within the bloodstream to the adrenal cortex, where it stimulates the secretion of corticosteroids. This is under normal biofeedback mechanism control, where high levels of corticosteroids in the bloodstream then inhibit the further release of CRF and ACTH (see Figure 7-3).

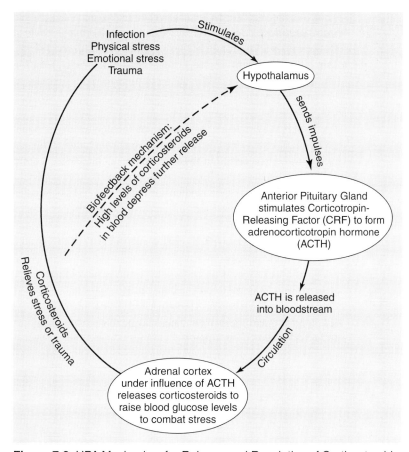

Figure 7-3 HPA Mechanism for Release and Regulation of Corticosteroids

If exogenous pharmacological corticosteroid drugs are used to treat diseases, then adrenal or HPA suppression can occur, causing the adrenal glands to atrophy, since they no longer have to work to produce these hormones. This means the body can't tell the difference between corticosteroids it has produced itself and those administered pharmacologically. The body just knows it has a higher level of hormones and tells itself to turn off its own production. It then becomes dependent on the pharmacological corticosteroids. As a result, pharmacological exogenously administered corticosteroids must be tapered down slowly to lower doses to give the body time to pick up production and regain internal regulation.

Corticosteroid Mechanism of Action

Corticosteroids have a variety of mechanisms of action, all related to blocking or diminishing the late-phase asthma responses by blocking the arachidonic acid cascade of metabolites (leukotrienes and prostaglandins). In addition, corticosteroids remove circulatory lymphocytes, monocytes, eosinophils, and basophils by moving them to lymph bone marrow and spleen. Less cells then reach the site of inflammation, and therefore there is less congestion. Corticosteroids also inhibit macrophage and leukocyte processing of antigens, so the ability of cells to respond to antigens is decreased, thus suppressing the immune response.

Corticosteroids also decrease the production of eosinophils, basophils, and monocytes. They have shown an additional beneficial effect, enhancing the responsiveness of the

CLINICAL PEARL

Corticosteroids are secreted daily by the adrenal cortex at the rate of about 10–30 mg/day. This isn't steady but is released in response to surgery, stress, infection, and emotion on a 24-hour diurnal rhythm cycle. The serum concentrations peak about 8:00 a.m. Night-shift workers have very different patterns or diurnal rhythms, and dosing time of exogenous pharmacological steroids may be reversed in their case.

β_2 receptors by increasing the responsiveness of adenyl cyclase in airway smooth muscle to catecholamines or β-agonists (see Chapter 5). Corticosteroids do not have a direct relaxing effect on bronchial muscle but do facilitate the effect of β-agonists, thereby enhancing the desired bronchodilation effects of β_2-adrenergic drugs given for the hyperreactive airways. Taking all these factors into account, corticosteroids clinically reduce airway inflammation, decrease airway obstruction, improve oxygenation, and increase the response to β-agonists (see Table 7-4).

The effect seen from corticosteroids is often time dependent. Although the cellular and biochemical effects of corticosteroids are immediate, clinical response takes longer. Increased responsiveness to β-agonists occurs within 2 hours, and β receptor density increases within 4 hours. Seasonal bronchial hyperresponsiveness (BHR) requires at least a week of therapy to reverse. Exercise induced bronchospasm (EIB) sensitivity decreases after 4 weeks of therapy.

Corticosteroid Use in Airway Remodeling

Corticosteroids prevent or suppress airway inflammation, which results in reduction of bronchial hyperresponsiveness and prevention and reduction of airway remodeling. Airway remodeling is important, because it is a change in the composition of the airway wall that occurs in some asthmatics. The structural changes in the airway result from long-standing airway inflammation. One of the consequences is persistent airway obstruction that might not be responsive to treatment. Based on this concept of airway remodeling, use of corticosteroids as an early anti-inflammatory intervention makes sense.

< CONTROVERSY >

Should drug therapy of asthma be disease-modifying and a primary prevention strategy, or should it simply produce symptomatic control?

Adverse Effects of Corticosteroids

Side effects of steroids can be considered short term and long term on the basis of duration of use and route of administration as systemic or topical. The most common side effects of short-term use include appetite stimulation, stomach irritation, headache, and mood changes. The mood changes can be a sense of well-being or a steroid psychosis. Steroids can exacerbate acne and can cause hypokalemia, hyperglycemia, and leukocytosis. The hyperglycemia causes what is called steroid diabetes. Once the steroids are discontinued, these side effects go away.

Long-term side effects include osteoporosis or bone changes that could lead to fractures; immunosuppression, which can lead to increased risk of infection; and myopathy of skeletal muscles. See Table 7-5 for corticosteroid side effects.

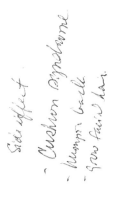

Table 7-4 Corticosteroid Effects on Inflammation

Effect
block arachidonic acid metabolites (leukotrienes and prostaglandins)
decrease monocytes, eosinophils, basophils
decrease lymphocytes and macrophages
inhibit late-phase inflammation
increase β_2 receptors and responsiveness

Table 7-5   Corticosteroid Side Effects

Category	Side Effect
immunologic	immunosuppression increased susceptibility to infections
cardiovascular	edema hypertension
CNS	euphoria insomnia
dermatologic	thin skin impaired wound healing bruising altered fat distribution
endocrinologic	diabetes cushingoid state
metabolic	electrolyte imbalance negative nitrogen balance
musculoskeletal	muscle weakness osteoporosis growth suppression
ophthalmic	glaucoma

CONTROVERSY

Controversy exists over the extent of effect corticosteroids have on children's growth, because of steroid-induced changes in bone growth and epiphyseal maturation. Several studies actually show improved growth rates for children switched to inhaled steroids from oral steroids. This could be due to better control of the asthma and less need for oral systemic steroids.

Oral and Parenteral Corticosteroid Administration

Sometimes oral steroids are given as pulse or burst doses, for example, 40 mg of prednisone orally per day for three days. Other times they are given on every-other-day regimens at two to three times the daily dose. Whatever the regimen, the lowest possible dose of steroid should be used to accomplish the therapeutic goal.

Corticosteroids often take days, not hours, to heal damaged airways. Although it's common to use parenteral administration, research results are ambivalent as to whether it is quicker acting than oral administration. Objective improvement takes a minimum of 6 to 12 hours, and maximum improvement may take longer than a week. Objective measures such as pulmonary function tests may show improvement 12 hours after administration. In the emergency room, corticosteroids are warranted for patients with a poor response to β-agonists over 1 to 2 hours. Because of the delayed onset, many clinicians initiate early corticosteroid use in order to lessen or prevent the late-phase inflammatory response.

℞   **Hydrocortisone** (Cortef) and **methylprednisolone** (SoluMedrol) are most commonly given by injection. Methylprednisolone's advantage is less fluid retention in patients with heart disease, because of fewer mineralcorticoid effects (again, see Table 7-3). After hospitalized patients improve in 48 to 72 hours, the IV dose is tapered to an oral dose for 2 weeks. If the patient was steroid dependent before hospitalization, tapering the dose to what it was before hospitalization is the goal.

Table 7-6 Comparison of Oral and Aerosol Corticosteroids

Characteristic of the Drug	*Oral*	*Aerosol*
HPA suppression	yes	no
Cushing's	yes	no
steroid dependence	high risk	low risk
local therapeutic effects	no	yes
risk to growth development in children	yes	no
ease of use	yes	no
cost	inexpensive	expensive
local airway reaction	no	yes

Inhaled Corticosteroids

[handwritten: poorly absorbed in bloodstream; stay on the airway]

The aerosol corticosteroids are chemically altered to minimize systemic toxicity and are available in metered dose inhalers (MDIs). Some aerosol steroids, such as triamcinolone, are poorly absorbed, and aerosols such as beclomethasone are inactivated quickly once absorbed. Inhalational or topical corticosteroids have advantages over oral or parenteral administration in terms of lessened systemic adverse effects. Topical side effects from aerosol administration include oropharyngeal fungal infections, with the most common being thrush (*Candida* yeast infection). Some patients may have changes in their voices and/or hoarseness from inhaled steroids. However, the minimization of systemic side effects via the inhalational route makes it ideal for treating airway inflammation (see Table 7-6, which provides a summary of advantages of aerosol and oral routes).

There is little advantage of one aerosol steroid over another when they are used in similar doses. Doses are usually classified as low, medium, or high (see Table 7-7 for comparative adult inhaled corticosteroid doses). Most inhaled steroids can be given twice daily. Doses should be adjusted to provide control with minimal side effects. Inhaled steroids have a different time course of response than oral steroids. Inhaled steroids produce symptom improvement in the first 1 to 2 weeks of therapy, with maximum improvement in 4 to 8 weeks. FEV$_1$ and PEFs may take 3 to 6 weeks for maximum improvement. The BHR improvement can take 1 to 3 months and continue over 1 year.

CLINICAL PEARL

Thrush (candidiasis) is treatable with liquid antifungal antibiotics that are swished in the mouth and swallowed. Using a spacer to reduce oropharyngeal deposition and rinsing the mouth with water or a mouthwash after taking the steroid MDI minimizes the occurrence of opportunistic fungal infections.

Table 7-7 Comparative Adult Inhaled Daily Corticosteroid Doses

Drug	*Low Dose*	*Medium Dose*	*High Dose*
beclomethasone dipropionate (Beclovent)	168–504 μg (4–12 puffs of 42 μg) (2–6 puffs of 84 μg)	504–840 μg (12–20 puffs of 42 μg) (6–10 puffs of 84 μg)	840 μg (>20 puffs of 42 μg) (>10 puffs of 84 μg)
budesonide turbuhaler (Pulmicort)	200–400 μg (1–2 inhalations)	400–600 μg (2–3 inhalations)	>600 μg (>3 inhalations)
flunisolide (Aerobid)	500–1000 μg (2–4 puffs)	1000–2000 μg (4–8 puffs)	>2000 μg (>8 puffs)
fluticasone (Flovent)	88–264 μg (2–6 puffs of 44 μg) or (2 puffs of 110 μg) (2–6 inhalations of 50 μg)	264–660 μg (2–6 puffs of 110 μg) (3–6 inhalations of 100 μg)	>660 μg (>6 puffs of 110 μg) or (>3 puffs of 220 μg) (>6 inhalations of 100 μg)
triamcinolone acetonide (Azmacort)	400–1000 μg (4–10 puffs)	1000–2000 μg (10–20 puffs)	>2000 μg (>20 puffs)

Table 7-8   Benefits of Daily Use of
Inhaled Corticosteroids

Benefit
fewer symptoms
fewer severe exacerbations
reduced use of quick-relief β_2 agents
reduction in airway remodeling
improved lung function
reduced airway inflammation

Benefits of Daily Corticosteroid Use

Corticosteroids are the most potent anti-inflammatory agents for asthma and are most effective inhalationally for long-term control of persistent asthma. They not only effect improvement in bronchial hyperresponsiveness over time but also prevent and reverse airway remodeling. This has led to thoughts that the drugs may improve long-term outcomes from asthma. Once corticosteroids are discontinued, however, the lung function returns to pretreatment values over a month or two. Because less drug is usually better in the long run, studies have looked at and determined that step-down dosing from oral corticosteroids to inhaled cortiscosteroids can be effective. There are many benefits of daily inhaled use. Table 7-8 lists these benefits.

STOP
& REVIEW

Do you start early or wait until later to administer corticosteroids? How do you decide what route to use? If using an inhaled bronchodilator in conjunction with an inhaled steroid, which do you give first and why?

www.prenhall.com/colbert

Get connected to the Web for a review of Cushing's syndrome, a condition that stimulates adrenal cortex hypersecretion. This is the same effect as could occur with long-term systemic steroid use.

Steroid Dependency

Steroid dependency can be classified into two forms. One is related to psychologic desire for the drug, and the other is related to physiologic steroid suppression of the normal functions of the hypothalamic pituitary adrenal axis (HPA). Psychologic dependence can occur because of the sense of well-being induced by these drugs as well as the effective symptom relief provided by them.

Withdrawing patients from steroids quickly can lead to physiologic adrenal insufficiency symptoms from HPA suppression. Steroid withdrawal syndrome consists of anorexia, nausea, vomiting, lethargy, headache, and hypotension. Ways to avoid steroid dependence include alternate-day steroid administration and aerosol use.

ANTIASTHMATICS

[handwritten: Intal   Tilade]

[handwritten margin notes: Mast cell stabilizer (horizontal striation); Cromolyn 4–6 wks to be effective]

℞ cromolyn and nedocromil sodium

Whereas corticosteroids are effective in treating an already established inflammatory process, mast-cell membrane stabilizers can impair or prevent the inflammatory process from ever beginning by preventing rupture of mast cells. Cromolyn (Intal) and nedocromil (Tilade), a chemical derivative with similar pharmacology, are similar drugs whose main difference is potency. For this reason, we will talk about the two drugs concurrently. They are used for allergic and nonallergic asthma and also for prevention of allergic rhinitis and exercise-induced bronchospasm (EIB).

Cromolyn is not a bronchodilator or inhibitor of action of the chemical mediators already released. Cromolyn's effect is prophylactic, and the drug must be used as a pretreatment. It is theorized that calcium influx into the mast cell is needed for microfilament contraction that will then expel the contents of (degranulate) the mast cell. Cromolyn works to inhibit calcium influx into the mast cell, and this prevents release of inflammatory mediators. This is why the drug is called a mast-cell stabilizer or mediator release inhibitor (MRI). By inhibiting release of inflammatory mediators, it blunts early- and late-phase asthmatic reactions to antigens, and it inhibits mast cell degranulation produced by immunologic and nonimmunologic mechanisms.

These drugs inhibit immediate early asthmatic reaction (EAR) to allergic challenge and EIB. Even though the following effects have not been associated with mast-cell mediator release, cromolyn has been shown to inhibit bronchoconstriction produced by inhalation of cold air, and ultrasonically nebulized water. These drugs also inhibit late asthmatic reactions (LAR) and prevent subsequent bronchial hyperresponsiveness (BHR). Long-term treatment can prevent the rise in BHR that is associated in some patients with pollen seasons.

CLINICAL PEARL

Cromolyn is not a bronchodilator and must not be used for acute reversal of bronchospasm. It must be used regularly for maximum effectiveness, even during symptom-free times.

CLINICAL PEARL

The drug ketotifen (Zaditen) is being investigated; it exhibits the same pharmacological activities as cromolyn. Its advantage is that it can be administered orally, yet its onset of activity still takes 4 to 6 weeks. Side effects include sedation and drowsiness. Overdosage include abdominal pain, confusion, bradycardia, hyperexcitability, tachycardia, tachypnea, and cyanosis.

Dosage Forms

Cromolyn and nedocromil are poorly absorbed from the GI tract, so they only work when deposited directly into the airways by aerosol administration and are not effective in oral forms. Cromolyn is available as a nebulized solution or as a microfine powder via a DPI device. Response and duration are both dose related. Cromolyn nebulized solution is compatible with β-agonist solutions, so they can be administered together. Nedocromil is only available as an MDI, and the prophylactic effect can take from 4 to 6 weeks to improve symptoms. The only way to know if the drug will work is to try it for 4 to 6 weeks and check the response. A positive response would be less frequency and/or severity of asthmatic episodes. Cromolyn may be an alternative for children who have side effects with theophylline.

Side Effects

Nedocromil and cromolyn are nontoxic drugs with no predeliction for tolerance. Following inhalation, cough and wheeze have been reported as well as bad taste and headache. Significant adverse side effects occur in less than 1 in 10,000 patients.

PROSTAGLANDINS

Physiology

Prostaglandins are present in almost all tissues, including the lungs. Prostaglandins are yet another group of chemical mediators that modulate airway function and pulmonary hemodynamics. Anything that promotes release of prostaglandins in the lung can alter ventilation perfusion disturbances. Some examples of these factors are presented in Table 7-9.

Some drugs inhibit prostaglandin synthesis in the body. These are commonly known as non-steroidal anti-inflammatory agents and include common medications such as ibuprofen, aspirin, and naproxen, which will be mentioned in the discussion of pain medications. Their inhibitory effect has been related to the induction of bronchospasm when used in some patients with asthma. It may be that aspirin-sensitive asthmatics differ from nonsensitive asthmatics by having a different reliance on the PGE mechanism than the β system to regulate airway tone.

Table 7-9 Factors That Affect Prostaglandin Release in the Lung

Factor
pulmonary embolism
lung edema
hypoxia
bradykinin
histamine
antigen–antibody reaction

Prostaglandins are classified on the basis of their chemical structure and categorized alphabetically. They are synthesized upon stimuli and released, not stored, once they are made. In addition, they have a very short half-life (minutes). The type of prostaglandin that dominates depends on the tissue location. In the lung, $PGF_2\alpha$ is the most common prostaglandin, and when stimulated and produced, it causes bronchoconstriction and increased mucus production.

PGE_1 and PGE_2 are also considered important in airway muscle tone and can cause bronchodilation. Prostaglandins are mentioned here because they may have future applications for therapy. Table 7-10 lists pulmonary effects of prostaglandins $PGF_2\alpha$ and PGE_1 and PGE_2 in the lung.

Table 7-10 Effects of Prostaglandins in Lung

	Airway	*Blood Vessels*
PGF_{2^a}	bronchoconstriction increased mucus secretion	contraction increased vascular resistance
PGE_1	bronchodilation	relaxation decreased resistance
PGE_2	bronchodilation	contraction increased resistance

LEUKOTRIENE MODIFIERS

Physiology

Leukotriene modifiers are the most recent group of medications to be available for asthma treatment and inhibit the leukotriene mediator cascade that leads to airway inflammation. Leukotrienes are potent mediators of inflammation involved in the pathogenesis of asthma. Leukotrienes are derived from arachidonic acid by the 5-lipoxygenase pathway. This pathway forms leukotrienes that cause contraction of airway smooth muscle, vasodilation, increased vascular permeability, increased mucus secretion, and decreased mucociliary clearance when they activate receptors. Three agents available are **zileuton** (Zyflo), **zafir-lukast** (Accolate), and **montelukast** (Singulair). Zafirlukast and montelukast are leukotriene antagonists. Zileuton is a 5-lipoxygenase inhibitor. They all work by preventing harmful effects of leukotrienes.

At this time, these drugs are considered alternatives to low-dose inhaled steroids, cromolyn, or nedocromil in patients with mild to persistent asthma; they are used for long-term control, not acute treatment. They are a logical drug choice on the basis of the role of leukotrienes in inflammation as previously discussed.

Zileuton's most significant effects are in the treatment of aspirin–sensitive asthma. It blocks decreased airway function and nasal, GI, and skin symptoms associated with aspirin sensitivity in asthmatics. This drug can cause elevated liver function in tests. Other side effects include headache, dyspepsia, and myalgia. Zileuton should not be used by pregnant women.

Zafirlukast is effective for allergen-induced asthma and early and late allergen responses. For best effects, the drug should be taken on an empty stomach. Theophylline or the antibiotic erythromycin decreases zafirlukast levels. Aspirin may increase zafirlukast levels. Drug interactions should be closely watched for with this drug. Side effects of zafirlukast include pharyngitis, headache, rhinitis, and gastritis. It may also decrease liver function.

Montelukast is the only leukotriene modifier the FDA has indicated for children 6 to 14 as well as 2 to 5 years old. Research results have shown that montelukast can decrease the number of puffs of β-agonists daily in children and increase the morning forced expiratory volume (FEV_1). It has also been shown to increase FEV_1 in adults. When used in combination with inhalational corticosteroids, montelukast decreases the dose of inhaled steroid needed. Side effects include fatigue, fever, nasal congestion, cough, dizziness, and rash.

TREATING UPPER AIRWAY CONGESTION

Any process that causes upper airway congestion will logically make it more difficult to breathe and therefore increase the work of breathing. In someone without lung disease, the increased work of breathing may be barely noticeable. However, in patients with lung disease, it may be overwhelming and contribute to overall decreased alveolar ventilation. Therefore, treatment of the common "head cold" is no trivial matter.

Allergic Rhinitis

Allergic rhinitis (runny nose) can be seasonal or perennial. It is characterized by an immunologic response that causes symptoms such as sneezing, rhinorrhea, nasal congestion, and pruritus. In addition to increasing the work of breathing, any upper airway congestion will increase airway resistance and the likelihood of the spread of infections. Because allergic rhinitis involves the degranulation of mast cells in the nasal passageways, one logical treatment would be to stabilize the mast cells.

Intranasal Medications

Intranasal mast cell stabilizers are used for allergic rhinitis and are administered before the onset of pollen season. Cromolyn is available intranasally (**Nasalcrom**) without a prescription and is effective for sneezing, rhinorrhea, and itching but not for preexisting nasal congestion. It must be given 3 to 4 times a day, and it takes 2 to 4 weeks to see full benefits.

Intranasal corticosteroids are also available. Intranasal corticosteroids inhibit cytokine release from nasal epithelial cells and inhibit leukotriene production. Intranasal corticosteroids also are beneficial in decreasing nasal congestion by decreasing function of mediators that affect vascular permeability. See Table 7-11 for common intranasal corticosteroids.

Intranasal corticosteroids can take 2 to 4 weeks to work, with 8 weeks an adequate treatment trial for efficacy. Maximum effects can take up to 6 months. Products differ in their side effects, not their efficacy, and include burning, stinging, irritation, and dry nose.

Antihistamine

Histamine is stored in tissue mast cells. In the lung, mast cells are located below the respiratory tract mucosa in connective tissue. Scientific efforts have been made to identify factors that cause release of histamine from mast cell storage sites. These efforts have told us

℞

CLINICAL PEARL

Intranasal cromolyn may be beneficial when visiting a friend with a cat or on other occasions of one-time exposure to a known allergen if used 15 to 30 minutes before exposure.

CLINICAL PEARL

Eye symptoms such as itching can also be a problem in allergic rhinitis. Ophthalmic corticosteroids or antihistamines are available for this indication.

Table 7-11   Intranasal Corticosteroids

R

Generic	Brand
beclomethasone dipropionate	Vancenase
	Beconase
budesonide	Rhinocort
flunisolide	Nasalide
fluticasone propionate	Flonase
triamcinolone	Nasacort
mometasone furoate	Nasonex

CLINICAL PEARL

Even drugs can cause histamine release. The itching frequently associated with narcotics such as morphine is due to histamine release, although it doesn't necessarily imply that the patient is allergic to the drug. The effects on histamine release by neuromuscular blocking drugs is one factor that influences the decision to use one drug over another.

CLINICAL PEARL

Histamine 2 receptors mediate actions of histamine on gastric secretion. Antagonists of this histamine are called H_2 blockers, not antihistamines, and drugs such as cimetidine (Tagamet) are H_2 blockers, not antihistamines.

CLINICAL PEARL

A histamine provocation test or challenge is based on this airway hyperactivity. This test can give information on an individual's response to therapeutic drugs as well as diagnostic information.

that the autonomic nervous system is involved through β, α, and cholinergic receptor sites on mast cells. Histamine production is influenced by nonspecific stimuli to tissue such as chemical stimuli, physical injury, or allergy. Cigarette smoke and dust are examples of substances that can cause histamine release (see Table 7-12 for more examples).

Histamine acts on two different receptors called histamine 1 and histamine 2. Histamine smooth muscle contraction is controlled by histamine 1 receptors. These receptors are activated by subepithelial irritant receptors, with a resultant increase in vagal activity. Drugs that antagonize histamine 1 receptors are called antihistamines.

Histamine release provokes airway obstruction. Airway obstruction can be due to mucosal edema and inflammatory cell infiltration with eosinophils. This can be influenced by release of local mediators. See Table for 7-13 for the pulmonary and systemic effects of histamine.

The mechanisms involved in the release of histamine and other mediators during allergic response are complex and consist of many steps. The antigen–antibody interaction triggers many of the steps. Therapy for histamine release has been directed toward prevention or inhibition of mediator release from storage sites and antagonism of airway response to mediators.

Drugs used to prevent the release of histamine from mast cells include β-agonists, methylxanthines, and cholinergic blockers, as discussed in Chapter 5. In addition, cromolyn and corticosteroids have a role in blocking histamine production, as discussed earlier in this chapter. Antihistamines block the action of histamine at histamine 1 receptors. They do not prevent or block the release of histamine at histamine receptors in the GI system. They are not useful in acute asthma treatment, since so many other mediators are released in acute asthma episodes as well. Antihistamines are basically used for allergic rhinitis. Antihistamines prevent the onset of symptoms better than they reverse symptoms already present.

Table 7-12   Factors That Influence Mediator Release from Mast Cells

Factor
antigen–antibody IgE reactions
mechanical tissue trauma
tissue hypoxia
drugs
dust
cigarette smoke

Table 7-13 Pulmonary and Systemic Effects of Histamine

Pulmonary	*Systemic*
increased airway resistance	vasodilation
decreased maximum expiratory flow rate	stimulates adenyl cyclase in mast cells
decreased diffusion capacity	release catecholamines from adrenal medulla
increased total lung capacity	increased vascular permeability
increased mucus production	
promote mucosal edema	

For predictable seasonal allergies, when would be the best time to start taking an antihistamine?

Side effects of antihistamines include dry mouth and throat, altered coordination, and sedation. Driving or the operation of dangerous machinery shouldn't occur under the influence of antihistamines, or anything else for that matter. Some patients experience excitation rather than the expected sedation. Antihistamines can induce their own metabolism, which may present as what appears to be tolerance to the drug with chronic use.

Like cephalosporin antibiotics, there are first- and second-generation antihistamines. First-generation antihistamines are sedating, and second-generation are less so. Second-generation antihistamines have antiallergic and anti-inflammatory effects. Improvement in symptoms with first-generation antihistamines occurs within 1 to 2 hours of the first dose, but maximum effects aren't seen for weeks.

Tolerance may develop in 2 to 3 weeks to the sedation effects. Decongestants are sometimes added to antihistamines for their stimulating effect to counteract sedation from antihistamines; see Table 7-14 for common antihistamines.

Decongestants

Nasal decongestants are α-adrenergic drugs with corresponding vasoconstrictive properties. It is the vasoconstriction that reduces the blood flow and therefore the swelling of the nasal passages in the inflammatory process. **Pseudoephedrine** (Sudafed) is used orally to treat nasal congestion. It should be used cautiously in patients with diabetes, heart disease, hyperthyroidism, or glaucoma. Owing to the vasoconstictive properties, blood pressure

CLINICAL PEARL
First-generation antihistamines are very effective at symptom relief. However, only about 30% of patients are satisfied with treatment, because of side effects.

CLINICAL PEARL
Regulations prevent some competitive athletes from taking oral stimulants such as decongestants. The OTC decongestant phenylpropanolamine is currently being phased out of the market because of its side effects.

Table 7-14 Common Antihistamines

First Generation	*Brand Name*
chlorpheniramine	Chlor-Trimeton
diphenhydramine	Benadryl
brompheniramine	Dimetane
Second Generation	
loratidine	Claritin
cetirizine	Zyrtec
fexofenadine	Allegra

should also be monitored. Topical decongestants such as nasal sprays can be used, but not too frequently, or rebound nasal congestion occurs. Topical decongestants are helpful for increasing absorption of intranasal corticosteroids.

SUMMARY

There are a variety of inflammatory pathways and mediators of inflammation. Anti-inflammatory drugs target these pathways to reduce the inflammatory response that leads to hyperactive airways, mucosal edema, and increased mucus production. Corticosteroids are one of the mainstays among anti-inflammatory drugs. They vary in pharmacology and cardiorespiratory therapeutic applications. They have very important physiological effects that must be balanced with their adverse effects. One method of achieving this balance is through careful attention to route of administration and dose and duration of use.

Antiasthmatic agents are used prophylactically to prevent the occurrence of the in-flammatory response; their role is different than corticosteroids. Antiasthmatics include leukotriene modifiers and mast-cell stabilizers.

Drugs that treat upper respiratory congestion are frequently used in combination with antiasthmatic and anti-inflammatory agents.

REVIEW QUESTIONS

1. The most common antibody involved in allergic asthma and rhinitis is:
   (a) IgG
   (b) IgE
   (c) IgF
   (d) IgT
   (e) IgB
2. Corticosteroids can be classified as:
   (a) mineralcorticoid
   (b) glucocorticoid
   (c) potassium sparing
   (d) glucose sparing
   (e) (a) and (b)
3. Routes used for corticosteroids include:
   (a) inhalational
   (b) oral
   (c) intranasal
   (d) parenteral
   (e) all of the above
4. Check which indication would be appropriate for the following drugs:
   prednisone   ___ acute asthma treatment
      ___ chronic asthma treatment

   cromolyn   ___ acute asthma treatment
      ___ chronic asthma treatment

   zileuton   ___ acute asthma treatment
      ___ chronic asthma treatment

5. Check which effect relates to each drug most closely.
   β-agonists   ___ block histamine release
      ___ block histamine production

   cromolyn   ___ block histamine release
      ___ block histamine production

   corticosteroids   ___ block histamine release
      ___ block histamine production

6. Describe the early and late phases of in-flammation and why they are important to pharmacotherapy.

7. Explain the role of the hypothalamic pituitary adrenal axis in terms the patient can understand.

8. List some factors that can influence mediator release from mast cells.

9. What are the important side effects of antihistamines?

10. A 57-year-old asthmatic presents with complaints of voice changes, hoarseness, white spots on throat and tongue, and a "funny taste in his mouth." What type of medication and route do you suspect may be causing these complaints? What would the proposed treatment and follow-up education consist of?

11. A patient with a history of severe late-phase asthma response is prescribed an inhaled short-acting bronchodilator, corticosteroid, and mast-cell stabilizer. Explain in lay terms when each of these drugs is indicated and highlight any special considerations concerning sequence, side effects, and what to expect as positive outcomes.

GLOSSARY

prostaglandin one of many hormone-like substances present throughout the body.

leukotriene group of biologically active compounds that regulate allergic and inflammatory reactions.

glucocorticoid one of two main groups of corticosteroids needed for stress response and utilization of carbohydrates, fat, and protein by the body.

corticosteroid any steroid hormone produced by the adrenal cortex.

mineralcorticoid one of two main groups of corticosteroids necessary for regulation of salt and water balance.

histamine vasodilator that mediates inflammation and allergic reactions.

antigen foreign material that stimulates the immune and inflammatory response.

chemical mediators initiators of the inflammatory process that are released in response to a stimulus.

www.prenhall.com/colbert

Use the address above to access the free, interactive Companion Web site created specifically for this textbook. Enhance your studying by viewing videos and animations, answering practice quiz questions, and reviewing an audio glossary and much more related to Chapter 7.

CHAPTER 8

Anti-Infective Agents

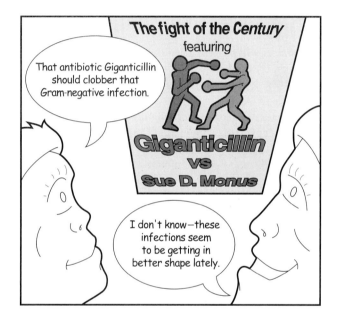

OBJECTIVES

Upon completion of this chapter you will be able to

- Understand the differentiation between Gram-positive and Gram-negative bacteria
- Discuss implications of antimicrobial sensitivies and resistance patterns
- Understand basic concepts of anti-infective therapy
- Identify the basic classifications of antibiotic, antiviral, antitubercular, and antifungal drugs
- Describe the role of aerosol anti-infective agents that may be administered directly into the lungs

ABBREVIATIONS

AIDS	acquired immunodeficiency syndrome	HIV	human immunodeficiency virus
ARDS	acute respiratory distress syndrome	MBC	minimum bactericidal concentration
CMV	cytomegalovirus	MIC	minimal inhibitory concentration

Main contributing author Catherine Hitt

MRSA	methicillin-resistant *Staphylo-coccus aureus*	PBP	penicillin-binding protein
PCP	*pneumocystis carinii* pneumonia	TB	tuberculosis
		WBC	white blood cell, or leukocyte

INTRODUCTION

With the discovery of penicillin in the 1940s, the antibiotic era began. Antibiotic availability and widespread use have been both a tremendous benefit and a burden to medical care. The beneficial effects are clear in the number of lives that have been spared from bacterial, viral, and fungal infections. The burden has presented itself with a vengeance in the last several decades with the evolution of pathogens that are able to resist the effects of many antibiotic agents.

This chapter will provide a general overview of the principles of antibacterial, antiviral, and antifungal chemotherapy. While this is a pharmacotherapy textbook, it is still important to review basic microbiological principles and apply them to drug therapy, so they will be reviewed here. Although protozoa and algae are also microorganisms, the limited contact health professionals have with them will limit their discussion in this chapter. In Chapter 14, we will look at the "big picture" and discuss the applications of anti-infective agents for particular respiratory indications such as pneumonias, tuberculosis, cystic fibrosis, bronchitis, COPD, and human immunodeficiency virus (HIV).

www.prenhall.com/colbert

In few other specialties do therapeutic approaches change as rapidly as in the case of anti-infective agents. Not only are new drugs marketed, but time-honored drugs lose their efficacy with repeated use and development of resistance among pathogens, as will be discussed later. After reading this chapter, look at the Web site for the most up-to-date list of anti-infective agents available, which is sure to be more updated than any textbook can be.

GENERAL PRINCIPLES OF ANTI-INFECTIVE THERAPY

Terminology

Chemotherapy is the application of a chemical agent that has specific toxic effects upon disease-producing organisms within a living animal. A chemotherapeutic substance derived from a living organism that kills microorganism growth is an **antibiotic.** Antibiotic is a general term derived from the Greek roots *anti-* (against) and *bios* (life). The term "antibiotic" was meant to distinguish between chemical therapeutic agents and those that come from living organisms such as penicillin. Nowadays, drugs are made mainly in the lab, and the terms are used interchangeably. Traditionally, antibiotics have referred to drugs for treating bacterial infections.

The Infectious Process

Before you make a decision about infectious pharmacological therapy, it's naturally important to make sure an infection is present. Signs and symptoms of an infectious process in the respiratory system can include subjective complaints of dyspnea, malaise, weakness, pain, and fatigue. Objective findings of fever, hypoxemia, elevated white blood cell (WBC) count, X-ray changes, and a dry or productive cough may also be present.

Once you have established the presence of an infectious process, you must now determine where it is located. Is it a respiratory or urinary tract infection? Is it a localized or systemic infection? Infections can be localized to a certain area such as the lungs or may become systemic and spread via the bloodstream throughout the body. Systemic infections cause hemodynamic, hematological, neurological, cellular, and of course respiratory changes. For this discussion, we are most interested in respiratory changes. These may include respiratory acidosis, tachypnea, hypoxemia, and even acute respiratory distress syndrome (ARDS). Systemic infections tend to require more aggressive treatment than local infections.

Empiric Therapy

Pathogens are disease-causing microorganisms. What complicates the picture is that a microorganism may be present and not pathogenic in one individual but pathogenic in another. Likewise, an organism in an individual may not normally be pathogenic, but changes in the person's immune system can make the same microorganism become a pathogen. Certain pathogens tend to be associated with certain sites of infection. See Table 8-1 for a list of pathogens common in respiratory infections. This knowledge can allow therapy to be **empiric.** Empiric implies that antibiotic therapy would be initiated on the basis of available data about the most likely cause of an infection in a given location (blood, skin, lungs, etc.).

The organism responsible for an infection may be a part of the patient's normal **flora.** The term implies that organisms share a symbiotic relationship with the host. When something is altered to change the symbiotic relationship, the organisms may flourish and become pathogenic. For example, fungal overgrowth may result secondary to antimicrobial use (e.g., a vaginal yeast infection during or following a course of antimicrobial therapy for sinusitis), or secondary bacterial infection may result from a primary viral infection (e.g., streptococcal pneumonia that develops following a primary infection with influenza). See Table 8-2 for a list of common flora found in a sputum sample.

What symptoms might lead you to suspect a pulmonary infection?

Table 8-1 Suspected Respiratory Infection Pathogens

Infection	*Suspected Pathogen*
pharyngitis	group A *Streptococcus*
bronchitis	*Haemophilus influenzae*
acute sinusitis	*Streptococcus pneumoniae*
chronic sinusitis	anaerobes, *Staphylococcus aureus*
pneumonia	
community-acquired	*Streptococcus pneumoniae*
	Haemophilus influenzae
hospital-acquired	anaerobes
	Gram-negative aerobic rods
otitis media	*Streptococcus pneumoniae*
epiglottitis	*Haemophilus influenzae*
croup	*Staphylococcus aureus*

Table 8-2   Common Normal Flora in Sputum Sample

Gram-Positive Cocci	Gram-Negative Bacilli	Gram-Negative Cocci
α-hemolytic *Streptococci* *Pneumococci* *Staphylococcus epidermidis*	*Haemophilus influenzae*	*Neisseria catarrhalis*

Bacteria Classification

To understand bacterial pathogens, it's important to understand basic bacteria classification. One of the broadest classes is based on bacteria's need for oxygen. If a bacterium needs oxygen to survive it is **aerobic.** If it does not it is called **anaerobic.** Fewer antibiotic options are available to treat anaerobic infections, and those infections can be more serious. Before you can determine which antibiotic should be used against a certain strain of bacteria, you must have a sample of the infected area tested in the laboratory, where it can be viewed under a microscope, allowing the bacteria to be further classified by the characteristic shape and staining properties. When you look under the microscope, bacteria can be round or rod shaped and exhibit certain individual shapes that act like fingerprints to help you identify bacterial type. See Figure 8-1 for the various types of bacteria according to shape.

Identification of Pathogenic Organisms

In clinical settings, the physician may elect to collect samples of secretions or fluids from the suspected site of infection for microbiological evaluation to identify the pathogen. Laboratory technicians then perform tests on these samples such as the **Gram stain** and **susceptibility testing** (petri disk and broth dilution) that can be used to guide treatment.

Gram Stain. The first test usually performed to classify bacteria is a Gram stain. Depending on their chemical makeup, microorganisms react differently when stained with colored dyes in a lab. Gram-positive bacteria stain purple, and Gram-negative stain pink upon completion of the Gram stain procedure.

The Gram stain determines the basic characteristics of the pathogen (e.g., bacterial or not, shape, Gram-positive, or Gram-negative). On the basis of this reaction, microorganisms are classified into broad categories as Gram-positive (sometimes shown as Gram (+)) or Gram-negative (Gram (−)). See Table 8-3 for representative Gram-positive and Gram-negative bacteria.

The Gram stain allows differentiation between bacterial cell types on the basis of chemical differences in their cell walls. Gram-positive cell walls are composed of a uniform

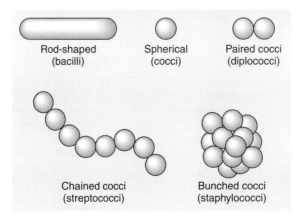

Rod-shaped (bacilli)

Spherical (cocci)

Paired cocci (diplococci)

Chained cocci (streptococci)

Bunched cocci (staphylococci)

Figure 8-1 Bacteria Morphology

Table 8-3 Representative Gram-Positive and Gram-Negative Bacteria

Gram-Negative Bacteria	Gram-Positive Bacteria
Pseudomonas	Clostridia
Bacteroides	Listeria
Campylobacter	Streptococci
Haemophilus	Staphylococci
Klebsiella	
Legionella	
Mycoplasma	

LEARNING HINT

Gram-negative infections, as a general rule, are harder to treat than Gram-positive infections. The cell wall is what maintains the integrity and therefore the life of the cell. Looking at Figure 8-2, you can see that the more layered Gram-negative wall may be tougher to destroy.

monolayer of peptidoglycans, while Gram-negative are composed of multiple layers, including an outer lipopolysaccharide/lipoprotein membrane and an inner peptidoglycan layer. In all bacteria, the cell wall functions to maintain the integrity of the cell, allowing for growth in different environments. It also serves as the target and mechanism of action for several classes of antibacterial agents (e.g., beta-lactams and glycopeptides). By knowing about the kind of cell wall, you are one step closer to customizing antibiotic treatment against the type of bacteria and type of infection. See Figure 8-2 for the differences between Gram-positive and Gram-negative cell walls.

Susceptibility Testing Methods. After an organism is identified, its susceptibility characteristics may be determined in order to guide antimicrobial therapy. If a microorganism is susceptible to an antibiotic, the antibiotic has a better chance of fighting the infection than if it is not susceptible. There are several methods by which microbial susceptibility may be determined. We will review disk diffusion and broth dilution methods.

Disk diffusion is a classic laboratory technique that provides qualitative information about susceptibility. The bacteria are cultured and grown on solid media (e.g., in a petri

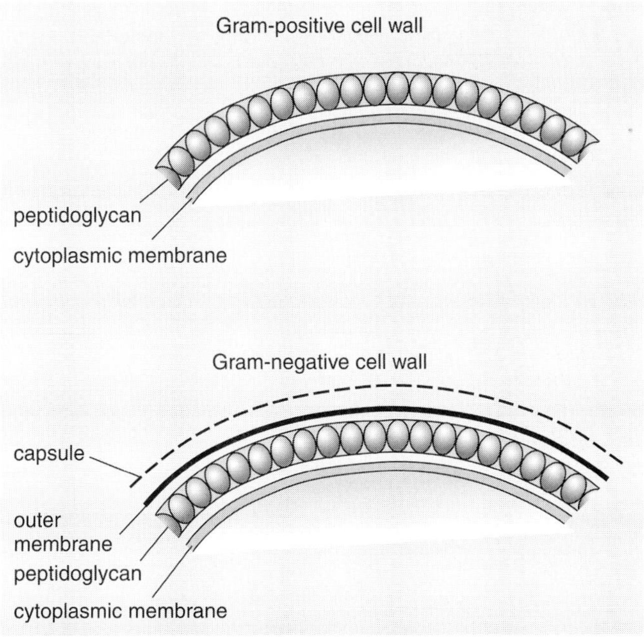

Figure 8-2 Bacterial Cell Walls

dish). Antibiotic-containing paper disks are then placed on the "lawn" of bacteria. After incubation, the areas without bacterial growth, known as the "zone of inhibition," are measured and compared with established standards to determine whether it is sensitive (the antibiotic will work), intermediate (the antibiotic may or may not work), or resistant (the antibiotic will not work). See Figure 8-3.

Broth Dilution. Broth dilution is a second, commonly used clinical method for determining bacterial sensitivity to an antimicrobial agent. This type of testing is more quantitative than the disk diffusion method; that is, it can more accurately identify the concentration of a drug needed to inhibit organism growth. The organism is placed in various test tubes containing defined concentrations of an antimicrobial agent and a liquid growth medium (see Figure 8-4). The test tubes are incubated for a designated amount of time and visually inspected for organism growth. The test tube with the lowest concentration of antimicrobial agent that inhibits the growth of the organism is referred to as the minimal inhibitory concentration, or MIC (tube #4 in Figure 8-4). The MIC does not provide information whether the organism is actually killed. The minimum bactericidal concentration or MBC determines this information. MBC determines its killing activity associated with an antimicrobial. The MBC is determined by taking a sample from each clear MIC tube and culturing it on agar plates. The concentration in which no significant bacterial growth is observed is the MBC.

The concentrations of the antimicrobial agent used in this method usually start several-fold higher than those concentrations that can safely be reached in the patient and are then serially diluted. If the MIC is identified at a concentration that cannot be achieved in the patient, then the organism is considered resistant. If the MIC is identified at a clinically achievable level, the organism is considered sensitive. If the MIC is identified at a level that may or may not be clinically achievable, the organism is considered intermediate.

CLINICAL PEARL

It's best to collect the sample of material from the infected area before an antibiotic is started, or you may not be able to grow and identify the pathogen. In patient care situations, antibiotics are often started before the results of that laboratory test are available. For serious infections, it's important to start an antibiotic as soon as possible and to adjust the drug or dose once a more precise diagnosis is available.

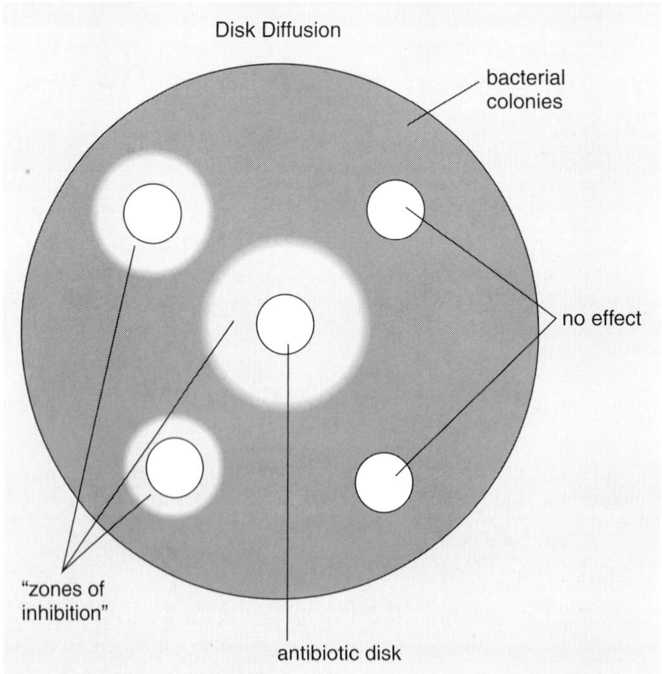

Figure 8-3 Disk Diffusion

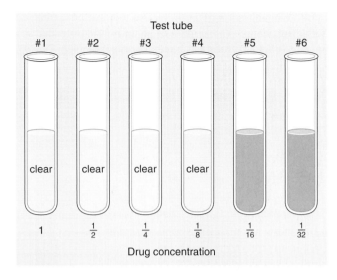

Figure 8-4 Broth Dilution

Mechanisms of Resistance

The development of so-called "super-bacteria" has been facilitated by the widespread misuse of antibacterial agents for infections of viral origin (e.g., common colds, influenza) and the continued use of broad-spectrum agents in the treatment of infections caused by single organisms, in which case a narrow-spectrum agent would do. Use of antibiotics effective against a wide range of microorganisms (**broad-spectrum** drug) can result in overkill if a drug effective against fewer microorganisms (**narrow-spectrum** drug) would be just as effective. Such use has resulted in selective evolution of bacteria that have adapted to become **resistant** to certain antibiotics, leaving physicians with limited options for the management of some infections. Viruses and fungi are also able to evolve into "super-pathogens" when exposed to antifungals and antivirals.

CLINICAL PEARL

Unlike Superman, these super-bacteria are not weakened by kryptonite.

Resistance to anti-infectives develops in many ways. One example is when the drug is destroyed by bacterial enzymes. Bacteria that produce the enzyme beta lactamase can make the antibiotics cephalosporins and penicillins inactive. Another method for resistance to occur is when some organisms develop enzymes that bind to the drug and prevent the drug from attaching to the binding site of the bacteria.

Resistance also develops when patients do not finish an anti-infective treatment. A rather common occurrence is patients who stop taking the drug once they begin to feel better. Think about this possible mechanism for resistance to occur. If you discontinue use of an antibiotic as soon as you feel better, the drug may have just destroyed enough of the weaker pathogens to give you symptomatic relief. However, there are still some minimal pathogenic bacteria remaining that haven't yet been killed and therefore represent a stronger strain. Now that the anti-infective has been prematurely discontinued, these stronger pathogens can multiply, and once they reach a certain level, the symptoms reappear. Now, however, when the drug is restarted it must contend with an overall stronger version of the pathogen.

STOP

& REVIEW

What would you tell a patient who says they quit taking their antibiotic after 2 days (prescribed for 7 days) because they now feel better?

Monitoring Anti-infective Therapy

Anti-infective treatment can be monitored by clinical or microbiological response. A clinical response would mean that the signs and symptoms of infection are gone as evidenced by declining WBC count and fever elimination. A microbiological response would mean the microorganism has been eliminated.

Following initiation of anti-infective therapy, it may be necessary to monitor drug levels for select agents. An example of an antibiotic class that is frequently monitored is the aminoglycosides. These agents have a narrow therapeutic index, meaning there is a fine line between therapeutic efficacy and toxicity.

What pulmonary signs and symptoms would you monitor to see if the antibiotic therapy is effective for a lung infection?

CLASSIFICATION OF ANTIBACTERIAL AGENTS

Bacteriostatic versus Bactericidal

There are many ways to classify antibacterials. The first way relates back to the lab test discussion. Antibacterial drugs are classified as either bacteriostatic or bactericidal. **Bacteriostatic** agents inhibit the replication of microorganisms and prevent the growth of the organisms without destroying them. **Bactericidal** drugs actively kill bacteria. Most antibiotics are bacteriostatic at low concentrations, but at higher concentrations, bactericidal activity is more likely to be present. See Table 8-4 for some common bacteriostatic and bactericidal drugs.

Broad versus Narrow

Antibacterials can also be classified according to whether they are broad spectrum or narrow spectrum. Broad-spectrum antibiotics are effective against a wider range of bacteria than are narrow-spectrum antibiotics. See Table 8-5 for an example of this classification system.

Based on Mechanism of Action

Just as there were multitudes of ways of classifying bacteria (aerobic/anaerobic, Gram-positive/negative), there are also multiple ways to classify antibacterial agents. One of the most commonly used antibacterial classifications is based on the mechanism of action of the anti-infective agent (see Table 8-6). While this seems most logical for pharmacology purposes, drugs are rarely selected clinically according to their mechanism of action.

Antibacterial Agents

For our discussions, we will give a brief description according to the following antibacterial drug classification: beta-lactams, quinolones, aminoglycosides, vancomycin, protein synthesis inhibitors, folate inhibitors, vancomycin, teicoplanin, metronidazole, dalfopristin/quinupristine, and oxazolidinones (see Table 8-7).

Beta Lactams

Beta-lactams include the following classes of drugs: penicillins, cephalosporins, monobactams (aztreonam), carbacephems (loracarbef), and penems (imipenem, meropenem). All beta-lactam antimicrobials act via inhibition of bacterial cell wall synthesis; to be effec-

Table 8-4   Antibacterial Classes

Bactericidal	*Bacteriostatic*
penicillins	erythromycin
cephalosporins	tetracyclines
vancomycin	

Table 8-5   Antimicrobial Spectrum Classification

Broad	*Narrow*
tetracyclines	penicillin
ampicillin	erythromycin
cephalosporins	vancomycin

Table 8-6   Anti-infective Classification Based on Mechanism of Action

Category	Mechanism of Action
I	inhibit the synthesis of the bacterial cell wall or activate enzymes that disrupt the bacterial cell wall (penicillins, cephalosporins, vancomycin, antifungals)
II	act directly on the cell membrane of the microorganism, causing leaking of the components of the cell (amphotericin B, nystatin)
III	inhibit protein synthesis by disrupting functions of the bacterial ribosomes (macrolides, tetracyclines)
IV	disrupt protein synthesis as well, but through a different process than category III (aminoglycosides)
V	alter the synthesis and metabolism of nucleic acid (rifampin, metronidazole, quinolones)
VI	inhibit metabolic processes fundamental to the microorganism (sulfonamides)
VII	inhibit viral replication by binding to viral enzymes needed to make DNA (acyclovir)

tively bactericidal, they require sensitive bacteria to be actively dividing. Their action is mediated through inhibition of enzymes that help build the bacteria's cell walls. These enzymes are generally referred to as penicillin-binding proteins (PBPs) and are located under the cell wall.

Bacteria have the ability to develop resistance to beta-lactam antimicrobials via a number of mechanisms. One such mechanism of resistance is the production of beta-lactamase (also known as penicillinase) enzymes, which destroy the beta-lactam ring, rendering the drug inactive. This is because an intact chemical beta lactam ring is necessary for the antibiotics' bactericidal activity.

Penicillins. The penicillins can be further subdivided into natural penicillins, penicillinase-resistant penicillins, aminopenicillins, extended-spectrum penicillins, and drugs combined with beta lactamase inhibitors. By changing the basic chemical structure, researchers have developed many penicillin derivatives. Combining a penicillin with a beta lactamase inhibitor may produce less resistance. Extended-spectrum penicillins are more active than natural penicillins and are more resistant to inactivation by Gram-negative bacteria. See Table 8-8 for commonly used penicillins.

Diarrhea is a main side effect of penicillins and most antibiotic classes. Otherwise penicillins have very little toxicity; however, 15% to 20% of people are allergic to this drug. The allergy can vary from an itchy, red, mild rash to wheezing and anaphylaxis.

Cephalosporins. Cephalosporins basically have the same mechanism of action as penicillins. They differ from penicillin in their antibacterial spectrum, resistance to beta lactamase, and pharmacokinetics. One of the advantages of some cephalosporins over penicillin is that they have a longer half-life, which allows for infrequent outpatient parenteral dosing for chronic infections. This keeps some patients from having to be hospitalized and allows them to be treated as outpatients.

CLINICAL PEARL

Penicillins are frequently used for prophylaxis to decrease the risk of infection in patients with conditions such as mechanical valves that may predispose them to infection. For example, some patients with a history of rheumatic heart disease take penicillin before a dental appointment to prevent a cardiac infection. That infection could occur as a result of bacteria being spread through the blood from the mouth to a vulnerable site such as the heart with dental manipulation.

Table 8-7   Antibacterial Classification

Beta lactams	Vancomycin
Aminoglycosides	Teicoplanin
Protein Synthesis Inhibitors	Dalfopristin/Quinupristin
Folate Inhibitors	Metronidazole
Quinolones	Oxazolidinones

Table 8-8 Commonly Used Penicillins

Type	Generic	Brand
natural penicillins	**penicillin G**	
	penicillin V	Veetids
aminopenicillins	**ampicillin**	Omnipen
	amoxicillin	Amoxil
penicillinase-resistant penicillins	**dicloxacillin**	Dynapen
	nafcillin	Unipen
extended spectrum penicillins	**piperacillin**	Pipracil
	ticarcillin	Ticar
drugs combined with beta lactamase inhibitors	**amoxicillin–clavulanate**	Augmentin
	ampicillin sulbactam	Unasyn
	piperacillin-tazobactam	Zosyn

The cephalosporins are generally divided into three or even four generations. Each generation is purported to be "better" than the last, or at least broader in coverage. First-generation cephalosporins are used for community-acquired infections in ambulatory patients and mild to moderate infections in hospitalized patients. Second-generation cephalosporins are used for otitis media in pediatrics and for respiratory and urinary tract infections in hospitalized patients. Third-generation cephalosporins are used in hospital-acquired infections. Because of their long half-life, they are also used for ambulatory patients. Fourth-generation cephalosporins are used for pneumonia, urinary tract infections, and skin infections. Cephalosporins have the same side effects as penicillins and are less toxic than many antibiotics. See Table 8-9 for some commonly used cephalosporins.

 Monobactams. **Aztreonam** (Azactam) is the only currently available antimicrobial in this new synthetic drug class. Aztreonam is available parenterally and has a wide spectrum of activity against Gram-negative organisms but little to none against Gram-positive or anaerobic microorganisms. An advantage of this drug is an unlikely cross-allergenicity with other beta lactams. Side effects include swelling at the injection site and nausea, vomiting, and diarrhea.

 Penems. There are currently two penems available for use in the United States, **imipenem** (Primaxin) and **meropenem** (Merrem). They are so similar in chemical class that they are frequently lumped together for discussion. They have the same pharmacological activity as other beta lactam antibiotics and are broad spectrum and active against many organisms that are resistant to penicillins, cephalosporins, and aminoglycosides. For this rea-

CLINICAL PEARL

A patient with a penicillin allergy has a 10% possibility of also being allergic to a cephalosporin antibiotic.

LEARNING HINT

As indicated in the class name, monobactams have one (mono-) beta lactam ring.

Table 8-9 Commonly Used Cephalosporins

Generation	Generic	Brand Name	Route
First	cephalexin	Keflex	po
	cefazolin	Ancef	IM, IV
Second	cefaclor	Ceclor	po
	cefoxitin	Mefoxin	IM, IV
	cefuroxime	Ceftin, Zinacef	po, IM, IV
Third	ceftriaxone	Rocephin	IM, IV
	ceftazidime	Fortaz	IM, IV
	cefoperazone	Cefobid	IM, IV
	cefixime	Suprax	po
Fourth	cefepime	Maxipime	IM, IV

℞

son, they are usually reserved for serious infections. Side effects include nausea, which may be related to the infusion rate, seizures, dizziness, and confusion.

Now that we have discussed the beta lactams in total, we can move on to another classification of antibacterials.

Quinolones

Quinolones are bactericidal. They block an enzyme responsible for DNA growth. Human cells do not have this enzyme, so the drug is specific for microorganisms. This drug class has been available for years as a quinolone selectively used for urinary tract infections caused by Gram-negative pathogens (**nalidixic acid** brand name NegGram).

There are many drug interactions with quinolones. These drugs should not be taken with antacids, since antacids may interfere with quinolone absorption. Quinolones may increase theophylline toxicity. Quinolones, like many antibiotics, are phototoxic, and patients should use sunscreen when taking them. Prolonged use of quinolones may cause **superinfection.** Superinfection is the appearance of a new infection with a different strain or species of microorganism during antibiotic treatment of a different infection. Usually the organism responsible for the superinfection is resistant to the antibiotic being given and is difficult to treat. Superinfections may appear 4 to 5 days after antibiotic initiation and require treatment with a different antibiotic and discontinuation of the current antibiotic. Superinfection can also occur with other anti-infective agents. Other quinolone side effects include nausea, dizziness, and an unpleasant taste.

Common fluoroquinolones include:

℞

- **ciprofloxacin** (Cipro)
- **levofloxacin** (Levoquin)

Aminoglycosides

Aminoglycosides are used in many serious infections for Gram-negative coverage. They are frequently used concurrently with another drug, such as ampicillin, to fight Gram-positive organisms. They are bactericidal and dosed on the basis of weight, renal function, and serum blood levels. Because they are ototoxic and nephrotoxic, they are not used for infections that could be treated with an alternative agent just as effectively. Aminoglycosides may increase muscle weakness because of a potential blockage of signals at the neuromuscular junction. Because of their systemic toxicity, they have applications for aerosol administration. Examples of aminoglycosides include:

℞

- **amikacin** (Amikin)
- **gentamicin** (Garamycin)
- **tobramycin** (Nebcin)

Vancomycin

℞

Vancomycin (Vancocin) is a bactericidal glycoprotein antibiotic. It binds to the cell walls of reproducing microorganisms and inhibits mucopeptide formation. The cell then becomes susceptible to lysis. Vancomycin is indicated for serious life-threatening infections caused by Gram-positive cocci. It is the most potent antibiotic available for infections caused by *Staphylococcus aureus* and *Streptococcus epidermidis.* It is frequently reserved for methicillin-resistant *Staphylococcus aureus* (MRSA). Hospitals closely monitor their vancomycin sensitivity patterns, since there are few alternatives should resistance become prevalent. Vancomycin can cause side effects with intravenous administration such as hypotension, nephrotoxicity, and ototoxicity. Rapid infusion can cause a histamine release and flushed skin, or what is called red neck syndrome (seriously). Vancomycin is monitored by serum drug levels.

Teicoplanin

Teicoplanin (Targocid) is a glycopeptide alternative to vancomycin currently unavailable in the United States. Resistance of enterococci to the glycopeptide vancomycin has made the search for an alternative drug such as teicoplanin important, which is why it deserves a brief mention.

Protein Synthesis Inhibitors

This classification includes macrolides and tetracyclines. Macrolides are commonly used to treat pulmonary infections. Erythromycin is in the macrolide class and may be bactericidal or static, depending on the organism's susceptibility and the drug concentration. Erythromycin may be synergistic with concurrent use of sulfonamides for *Haemophilus influenzae*. Erythromycin causes stomach distress and diarrhea, although the newer macrolide azithromycin causes less of this. Erythromycin interacts with theophylline to decrease theophylline metabolism, so doses of theophylline need to be adjusted when erythromycin is used concurrently. Since macrolides are commonly used for respiratory infections, this interaction should be closely monitored. Common macrolides include:

- **erythromycin** (E-mycin)
- **clarithromycin** (Biaxin)
- **azithromycin** (Zithromax)

Tetracyclines

The tetracyclines have been available for approximately 50 years and have a relatively broad spectrum of activity, including Gram-positive and Gram-negative aerobic and anaerobic bacteria as well as mycoplasmas, some mycobacteria, chlamydia, and spirochetes. They are produced by soil organisms and are bacteriostatic. Uses include acne, Rocky Mountain Spotted Fever, Lyme disease, and as part of a treatment regimen for peptic ulcer disease.

Tetracycline cannot be taken with antacids, iron, or dairy products, because they will bind with each other and not be absorbed. Pregnant woman and children under the age of nine shouldn't take tetracycline, because permanent tooth discoloration could result. Common tetracyclines include:

- **doxycycline** (Vibramycin)
- **minocycline** (Minocin)

Folate Inhibitors

Sulfonamides are classic examples and are considered bacteriostatic. They block a step in the synthesis of folic acid and destroy bacteria. The most common side effects are rash, drug fever, and blood complications. Their main use is the treatment of uncomplicated urinary tract infections. Sulfonamides are frequently used in combination with trimethoprim for *pneumocystis carinii*. This will be discussed more in Chapter 14. Common sulfonamides include:

- **sulfamethoxazole trimethoprim** (Bactrim, Septra)
- **sulfamethoxazole** (Gantanol)
- **sulfisoxazole** (Gantrisin)

Oxazolidinones

Linezolid (Zyvox) is the only oxazolidinone being clinically researched at present. The oxazolidinones are synthetic agents with a novel mechanism of action of inhibiting the bacterial translation (synthesis of essential proteins) process. This class is mainly bacteriostatic and active against primarily Gram-positive agents. Stay tuned to the Web site for updated information on this promising new drug.

Dalfopristin/quinupristine

℞   **Dalfopristin/quinupristine** (Synercid) is a parenteral product comprised of two drugs from the chemical class called streptogramin. Both are bacteriostatic against Gram-positive bacteria. They can be bactericidal against staphylococci, including the methicillin-resistant strains. They may have a role in infections associated with vancomycin-resistant enterococcus.

Metronidazole

℞   **Metronidazole** (Flagyl) is a synthetic drug with an anaerobic spectrum of activity. It is part of one antibiotic treatment for peptic ulcer disease. Side effects include a metallic taste and intolerance to alcohol. Patients on metronidazole should not drink alcohol for up to 3 days after discontinuing the drug, to prevent adverse effects of nausea and flushing that may result from the combination. This is similar to the reaction alcoholics have if prescribed the alcohol deterrent disulfuram (Antabuse) as an aid to alcoholic recovery.

Antitubercular Agents

Tuberculosis (TB) is a disease usually confined to the lungs. For this reason, it is an important part of this book and will be elaborated upon more in Chapter 14; we will merely introduce it here. TB can be symptomatic or asymptomatic, but it is a chronic disease requiring months of treatment with the appropriate anti-infective.

Drug-resistant TB can occur because of suboptimal treatment of tuberculosis. At diagnosis, most TB is susceptible to the chosen drug, but because of the long duration of treatment needed and resultant noncompliance with drugs, resistant TB often develops. This has the potential to become a public health emergency, especially since there are currently no new drugs for TB in clinical research trials.

TB drugs are categorized as first-line primary drugs and secondary retreatment agents. Primary agents are bactericidal, and second-line drugs are bacteriostatic and used only in combination with first-line drugs when resistance is present. Second-line drugs are secondary because they are more toxic (see Table 8-10 for a list of drugs used to treat TB).

Isoniazid can cause liver toxicity, which is enhanced when alcohol is used concurrently. Patients frequently complain of a peripheral neuropathy with isoniazid or ethionamide. Ethambutol may cause optic changes.

Antivirals

Viruses are the most common infectious agents in humans. A virus is an obligate parasite, which means it can only live and replicate in a living host cell. This makes it difficult to kill the virus without harming the host cell. Because this is a different situation than with

CLINICAL PEARL

Rifampin can cause urine, feces, saliva or sputum, and tears to be colored red-orange. Patients should be warned to expect this and should be cautioned about staining soft contact lenses. Is it any wonder compliance may not be good with TB drugs, considering these side effects?

Table 8-10   Drugs Used to Treat TB

		Generic	*Brand Name*
Primary		**isoniazid**	INH
		rifampin	Rimactane
		pyrazinamide	Tebrazid
		ethambutol	Myambutol
Secondary		**streptomycin**	Streptomycin
		cycloserine	Seromycin
		ethionamide	Trecator-SC

℞

bacteria, different drugs are needed to treat viruses than bacteria. Viruses are classified by whether they contain RNA or DNA. RNA viruses cause diseases such as influenza, polio, HIV, rabies, and encephalitis. DNA viruses cause adenovirus respiratory disease, papilloma warts, herpes simplex, and Epstein–Barr mononucleosis.

Immunization has been the mainstay treatment of many of the viral infections such as influenza, measles, mumps, polio, and rubella. Only recently have more antiviral drugs become available for diseases such as the common cold and flu. Viral infections are classified by their severity, length of time present, and body parts affected. Infections such as the common cold and influenza can be acute and quickly resolve, or they can be slow and have a progressive course, as with HIV. Viral infections can be local and just affect the respiratory tract, for example, or generalized and spread throughout the blood stream. Some viruses can be dormant and then under certain conditions reproduce again. This is called latency and implies that a disease may surface years after transmission or after the initial breakout.

Antivirals to Treat Herpes.

Herpes is a DNA virus that can cause the vesicular skin eruption most people know as fever blisters or cold sores. It can also cause genital herpes, which can be spread by sexual contact with an infected person. The main drugs to treat herpes are **acyclovir** (Zovirax) and **famciclovir** (Famvir). These drugs interfere with viral DNA and inhibit viral replication. They are also used to treat postherpetic neuralgia, or shingles.

Antivirals for Influenza.

Influenza or "the flu" is a common viral infection due to different strains of the influenza virus. Certain patients are at higher risk for complications from influenza. These include the elderly, diabetics, and patients with cardiac, renal, and respiratory problems. Influenza agents include **amantadine** (Symmetrel), **rimantadine** (Flumadine), **zanamivir** (Relenza), and **oseltamivir** (Tamiflu). Amantadine and rimantadine have been available for years. They are effective against Influenza A virus; however, their use is limited by CNS side effects.

Zanamivir and oseltamivir have recently been marketed as drugs to cut the duration of the flu by at least 1 day and maybe 3. These two drugs are called neuraminidase inhibitors. They are indicated for treatment of both influenza A and influenza B. Zanamivir is available as an inhaled medication delivered by a breath-activated diskhaler. It has been associated with adverse respiratory effects in patients with airway disease.

Antivirals to Treat Respiratory Syncytial Virus.

Ribavirin is an antiviral with inhibitory activity against respiratory syncytial virus (RSV), influenzas A and B, and herpes simplex. Although its mechanism is not known for sure it inhibits essential nucleic acid formation in viral particles. RSV is a pathogen causing bronchiolitis and pneumonia and is a major cause of acute respiratory disease in children. Severe cases of RSV are treated with aerosolized ribavarin (Virazole). Ribavirin is administered through a small particle aerosol generator (SPAG) for 12 to 18 hours daily for 3 to 7 days. Since aerosolized ribavirin can escape into the air around the patient, visitors and staff may get exposed to the drug, and because of its teratogenicity, this is a concern. It should not be mixed together with any other aerosol medications. See Table 8-11 for common antivirals to treat herpes, influenza, and RSV.

Antivirals to Treat Acquired Immunodeficiency Syndrome (AIDS).

AIDS is a progressively fatal disease caused by the human immunodeficiency virus (HIV). Treatment of HIV comprises several different drugs to suppress the virus. In addition, several HIV vaccines are undergoing clinical testing. AIDS depresses the immune system and allows infections to develop. These can include malignant herpes simplex virus, cytomegalovirus (CMV), Kaposi's sarcoma, and commonly *Pneumocystis carinii,* which leads to severe pneumonia in many AIDS patients. Because of the relationship to the respiratory system, AIDS and *Pneumocystis carinii* pneumonia (PCP) will be discussed in depth in Chapter 14. In addition, periodic updates and new drugs will be posted on the Web site.

Table 8-11   Common Antivirals

Disease	Generic	Brand Name
herpes	**acyclovir**	Zovirax
	famciclovir	Famvir
influenza	**zanamivir (inhaled)**	Relenza
	oseltamivir	Tamiflu
	amantadine	Symmetrel
	rimantidine	Flumadine
RSV	**ribavirin**	Virazole

Antifungals

A fungus is reproduced by spores, has a rigid cell wall, and has no chlorphyll. Fungi include mushrooms, yeasts, and molds. Fungi have ergosterol instead of the cholesterol in human cells. Antifungals work by preventing the making of ergosterol, which is a building block for the cell membranes. Fungal infections are most likely to develop in patients with an impaired immune system. In addition, antibiotics can destroy the body's natural flora, which can result in an opportunistic fungal infection.

Some examples of fungal infections include ringworm, athlete's foot, or jock itch, all of which can be treated with topical antifungal creams. More serious fungal infections can include histoplasmosis within the lung and candida albicans (thrush) of the oral cavity. These can progress to systemic infections.

Nystatin (Mycostatin) is an antifungal agent available orally and as a topical cream; it is used to treat candida albicans and skin fungal infections. **Miconazole** (Monistat) is a topical cream used for vaginal yeast infections. Miconazole can also be administered IV for systemic fungal infections. Other systemic antifungal infections include **amphotericin B** (Fungizone), **fluconazole** (Diflucan), and **ketoconazole** (Nizoral).

When given systemically, amphotericin B is a highly toxic drug that requires close monitoring. Toxicity can include renal and liver damage, which may manifest itself as patient fatigue, anorexia, nausea, vomiting, jaundice, or dark urine. See Table 8-12 for the common antifungal agents.

Table 8-12   Common Antifungals

Generic	Brand Name	Indication/Route
nystatin	Mycostatin	local skin candidiasis oral thrush
miconazole	Monistat	vaginal yeast IV systemic
amphotericin B	Fungizone	IV systemic
fluconazole	Diflucan	oral thrush IV systemic
ketoconazole	Nizoral	local scalp shampoo po for systemic

AEROSOL ANTI-INFECTIVE THERAPY

Rationale

Most pulmonary infections are treated with systemic antimicrobials administered either orally or parenterally. If pulmonary tissue is damaged or full of exudates, diffusion of systemically administered agents may be impaired. Because of this, there may be a role for aerosolized antiinfective agents, but thus far they still remain a relatively unproven therapy.

Another rationale for topical local anti-infective therapy delivered by aerosolization is fewer side effects and direct deposition at the infected site. Some of the aerosolized agents used include gentamicin, tobramycin, ribavirin, and pentamidine.

As logical as this route may sound, there are some disadvantages. Most of the aerosolized anti-infective agents can cause bronchospasm. Pretreating with a bronchodilator may be advantageous. In addition, some of these agents require specialized equipment to create and deliver the aerosol. It is also difficult to know exact dosing requirements, since penetration and potential antimicrobial inactivation occur when drugs are deposited in the mucus. Lack of information on the pharmacokinetics of aerosol-delivered drugs makes it difficult to predict effectiveness. Unintended exposure of the aerosols to the healthcare deliverer and others can have potential hazards.

Few studies have been done looking at anti-infective aerosol administration, and those that have been done have primarily targeted the cystic fibrosis patient population. Other diseases that may lend themselves to aerosol-route treatment include tuberculosis, pulmonary aspergillosis, and coccidiomycosis. The commonality among these diseases is the presence of a cavitating lesion that makes it difficult for antibiotics to penetrate systemically. Based on the rationale for penetration, it may make sense to use combination aerosol and systemic therapy to maximize efficacy.

Chapter 14 will discuss the use of aerosolized ribavarin for RSV, pentamidine for PCP, and other aerosolized anti-infective agents to treat various pulmonary infections.

SUMMARY

Healthcare practitioners must be able to identify signs and symptoms of infection and be familiar with medical indications for antibiotics. Just as important, if not more important, is knowledge of indications *not* to use antibiotics. Currently available drugs to prevent or treat infection come in several different classifications and vary in their degree of effectiveness against different microorganisms. Several factors are involved in appropriate antibiotic drug selection, some of which require incorporation of microbiological principles and effective patient monitoring of signs and symptoms. This chapter provides a foundation for applying these drugs to clinical practice in the treatment of respiratory infectious diseases covered in Chapter 14.

REVIEW QUESTIONS

1. Bacteria are classified on the basis of:
   (a) dilution of serum
   (b) staining properties
   (c) need for water to survive
   (d) location in the body
   (e) resistance patterns
2. Beta lactam antibiotics include:
   (a) penicillins
   (b) cephalosporins
   (c) monobactams
   (d) carbapenems
   (e) all of the above
3. Antivirals for flu treatment:
   (a) replace vaccination
   (b) are only administered IV

   (c) are most effective 3 days after flu presentation
   (d) may decrease the duration of the flu
   (e) also treat RSV
4. Viruses:
   (a) are the least common infectious agents in humans
   (b) are classified by cell wall type and shape
   (c) are responsible for symptomatic TB
   (d) can be dormant or latent
   (e) inhibit further viral replication
5. White blood cell (WBC) count elevation:
   (a) is always associated with an infection
   (b) equals normal flora in sputum

(c) can be present without an infectious process

(d) determines the need for bactericidal or bacteriostatic therapy

(e) is always associated with TB

6. How do a bactericidal and a bacteriostatic antibiotic differ?

7. Why is resistance a problem with antibiotics?

8. Describe the role of empiric antimicrobial therapy.

9. How would you explain the difference between a broad-spectrum and a narrow-spectrum antibiotic?

CASE STUDY

A 68-year-old gentleman is hospitalized for possible pneumonia. His past medical history is significant for three outpatient courses of antibiotics over the last 2 months with tetracycline, erythromycin, and levofloxacin. However, he has stated that on some occasions he stopped taking the antibiotic prematurely because he felt better, and on other occasions he discontinued antibiotic use owing to an upset stomach. What type of education would you give this patient? What signs and symptoms would you expect with his pneumonia? What lab and diagnostic tests would confirm the pneumonia? Finally, why may this patient be more difficult to treat with anti-infective agents?

GLOSSARY

aerobic   refers to bacteria that need oxygen to survive.

anaerobic   refers to bacteria that don't need oxygen to survive.

antibiotic   substance that destroys or inhibits the growth of other microorganisms.

bactericidal   refers to drugs that kill bacteria.

bacteriostatic   inhibiting of bacterial growth.

broad spectrum   antibiotic classification system based on bacteria type that the drug is effective against.

chemotherapy   prevention or treatment of disease by use of chemical substances.

empiric   antimicrobial therapy begun before a specific pathogen has been identified.

flora   normal harmless microbial content of the body.

gram stain   method of staining bacterial cells, used to identify the type.

narrow spectrum   antibiotic classification system based on bacteria type that the drug is effective against.

pathogen   disease-producing microorganism.

resistance   degree to which a disease-causing organism remains unaffected by antibiotics.

superinfection   new infection that complicates an existing infection because of antibiotic resistance to drugs used.

susceptibility test   a lab microbiology test that establishes the drug sensitivity of a bacterium.

www.prenhall.com/colbert

Use the address above to access the free, interactive Companion Web site created specifically for this textbook. Enhance your studying by viewing videos and animations, answering practice quiz questions, and reviewing an audio glossary and much more related to Chapter 8.

CHAPTER 9

Cardiac and Renal Agents

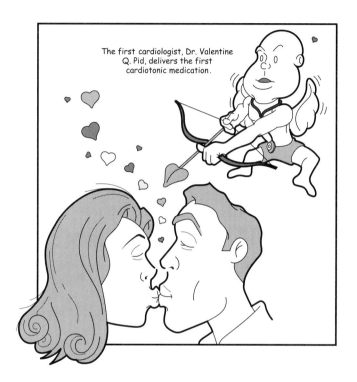

The first cardiologist, Dr. Valentine Q. Pid, delivers the first cardiotonic medication.

OBJECTIVES

Upon completion of this chapter you will be able to

- Define key terms related to cardiac and renal agents
- Relate cardiovascular physiology to pharmacological treatments
- Describe pharmacological effects of antiarrhythmics, inotropes, diuretics, and vasodilators
- Understand the role of pharmacological therapy for arrhythmias, congestive heart failure, myocardial infarction, and angina

ABBREVIATIONS

Ca	calcium	CHF	congestive heart failure
CO	cardiac output	SA	sinoatrial
ACE	angiotensin-converting enzyme	AV	atrioventricular
ADH	antidiuretic hormone	Na	sodium

K	potassium	CCB	calcium-channel blocker
MI	myocardial infarction	CEB	calcium entry blocker
PVCs	premature ventricular contractions	BPH	benign prostatic hypertrophy
		UTI	urinary tract infection
ECG	electrocardiogram	PAT	paroxysmal atrial tachycardia
ACh	acetylcholine		

INTRODUCTION

The heart, lungs, and kidneys are intricately related, which explains the need for and cohesiveness of a textbook on cardiopulmonary pharmacotherapy. For example, patients with chronic lung disease often have chronic hypoxemia. The heart must compensate for the low levels of oxygen by several mechanisms that all increase the cardiac workload. Over time, this can lead to heart disease secondary to the underlying lung disease.

In addition, the renal system is intricately related to the heart and lungs. The kidneys' regulation of fluid balance can affect the fluid volume and thus the pressures within the cardiovascular system. Too much fluid retention can build up and eventually back up into the lungs and severely impair vital diffusion of oxygen. If the kidneys do not maintain proper acid–base or electrolyte balance, serious cardiac arrhythmias may develop.

If the lungs do not maintain adequate oxygen levels, the heart may not function properly, and cardiac output may decrease. Because the kidneys require adequate blood supply (perfusion) in order to function properly, they may be severely affected. As you can see, any dysfunction in the heart, lungs, or kidneys may have major implications for the other systems.

The cardiovascular system's primary role is to ensure the vital circulation of blood throughout our bodies. To accomplish this, three basic components are required. You first need a strong functioning pump (heart) to generate the pressure needed to push the blood through the system. Second, you need a piping system (vessels) to transport the blood and appropriately handle and react to changes of pressures within the system. Finally, you need the blood itself to flow freely through blood vessels and clot when the need occurs. This chapter will focus on pharmacologic agents that will ensure proper functioning of the heart and related systems. The following chapter will focus on drugs that affect the blood vessels and blood itself.

This chapter will discuss the most common cardiopulmonary and renal pharmacotherapy. The emphasis will be on the treatment of the most common cardiac conditions: congestive heart failure (CHF), cardiac arrhythmias, myocardial infarction (MI), and angina. Pharmacological classes discussed will include antiarrhythmics, inotropes, vasodilators, and diuretics.

CARDIOVASCULAR OVERVIEW

Basic Terminology

For the heart to function optimally, it must maintain an appropriate rate, rhythm, and force of contraction. Pharmacologic agents for the heart can either positively or negatively affect these three variables. **Chronotropic** drugs affect the rate of the heart and can either increase its rate (positive chronotropic) or decrease its rate (negative chronotropic). **Inotropic** drugs affect the force of contraction and again can be either positive or negative. **Dromotropic** drugs alter the rhythm or electrical conduction through the heart muscle. A positive dromotropic drug enhances the electrical conduction of signals in certain parts of the heart, whereas negative dromotropic drugs will slow conduction.

LEARNING HINT

To remember the difference between the right and left heart, try to associate the letter R in "right" with the following: The right heart has the tricuspid valve and receives deoxygenated blood from the veins. Also, the right heart pumps into the respiratory system. The left therefore must have the mitral valve and pumps oxygenated blood throughout the body.

Cardiac Circulation

The heart is divided into four chambers (two ventricles and two atria). The atria sit above the ventricles and are reservoirs that allow blood to flow into the ventricles when the valves open between them. The tricuspid valve separates the right atrium and right ventricle. The mitral valve separates the left atrium. The heart can be considered to be two separate pumps. The right side of the heart receives deoxygenated blood from all parts of the body and pumps this blood through the pulmonary system to become oxygenated. The left side of the heart receives the oxygenated blood and pumps it throughout the body (see Figure 9-1, which shows the cardiac circulation).

The heart's contractility is what supplies the pressure to force blood through the various vessels and supply perfusion throughout the body. The heart is functionally comprised of cardiac muscle. The heart, like any muscle, needs to be supplied with oxygen and vital nutrients to function properly. The coronary arteries supply blood to the heart, and coronary veins carry away the metabolic waste products.

How do you think blockage of coronary arteries will affect the heart's contractility?

Cardiac Conduction

For the heart to pump blood effectively it must contract in a highly integrated and coordinated fashion. The right and left atria must contract at the same time, sending blood into the right and left ventricle, respectively. There must next be a slight contractile pause to allow

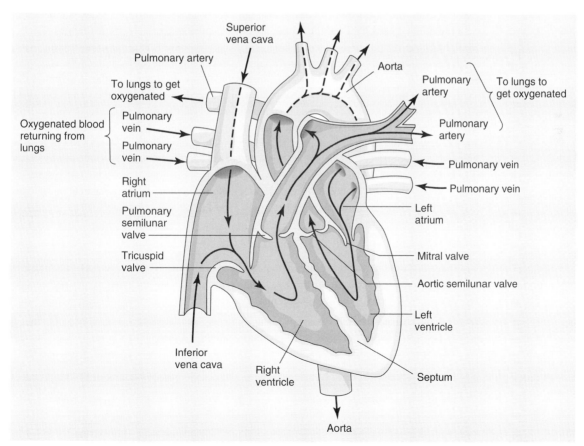

Figure 9-1 Cardiac Circulation

the ventricles adequate filling time. Then, the ventricles must contract simultaneously, the right sending its deoxygenated blood into the pulmonary system and the left sending its oxygenated blood through the aorta and out to the entire body.

www.prenhall.com/colbert

Get connected to the Web to see an animation of this coordinated cardiac conduction system.

Both electrical and mechanical properties of the heart are relevant to cardiovascular pharmacology. The heart muscle contraction and subsequent pumping represents a mechanical action. However, this mechanical action must be initiated by an electrical response. Muscle contraction is electrically characterized by a change in action potential, which is the basis for electrocardiogram (ECG) monitoring. In the heart, an intricate electric **conduction** system maintains regular rate and rhythm.

Cardiac activity depends on generation of an electrical impulse in the sinoatrial (SA) node, which is considered the normal pacemaker for the heart. The SA node is innervated by both parasympathetic and sympathetic nerves which set the heart rate. In review, the sympathetic nerves release norepinephrine (NE) and cause adrenergic responses, and the parasympathetic releases acetylcholine (ACh) and causes cholinergic responses. NE increases heart rate and force of contraction, and ACh causes the opposite, so a balance is maintained. See Table 9-1 for the adrenergic and cholinergic effects on the heart.

The SA node paces the heart by depolarizing and stimulating the conducting nerves of the heart. The impulse then spreads through the atria. After the atria contract, the electrical impulse now travels to the node between the atria and the ventricles, called the atrioventricular or AV node. There is a slight delay (approximately .20 seconds) to allow the ventricles to fill with blood. The impulse then travels through the bundle of His, located in the septal wall between the ventricles, and branches into the right bundle branch, going to the right ventricle, and the left bundle branch, going to the left ventricle. The bundle of His consists of a thick bunch of conducting nerve fibers that carry current to the end of the conduction system, or the Purkinje fibers. From there, conduction proceeds through the Purkinje conduction system located throughout the ventricular muscle, depolarizing the ventricles, thus causing contraction. See Figure 9-2, which shows the electrical pathway of conduction through the heart.

Ion Influence

Now that we've discussed the mechanics of myocardial contraction, we can look at the physiologic processes that start it. The cardiac **action potential** is related to contraction and relaxation of the heart. This action potential is controlled at the cellular level by ions trans-

Table 9-1   Adrenergic and Cholinergic Effects on the Heart

Sympathetic–Adrenergic	*Parasympathetic–Cholinergic*
↑ HR	cardiac slowing
↑ force of contraction	↓ force of contraction
↑ automaticity	↓ automaticity
↑ AV conduction	inhibition of AV conduction

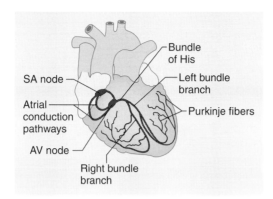

Figure 9-2 Electrical Conduction Through the Heart

porting in and out of cells. Different ionic currents generate different phases of the action potential. In each of the phases, an electrical gradient occurs between the inside and the outside of the cell membrane. Cells cycle between resting, activation, and inactivation states.

Specifically, the pacemaking and conduction throughout the heart are driven by action potentials that are dependent on sodium (Na), calcium (Ca), and potassium (K) activity, and their passages through certain ionic channels within the membranes of the myocardial cells. Potassium moves out of the cell while sodium moves in for a process called depolarization, which precedes the mechanical contraction. The muscle must now return to its resting potential or repolarize, with potassium moving back into the cell and sodium back out. In addition, calcium is needed for the actual muscle contraction to occur. Calcium influences actin and myosin, which control cardiac cell length and muscle contraction.

Some ionic channels cannot be reactivated or opened until a certain phase of the action potential occurs. The time when cells can't be excited after electrical stimulation is called the **refractory period.** Some cardiac cells must wait for a stimulus, while others have spontaneous self-excitability capabilities. During some phases, there are different levels of refractoriness present, which means electrical stimulation cannot occur or can occur only with a very strong stimulus. Different tissues depend on different ions, have differences in recovery of tissue excitability, and are affected differently by drugs that influence their conduction properties.

Can you explain why it is important to monitor levels of the ions (electrolytes) sodium, potassium, and calcium through lab tests?

The ECG Tracing

Electrocardiograms (ECGs) record electrical activity of the heart as deflection points represented by the letters P, Q, R, S, and T. Each of these letters represents either the depolarization or the repolarization process that occurs within various parts of the heart (see Figure 9-3, which shows a normal ECG tracing).

The P wave represents the atrial depolarization, which is normally followed by the mechanical contraction of the right and left atria. The QRS complex shows ventricular depolarization, which is followed by the mechanical contraction of the right and left ventricle. The T wave shows the repolarization (back to resting potential) of the ventricles so that they are ready for another stimulus. The atria must also return back to resting or repolarize, and this normally occurs at the same time the ventricles are depolarizing. Since the ventricles are much larger and generate a greater electrical deflection (QRS), you normally do not see the small deflection of atrial repolarization hidden in the QRS complex.

LEARNING HINT

The interval from the beginning of the P wave to the beginning of the QRS shows how long the impulse takes to travel from the atria to the ventricle. If that interval is too long, an atrioventricular conduction problem exists.

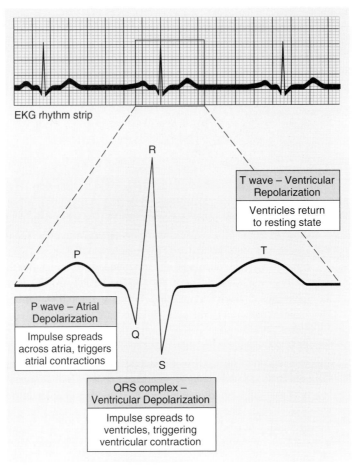

Figure 9-3 Normal ECG Tracing
Note: Atria repolarization normally occurs during QRS

www.prenhall.com/colbert

A normal ECG is presented in the Web site as well as tracings corresponding to the common arrhythmias.

Arrhythmias

Any deviation from the normal ECG tracing is termed an **arrhythmia.** The mechanisms of cardiac arrhythmias include disorders of automaticity and/or conduction. Automaticity is normal when pacemaker activity originates in the SA node. Arrhythmias mainly occur because the pacemaker originates somewhere other than the SA node (abnormal automaticity) or the impulse doesn't follow normal conduction pathway and abnormal conduction occurs. When the SA node is altered and conduction is interrupted, other areas become excitable. Nonautomatic cells can now become automatic and fire, thus causing a contraction to occur out of sequence and adversely affect cardiac output.

Cells can become excited if there is an oxygen deficit, as in ischemia or infarction, or if an electrolyte imbalance occurs. Since those conditions can be transient and unpredictable, it explains why arrhythmia occurrence can be variable. Arrhythmias can occur in hearts with abnormal function or even in a normally functioning heart if influenced adversely by exercise, diet, or electrolyte changes.

Arrhythmias are diagnosed and treatment decisions are made on the basis of objective ECG data and subjective patient clinical signs and symptoms. By pharmacologically affecting cardiac conduction and the autonomic nervous system, drugs can assist in managing arrhythmias. Arrhythmias, regardless of where they originate, may cause no symptoms or may be life threatening. Sometimes arrhythmias are rated according to their outcome potential as benign, potentially malignant, or malignant. This objective rating helps in making individualized decisions about whom to treat and with what drug to treat and what the benefit risk is. Since underlying arrhythmias are variable by nature, **proarrhythmias** or arrhythmias induced by drugs can be difficult to diagnose, so awareness among healthcare professionals is important. Antiarrhythmic treatment is warranted when hemodynamic compromise occurs, when an increase in myocardial oxygen demand occurs, or when the arrhythmias may lead to malignant ventricular arrhythmias.

Sites of Arrhythmias

Arrhythmias can develop in the atria or ventricles. They can happen in the critical care unit or while sitting at home in the recliner. Arrhythmias requiring drug treatment can be divided into supraventricular (above the ventricles) and ventricular on the basis of where in the heart the arrhythmias originate. The common supraventricular arrhythmias are atrial fibrillation or flutter, paroxysmal supraventricular tachycardia, and autonomic atrial tachycardias. The ventricular arrhythmias include premature ventricular contractions (PVCs), ventricular tachycardia, torsade de pointes, and ventricular fibrillation.

> **CONTROVERSY**
>
> As more mechanical technological advances like pacemakers occur in the treatment of arrhythmias, fewer pharmacological antiarrhythmics will be used. This is good news, since many prescribers are concerned about antiarrhythmic drugs' side effects, toxicity, and potential to cause additional arrhythmias.

Potential arrhythmia outcomes can range from mild discomfort to sudden death. Recurrence of the arrhythmia is best documented by ECG or holter test cardiac monitoring and should include not only time but frequency of recurrence and any related activity. Symptoms tolerance, blood pressure, heart rate, side effects, quality of life, and economics are all considered in the benefit–risk decision to use an antiarrhythmic drug.

ANTIARRHYTHMIC AGENTS

Therapeutic Goals

Goals for drugs used for cardiac arrhythmias are to restore and maintain normal sinus rhythm where the electrical impulse to begin cardiac conduction should occur at the SA node. In addition, antiarrhythmic treatment attempts to suppress those excitable areas of the heart that fire outside of the normal conduction pathway and impair cardiac output. These areas are referred to as ectopic foci. Finally, antiarrhythmic agents attempt to control ventricular rate and optimize cardiac output.

Mechanism of Action

Antiarrhythmics' mechanism of action is both pharmacological and electrophysiological. They basically work to alter conduction through atria or ventricles. They may do so in several ways. One way is to depress automatic properties of abnormal pacemaker cells. The drugs can accomplish this electrophysiologically by affecting depolarization and the threshold level of these excitable cells. Another way is to alter conduction characteristics within the heart by either facilitating or depressing conduction.

Antiarrhythmic Drug Classification

Antiarrhythmic drugs are classified into four classes, with subclasses for Class I (see Table 9-2). This classification is based on electrophysiologic actions in vitro (in the lab), where the different drug classes affect different phases of the action potential or ionic channels. These drugs affect calcium and sodium channels, prolong the repolarization phase, or block β-adrenergic activity, and they are classified accordingly.

It's important to notice that some of the most useful drugs for treating arrhythmias are not in this classification (i.e., atropine for bradycardia, epinephrine for asystole); these will be covered in detail in chapter 15 on advanced cardiac life support (ACLS).

In addition, this classification doesn't have a place for all drugs (such as digoxin). Adding to the confusion, drugs in the same class don't necessarily have the same medical indications or treat the same arrhythmias, and therefore drugs within each class cannot necessarily be substituted for each other. For example, the antiarrhythmic bretylium (class III) may be effective for ventricular fibrillation but not ventricular tachycardia. Many drugs also have properties of more than one antiarrhythmic class. We will discuss each class separately to attempt to sort this all out. This does validate that what happens in the lab (**in vitro**) does not always translate directly to what happens in the human body (**in vivo**).

℞

Class I—Na-Channel Blockers. **Procainamide** (Pronestyl) and **quinidine** (Quinaglute) are both classified as I A drugs. Class I A drugs are sodium-channel blockers. By blocking the sodium channel of the muscle cell, they prevent depolarization and thus decrease excitability and contraction outside of the SA node. These drugs have little effect on SA node automaticity. They are often used interchangeably to treat supraventricular arrhythmias such as atrial fibrillation and flutter and paroxysmal atrial tachycardia (PAT). In addition, they can both be used to treat ventricular tachycardia. This is useful, because they

Table 9-2 Antiarrhythmic Drug Classes

Class	*Function*	*Generic*	*Brand Name*
I A	Na-channel blockers	quinidine procainamide	Quinaglute Pronestyl
I B	Na-channel blockers	lidocaine mexiletene tocainide	Xylocaine Mexitil Tonocard
I C	Na-channel blockers	moricizine flecainide propafenone	Ethmozine Tambocor Rythmol
II	β-adrenergic blockers	propranolol esmolol	Inderal Brevibloc
III	drugs to prolong repolarization	amiodarone bretylium sotalol	Cordarone Bretylol Betapace
IV	Ca-channel blocker	verapamil	Isoptin

both have side effects that frequently lead to discontinuation and the need for an alternate drug. Quinidine can cause diarrhea, thrombocytopenia, and cinchonism. Cinchonism consists of headache, blurred vision, tinnitus, confusion, and nausea.

Quinidine also has secondary vagal blocking effects, which are opposite from the primary effect of decreasing excitability, which can be problematic clinically. This means that quinidine may have an additive effect with anticholinergics.

Procainamide can cause leukopenia, hypotension, and a dermatological butterfly-like rash on the face called lupus. Procainamide may potentiate neuromuscular blocking drugs.

℞ **Lidocaine** (Xylocaine) is a Class I B drug given systemically for ventricular arrhythmias such as premature ventricular contractions (PVCs), ventricular tachycardia, and fibrillation. Major side effects involve the CNS and include confusion, dizziness, disorientation, and respiratory depression. Lidocaine doses should be adjusted in patients with liver impairment and congestive heart failure. Other class I B drugs include **phenytoin, mexiletene, and tocainide.**

℞ Class I C drugs, such as **propafenone** (Rhythmol), may have some Class II effects. Class I C drugs slow conduction velocity more than the other agents. Class I C drugs can cause a negative inotropic effect on the heart. Side effects of propafenone include blurred

℞ vision, dizziness, somnolence, and paresthesias. Other Class I C drugs include **moricizine** and **flecainide.**

LEARNING HINT

Remember a previous learning hint that you have one heart (β_1) and two lungs (β_2)? Therefore, if the beta blocker for the heart condition also binds with and blocks the β_2 receptors in the lungs, bronchoconstriction may occur.

Beta Blockers—Class II. Beta blockers are Class II antiarrhythmics and mainly work because of their antiadrenergic effects. Beta blockers slow conduction through the AV node and inhibit sympathetic neurotransmission. They result in decreases in heart rate (negative chronotropic), myocardial contractility (negative inotropic), blood pressure, and myocardial oxygen demand. Class II agents primarily treat supraventricular tachycardias. Beta blockers are also considered to have a membrane-stabilizing effect on the heart. Beta blockers decrease the likelihood of sudden death due to arrhythmias after a myocardial infarction (MI). In patients who may be prone to bronchoconstriction, the benefit versus the risk of using the drug for this indication must be considered. Other side effects to consider in this benefit–risk assessment are heart failure, depressed AV conduction, and hypotension.

℞ Examples of beta blockers include **propranolol** and **esmolol.**

℞ ***Class III—Drugs to Prolong Repolarization (Potassium-Channel Blocker).*** **Amiodarone** (Cordarone) is a Class III drug, but it really has electrophysiological characteristics of all classes of antiarrhythmics. Amiodarone reduces automaticity of the SA node and ectopic foci, reduces conduction velocity, and increases the refractory period. It is used to treat recurrent ventricular fibrillation, unstable ventricular tachycardia, and atrial fibrillation. It can be both very effective and very toxic. It has a very long half-life and can take weeks to control arrhythmias. Side effects include reversible corneal deposits, hypo- or hyperthyroidism, pulmonary fibrosis, and photosensitivity. Some patients taking amiodarone get a bluish color tone to the skin that is not to be confused with cyanosis. Amiodarone can interact significantly with other cardiac drugs, especially with the blood thinner coumadin.

℞ Another Class III drug is **bretylium** (Bretylol). It prevents release and reuptake of neurotransmitters and prolongs the action potential and is also used to treat ventricular fibrillation and tachycardia. Bretylium can cause hypotension or hypertension. Arrhythmias may worsen before they improve with bretylium; it can cause an initial increase release in norepinephrine that may increase the heart rate.

℞ **Sotalol** (Betapace) is yet another drug option in Class III. Sotalol also has some class II properties. It slows heart rate, decreases AV nodal conduction, and increases AV nodal refractoriness. It is used as an option to treat atrial fibrillation.

R

Class IV—Calcium-Channel Blockers. Calcium channel blockers are Class IV antiarrhythmics. The terms calcium-channel blocker (CCB) and calcium entry blocker (CEB) are used synonymously. There are two types of calcium-channels in the SA and AV node. Not all calcium-channel blockers work at the same receptor sites, because the chemical structures and pharmacologies of the drugs are different. **Verapamil** (Calan) is the main calcium-channel blocker used for supraventricular tachycardiac arrhythmias. It reduces automaticity of the SA node and ectopic foci, reduces conduction velocity, and increases the refractory period. Side effects are bradycardia, hypotension, heart block, heart failure, dizziness, and constipation. Verapamil is also used for the treatment of angina and hypertension.

Now that you have been introduced to the different classes of antiarrhythmic drugs, it's important to compare them. See Table 9-3 for the effects of antiarrhythmic drugs on cardiovascular functioning. The four classes of antiarrhythmic drugs each have characteristic electrophysiologic, autonomic, contractility, and hemodynamic effects on the heart. Some of these effects are desirable, and others may explain patient intolerance to the antiarrhythmic. Notice from the table that some effects change over time. If a patient needed an antiarrhythmic that would increase vagal activity, this table might suggest that the best drug option would be a Class IV calcium-channel blocker. This is an example of how a table like this can be used clinically to make prescribing decisions.

Digoxin

R

Digoxin is an unclassified antiarrhythmic that inhibits the sodium/potassium exchange pump in the heart, which then leads to increased intracellular sodium and calcium. The increased total calcium available for release by the action potential will cause an increase in the contractility of the heart. Digoxin has a half-life of 36 hours or longer, so frequently a loading dose is used.

Digoxin is often given before quinidine in patients with atrial fibrillation, since the ventricular rate may increase as quinidine facilitates AV conduction. Digoxin doesn't convert atrial fibrillation to normal sinus rhythm, but it slows the ventricular rate. Some side effects of digoxin include anorexia, visual disturbances, and fatigue. Serum levels of digoxin can guide dose adjustments. Drug interactions occur with drugs that affect serum electrolytes.

CLINICAL PEARL
Digoxin will further be discussed in the treatment of congestive heart failure, where the prolongation of the PR interval (more filling time) coupled with the increased myocardial contraction both help treat the disease.

Adenosine

Adenosine (Adenocard) is an unclassified antiarrhythmic used for superaventricular tachycardia. It slows conduction through the AV and SA nodes. The drug is used intravenously and has a very short half-life. Side effects include transient facial flushing and dyspnea. It

Table 9-3   Effects of Antiarrhythmic Drugs on Cardiovascular Function

Category	Effect	Class 1A	Class 1B Class 1C	Class 2	Class 3	Class 4
electrophysiologic	automaticity (chronotropic)	↓	↓ or 0	↓	↑ then ↓	↓
	effective refractory period	↓ AV node ↑ ventricle	↓	↓	↑	↑
	conduction (dromotropic)	↓	0 1B ↓↓ 1C	↓	0	0 or ↓
autonomic	vagal	↓	0	↓	0	↑
	sympathetic	0	0	↓	↓	0
contractility	inotropic	↓	0	↓	↑ then ↓	↓
hemodynamic	cardiac output	↓	0 or ↓	↓	↑ then ↓	↓
	blood pressure	↓	0 or ↓	↓	↓	↓

should be cautiously used in asthmatics. Theophylline will block the electrophysiologic effects of adenosine.

Proarrhythmia

Decreased use of antiarrhythmics in the last few years is due to increased awareness of the proarrhythmic activity of these drugs. "Proarrhythmic" means that the drugs may cause arrhythmias, which is not the desired outcome when you are giving them to decrease arrhythmias. Arrhythmias can even be a sign of antiarrhythmic drug toxicity. If that is the case, it is an indication to change a drug dose rather than add a new antiarrhythmic to treat a symptom of antiarrhythmic toxicity. The antiarrhythmic digoxin is an example of a drug that can cause arrhythmias when given in toxic doses.

Have you ever thought of this drug paradox? Administered appropriately and monitored appropriately, drugs can save lives. Administered inappropriately or monitored inappropriately, they can take lives. You may think that you aren't too involved with cardiovascular drugs, but statistics on heart disease tell us differently. How would you know if a patient on digoxin with arrhythmias had digoxin-induced arrhythmias or not?

While it would be nice to have a cookbook approach to arrhythmias, from the information presented so far you can see why this is not possible. Likewise, it is not possible to have a black-and-white table that matches type of arrhythmia with drug or antiarrhythmic drug class. The most specific antiarrhythmic drug use information that matches arrhythmia with drug is found in the ACLS guidelines, which will be covered in Chapter 15.

CONGESTIVE HEART FAILURE

Definition

Congestive heart failure (CHF) is one the more common cardiac diseases. Congestive heart failure occurs when ventricles are not able to pump enough blood to supply the body. The loss of contractility or pump efficiency makes the blood volume increase within the heart, and the heart eventually enlarges. This means that less blood gets to other parts of the body where it is needed and also causes the kidney to change fluid regulation. The kidney, sensing a lack of perfusion, retains fluid to increase vascular volume to attempt to increase perfusion. This now puts more stress on the heart and exacerbates the CHF and edema. As a result, edema occurs in the gravity-dependent extremities such as the ankles, and if CHF is left untreated, the fluid builds up within the lungs and can result in pulmonary edema.

CHF can be right- or left-sided heart failure, and symptoms may vary for each. Since drugs can cause CHF by inhibiting myocardial contractility or expanding plasma volume, drug-induced CHF must be ruled out before treatment occurs.

Drugs to Treat CHF

Pharmacological treatment for CHF consists of removal of sodium and water with diuretics, increasing contraction of the heart with positive inotropic activity, and decreasing vascular resistance with vasodilators. **Afterload** is the force against which the heart must pump, and **preload** is the amount of blood in the ventricles before contraction. When volume increases secondary to sodium and water retention, the preload increases. Afterload increases can be caused by peripheral vasoconstriction. By decreasing preload and afterload, vasodilators can be effective treatment for CHF. In essence, they open up the pipes (vessels), thus decreasing the resistance to blood flow. Basically, heart failure drugs improve heart contractility and decrease the heart's work (see Figure 9-4).

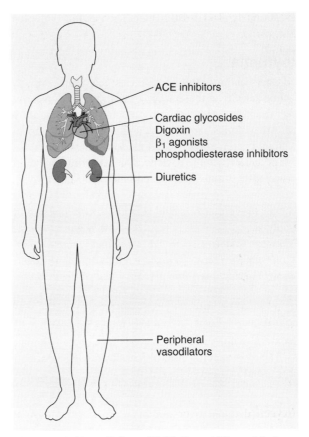

Figure 9-4 Heart Failure (CHF) Drugs' Sites of Action

Digoxin as an Inotrope

Digoxin is one of the oldest inotropic drugs known to man. Inotropes increase the peak tension produced by the heart during systolic contraction. This allows the heart to more effectively pump blood. As mentioned previously in this chapter, digoxin increases calcium availability for contracting, which leads to enhanced force of contraction.

Digoxin has both mechanical and electrical effects in the heart. Digoxin's electrical effects occur because an increase in parasympathetic stimulation in the heart decreases firing in the AV node (negative dromotropic effect). This is beneficial, because it allows for more effective ventricular filling time. Concurrently, the mechanical action of digoxin increases cardiac contractility, so the heart will pump stronger. This increased cardiac contractility coupled with better filling volume results in increased ventricular ejection, increased cardiac output, and increased renal blood flow. This also results in decreased compensatory sympathetic and renal response, because the kidneys now are better perfused.

$\diamond$ CONTROVERSY $\diamond$

Digoxin's use for CHF goes in and out of favor depending on the latest research. Research results differ as to whether the drug increases survival or just improves quality of life.

ACE Inhibitors for CHF

Angiotensin-converting enzyme (ACE) inhibitors decrease blood levels of angiotensin II. Angiotensin II is a vasoconstrictor, and therefore blocking its production induces vasodilation. Angiotensin II also promotes sodium retention and increases norepinephrine release. Because vasoconstriction increases systemic vascular resistance in heart failure and causes an increased workload, promoting vasodilation by inhibiting angiotensin II is beneficial.

ACE inhibitors have no direct positive inotropic effects, but they decrease aldosterone secretion, salt and water retention, and vascular resistance. ACE inhibitors decrease afterload and alter structural changes in the congested heart by remodeling. They decrease symptoms and are shown to prolong life in patients with CHF. ACE inhibitors probably have fewer potential side effects than digoxin, and these include dry nonproductive cough, worsening of renal function, proteinuria, and hyperkalemia. The increased potassium can be beneficial when ACE inhibitors are used concurrently with a diuretic for CHF, which may lower serum potassium levels.

Dobutamine for CHF

℞ β_1-agonists, such as **dobutamine,** are used for acute patients with congestive heart failure. Dobutamine is a β_1-agonist with some β_2-adrenergic activity that was developed because the β_1-agonist isoproterenol caused too many arrhythmias. Dobutamine increases cardiac output and decreases left ventricular filling pressure. Since dobutamine increases cardiac output without increasing oxygen demand or decreasing coronary blood flow by tachycardia, it is useful in heart failure after MI. There are no endogenous catecholamines released by dobutamine administration, so it has advantages relating to myocardial oxygen demand over norepinephrine and dopamine. It is only available for intravenous administration.

Dopamine for CHF

℞ **Dopamine** is a precursor of norepinephrine and releases endogenous norepinephrine. Depending on the dose, dopamine stimulates dopaminergic, β_1-, and α-adrenergic receptors. Dopamine affects dopamine receptors at low doses to improve renal blood flow. At high doses, it acts as an inotrope by stimulating β receptors. Dopamine infusions should not be abruptly discontinued.

Nitroprusside for CHF

℞ Intravenous **nitroprusside** dilates both arterial and venous vessels, so it decreases afterload and preload. The drug is not stable in the presence of heat or light, which is a disadvantage in its use. The main side effect is hypotension, which will decrease cardiac output.

Beta Antagonists for CHF

CLINICAL PEARL
Many cardiac problems are attributable to poor health habits or bad genes or a combination of both. It is easy for patients to think medications for heart problems are magic bullets and will allow them to ignore diet and exercise. Diet and exercise are important treatment components of cardiovascular disease.

Beta blockers are also used occasionally for CHF, even though it seems a contradiction in terms to have the choice of both an agonist and an antagonist for the same disease. Beta blockers may be beneficial in CHF by slowing the heart rate to allow more time for complete ventricular filling, reducing myocardial oxygen demand, and controlling blood pressure. Since the body's normal physiologic response to decreased cardiac output is activation of the sympathetic nervous system, the use of beta blockers may make ℞ sense. **Carvedilol** (Coreg) is a beta blocker with alpha-blocking and therefore vasodilator properties.

Vasodilators for CHF

Vasodilators can greatly reduce the afterload forces upon the heart. Three classes of vasodilators are used. Vasodilators decrease afterload by:

- dilating arterial vessels (hydralazine)
- dilating venous vessels and decreasing preload (nitrates)
- affecting both arterial and venous vessels (ACE inhibitors)
- dilating arterial vessels (calcium-channel blockers)

 Hydralazine, the prototype arteriole dilator, is especially beneficial in reducing pulmonary vascular resistance in patients with severe pulmonary hypertension. Hydralazine can cause some fluid retention, which may result in the need for increased diuretic doses. It can also cause a reflex tachycardia, which may benefit from concurrent use of a beta blocker.

Nitrates complement hydralazine and are used topically or orally. The vasodilator nitroglycerin dilates arterioles (reducing afterload) and increases efficiency by affecting venous return (reducing preload returning to heart). By decreasing afterload and preload simultaneously, it increases cardiac output by decreasing systemic vascular resistance, and it relieves ventricular congestion through decreased venous return.

As already described, ACE inhibitors inhibit the angiotensin-converting enzyme. That enzyme is responsible for degradation of bradykinin and other vasodilators. Beneficial effects of lower pulmonary capillary wedge pressure and systemic vascular resistance result, as well as an increased cardiac index. While hemodynamic tolerance occurs with other vasodilators, ACE inhibitors usually produce a greater response with time.

Calcium-channel blockers can cause afterload reduction by dilating arterial vessels and therefore relieve CHF symptoms. They do not affect preload. Not all calcium-channel blockers are equally effective for CHF. Use of these drugs is limited by their negative inotropic effect.

Phosphodiesterase Inhibitors for CHF

Phosphodiesterase inhibitors increase cAMP levels by inhibiting its breakdown by the enzyme phosphodiesterase. This results in increased vascular smooth muscle relaxation and increase in heart contractility. Examples of phosphodiesterase inhibitors include **amrinone** (Inocor) and **milrinone** (Primacor). Both are available for parenteral administration. The main side effects are arrhythmias and hypotension.

Diuretics for CHF

The drug class most all physicians prescribe and agree on for CHF is diuretics to get rid of excess volume that increases the workload of the heart. The risk of diuresis in CHF is volume depletion and decreased cardiac output. Diuretic side effects can include azotemia, dehydration, hypokalemia, hyponatremia, hypochloremic alkalosis, hypomagnesemia, hyperglycemia, and hyperuricemia. Despite the risk of hypokalemia, not all patients will require potassium supplements. Automatically initiating potassium concurrently with a diuretic is therefore not recommended. Hyperkalemia can be just as dangerous as hypokalemia.

IV diuresis is quicker but not necessarily more efficient. Diuretic doses are usually given early in the day to prevent nocturnal diuresis. Objective monitoring of diuretics in CHF would include weight loss, and decrease in edema and breath sounds associated with pulmonary edema. Because different diuretics may have different mechanisms of action, as discussed later, combination use of two diuretics concurrently may be rational. See Figure 9-5 for a breakdown of the drugs used to treat CHF.

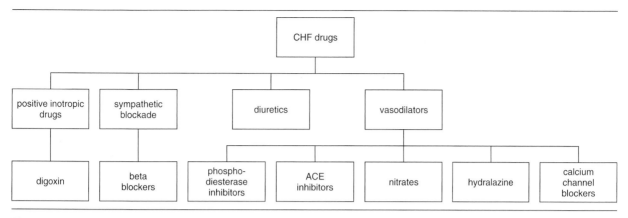

Figure 9-5   Subgroups of Drugs for CHF

RENAL PHARMACOLOGY

Renal Physiology

To understand renal pharmacology, it is important to review the basics of renal physiology. Kidneys rid the body of waste products through filtration of the blood. In addition, the kidneys maintain fluid and electrolyte and acid–base balance. The kidney is primarily thought of as an excretory organ; it also plays an important role in drug elimination.

The functional unit of the kidney is the nephron, which is comprised of the glomerulus, proximal convoluted tubule, the loop of Henle, the distal convoluted tubule, and the collecting duct. As blood is filtered in the glomerulus, it then drains into the tubular systems, where parts of the filtrate can be reabsorbed back into the blood via the peritubular capillary system. The filtrate remaining in the tubular system is excreted via the urine. See Figure 9-6 for an illustration of the nepron.

Electrolytes or salts that are filtered are usually reabsorbed at a certain site along the kidney. Electrolytes regulate acid–base balance and affect neuromuscular activity. Blood volume is regulated by sodium and water reabsorption, which are affected by osmosis and concentration gradients and influenced by antidiuretic hormone (ADH) and aldosterone. Renal secretion of electrolytes is also important in helping to control the acid–base balance of the body.

Diuretics basically do not allow sodium to be reabsorbed back into the peritubular capillary system (bloodstream). If sodium stays within the tubular system, it draws water via osmosis into the tubular system, which is then excreted as increased urine output.

All diuretics increase salt and water excretion, but the effect diuretics have on other ions depends on the diuretic. Diuretics are classified according to the site in the nephron where they work. Since the mechanisms of reabsorption of sodium and water and chloride and potassium are different in each of the segments of the kidney, diuretics acting on different segments have different mechanisms.

Specific Diuretics

The three main groups of diuretics, based on their site of action within the nephron are the thiazide, loop, and potassium-sparing diuretics. The thiazide diuretics increase the excretion of sodium and therefore water at the distal convoluted tubule. Examples of thiazide diuretics include:

- **chlorothiazide** (Diuril)
- **hydrochlorothiazide** (HydroDiuril)

LEARNING HINT

To get a visual picture, imagine the tubular system as PVC piping—you know, the white plastic kind used for drains like under your sink. Now wrap red yarn all around it to represent the peritubular capillary system. What stays in the pipe gets excreted from the body via urination or goes down the drain. What gets "reabsorbed" (via capillary diffusion) goes into the red yarn to be re-circulated in the bloodstream.

℞

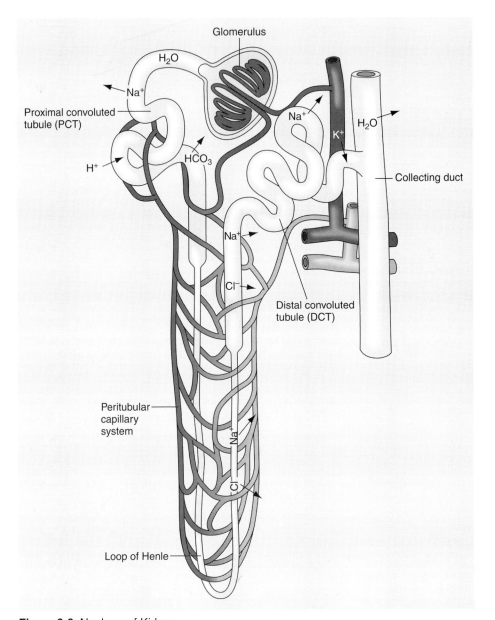

Figure 9-6 Nephron of Kidney

Loop diuretics increase sodium and water excretion at the proximal and distal tubules and the loop of Henle by blocking reabsorption of sodium into the bloodstream. These are the most potent diuretics. Examples of loop diuretics include:

℞
- **Bumetanide** (Bumex)
- **Furosemide** (Lasix)

Potassium-sparing diuretics do not allow potassium to be excreted along with the sodium as thiazides or loop diuretics do. The excessive loss of potassium leading to hypokalemia can have serious cardiac effects. Patients on thiazide or loop diuretics may be given potassium supplements or may take a potassium-sparing diuretic alone or in combination with other diuretics. Potassium-sparing diuretics include:

- **amiloride** (Midamor)
- **spironolactone** (Aldactone)
- **triamterene** (Dyrenium)

Other Renal Medications

Other renal medications primarily include drugs used to treat urinary tract infections (UTIs), urinary analgesics, and benign prostatic hypertrophy (BPH). Systemic antibiotics and sulfonamides are primarily used to treat UTIs. Urinary analgesics are indicated for burning and painful urination. BPH is common in men over age 50 and occurs when the prostrate enlarges, making urination difficult. BPH drugs inhibit the enzyme that leads to hormonal changes to enlarge the prostrate. The main drug in this category is finasteride (Proscar), which must be given for 6 to 12 months to see if it is effective in prostrate size reduction.

SHOCK MANAGEMENT

Shock is a potentially fatal condition in which tissues are poorly perfused. Treatment consists of oxygenation, blood pressure support, and maintaining acid–base balance. Different kinds of shock, such as cardiogenic or hypovolemic, may be treated differently. Some of the same drugs discussed for CHF are used for shock. Vasopressors (agents that vasoconstrict) improve cardiac function by stimulating adrenergic receptors. When peripheral vasoconstriction occurs, blood is shunted to the heart and lungs. You will find more on the treatment of shock in the chapter on advanced cardiac life support (ACLS).

Does it seem odd that a vasoconstrictor would be used to treat a condition characterized by poor tissue perfusion? The price paid for this may be ischemic damage peripherally. Can you understand why?

ANGINA

Angina Pathophysiology

Angina or chest pain is a symptom of myocardial ischemia, or lack of oxygen, which occurs when oxygen supply and demand in the heart are unbalanced. The heart, like any muscle, needs oxygen and vital nutrients to function; these are supplied by the coronary arteries. Coronary blood flow is closely related to myocardial oxygen consumption. It is regulated physiologically by physical factors and vascular, neural, and humoral control. If the heart cannot respond to changes in demand or supply through increased blood flow because of occlusion of a coronary artery, a heart attack occurs. Drug therapy of angina is aimed at decreasing consumption of oxygen by the heart or increasing the delivery of oxygen to the heart. How much oxygen the heart needs is determined by contractility, rate of contraction, and the heart wall tension.

Pharmacologic Treatment of Angina

Pharmacological treatment of angina is aimed at pain relief and prevention of recurrent pain. **Nitroglycerin** administered sublingually is used for quick relief, since drug absorption is fast through this route. Nitrates such as nitroglycerin reduce preload and afterload by dilating both veins and arteries, thus decreasing cardiac workload. Prophylactic treatment of angina is given by calcium entry blockers, beta blockers, or nitrates. Since myocardial ischemia can result from different mechanisms, it makes sense to use antianginals that work by different mechanisms.

See Figure 9-7 for a breakdown of the drug groups to treat angina.

Beta Blockers as Antianginals

β receptors are connected to adenyl cyclase by a G protein. When a β-agonist binds with the receptor, the G protein tells adenyl cyclase to make cyclic adenosine monophosphate (cAMP). The new molecule then acts like a messenger in the cell and can cause hyperpolarization of some parts of the heart. This can be a problem if the heart is damaged or hypoxic. β receptor activation can also cause cardiac metabolism to increase and require more oxygen.

Beta blockers decrease myocardial oxygen consumption by decreasing heart rate, contractility, blood pressure, and afterload, especially during exercise. They also decrease catecholamines in the ischemic heart. For these reasons, beta blockers used in myocardial infarction patients can limit infarct size and decrease the incidence of arrhythmias. Beta blockers are used for prophylaxis of angina to decrease frequency and severity of attacks.

Beta blockers can cause bradycardia and exacerbation of chest pain on drug withdrawal unless a drug taper is scheduled. Beta blockers are contraindicated in patients with bronchial asthma or pulmonary disease that is due to induced bronchoconstriction. If a beta blocker is needed for angina in a patient with bronchial constriction, a selective β_1-agent is preferred. In addition to their β receptor selectivity, beta blockers differ in their duration of action, pharmacokinetics, and price.

Calcium-Channel Blockers as Antianginals

Calcium-channel blockers inhibit the calcium influx into muscle that initiates contraction. They are also vasodilators, since they act directly on vascular smooth muscle. As noted in the antiarrhythmic section of this chapter, they also decrease contractility, AV conduction, and automaticity.

Since calcium-channel blockers decrease myocardial oxygen demand by reducing afterload, contractility, and heart rate, you might expect this drug class to have the same benefits in an acute MI as beta blockers. While studies in lab and animal data do show this, clinical conditions do not, which is always the dilemma when evaluating medical literature. Within the calcium-channel blocker class, drugs differ in how much vasodilation and cardiac suppression individual agents cause. See Table 9-4 for comparison of Calcium-Channel Blockers.

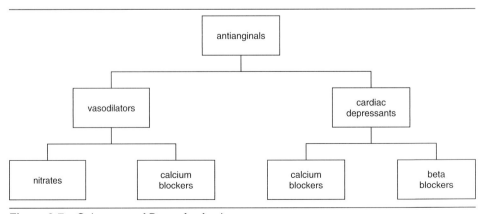

Figure 9-7   Subgroups of Drugs for Angina

Table 9-4   Comparison of Calcium-Channel Blockers

	Diltiazem	*Nifedipine*	*Verapamil*
coronary vasodilation	+++	+++	++
peripheral vasodilation	+	+++	++
contractility	0	↑↓	↓

Nitroglycerin as an Antianginal

Nitroglycerin works like the naturally occurring vasodilator endothelium-derived relaxing factor to relax smooth muscle (vascular and nonvascular). It works to increase cGMP formation by the release of nitric oxide from nitrates. Relaxation is probably due to cAMP activation of protein kinase. Relaxation causes a decrease in heart-wall tension and reduction of preload, with a lesser decrease in afterload. Nitroglycerin causes a reflex tachycardia, which can outweigh its beneficial effects. This is why combination use of nitrates and beta blockers, which slow the heart rate, can be beneficial.

Venodilation also causes orthostatic hypotension and headache. Since it affects nonvascular smooth muscle, relaxation of the bronchi and other smooth muscles can occur. Since heart pain and heartburn symptoms can be very similar, a response to nitroglycerin may not allow you to distinguish cardiac from GI pain. Chronic administration of nitrates can lead to tolerance and lessened effects, as discussed in Chapter 1. This is prevented by a daily nitrate-free interval, such as removing a topical patch at night or not taking the last oral dose after 7:00 p.m. at night. See Table 9-5 for an Antianginals comparison.

Table 9-5   Antianginals Comparison

	Contractility	*Afterload*	*Preload*	*HR*
calcium channel blockers	↓	↓		
β-adrenergic blockers	↓	↓		↓
nitrates		↓	↓	↑

MYOCARDIAL INFARCTION

Treatment goals for acute MI are to save the myocardium, preserve left ventricular function, and reduce the risk of complications. Treatment strategies used include reperfusion therapy and antithrombosis and anti-ischemic therapy. Some of the same drugs discussed in the angina section are used for MI. The reperfusion therapy and antithrombosis therapies will be discussed in the next chapter.

ACE Inhibitors After MI

ACE inhibitors used post-MI in patients with reduced left ventricle function cause decreased mortality if used within the first 2 weeks post-MI. For every 1,000 patients treated, five lives would be saved by doing so. This kind of cost–benefit decision-making is often used when prescribing medications. Obviously, if you were one of the five whose life was saved, the cost of the drug would be worth the benefit. For the other 995 patients, though, drug costs can be expensive without the benefit. Good medical studies are designed to provide information as specific as possible to identify those who would actually benefit from drug therapy.

SUMMARY

To facilitate a complete understanding of complex drug classifications for heart and kidney medications, this chapter related cardiac and renal physiology to pharmacology and explored the interrelationships of the cardiovascular, respiratory, and renal systems. Various agents to treat various cardiac arrhythmias, congestive heart failure, myocardial infarction, and angina were discussed, with emphasis on their mechanisms of action. Several of the medications had multiple indications and multiple mechanisms of action, with ACE inhibitors being a classic example. Cardiovascular agents demonstrate that drug use is frequently controversial and always requires a balance between efficacy and toxicity. Keep this in mind as you continue on to yet more cardiovascular pharmacotherapy in the next chapter.

REVIEW QUESTIONS

1. A 68-year-old patient was started on digoxin for CHF yesterday. Today he is complaining of swollen ankles and respiratory difficulty. Auscultation reveals diffuse crackles suggesting lung fluid. What could be possible causes?
   (a) positive inotropic effect
   (b) subtherapeutic digoxin level
   (c) new-onset asthma triggered by digoxin
   (d) diuresis

2. Match diuretic drug name with class:
   thiazide   furosemide
   loop   triamterene
   K-sparing   chlorothiazide

3. Match term with cardiac function:
   chronotropic   rate
   inotropic   rhythm
   dromotropic   force of contraction

4. Arrhythmias can occur:
   (a) in normal hearts
   (b) in abnormal hearts
   (c) with symptoms
   (d) without symptoms
   (e) all of the above

5. Vasodilators for CHF may include:
   (a) digoxin
   (b) propranolol
   (c) hydralazine
   (d) atropine
   (e) all of the above

6. What are some of the issues to consider when considering whether or not to use an antiarrhythmic?

7. Explain the rationale for combination use of nitrates and hydralazine for CHF.

8. Describe different mechanisms of action for antianginals as they relate to mechanisms of cardiac ischemia.

9. Describe how antiarrhythmics differ from each other.

10. What is a proarrhythmia?

CASE STUDY

An elderly female presents to the ER with complaints of shortness of breath and pedal edema (swollen ankles). Breath sounds show diffuse crackles, suggesting pulmonary congestion. She is being treated with a diuretic and vasodilator. What potential medical problems may she have? What is the role and pharmacological effect of a diuretic and vasodilator for the medical condition you have hypothesized? What would be some side effects to watch for? What are other drug options if her current therapy isn't effective?

GLOSSARY

arrhythmia   any deviation from the normal ECG tracing.

afterload   force against which the heart must pump, including tension that develops in ventricular wall during systole.

preload   filling pressure of the heart during diastole.

conduction   transmission of electrical impulses through fibers in the heart, causing heart muscle contraction.

vasodilator   a drug that selectively dilates blood vessels.

inotropic   affecting force or energy of cardiac conduction.

chronotropic   affecting time or rate of cardiac contractions.

dromotropic   a drug that alters rhythm or electrical conduction of the heart.

action potential   change in membrane voltage that occurs with cardiac conduction.

proarrhythmia   arrhythmia induced by antiarrhythmic drugs.

refractory period   period of time before a new action potential can be initiated.

www.prenhall.com/colbert

Use the address above to access the free, interactive Companion Web site created specifically for this textbook. Enhance your studying by viewing videos and animations, answering practice quiz questions, and reviewing an audio glossary and much more related to Chapter 9.

CHAPTER 10

Blood Pressure and Antithrombotic Agents

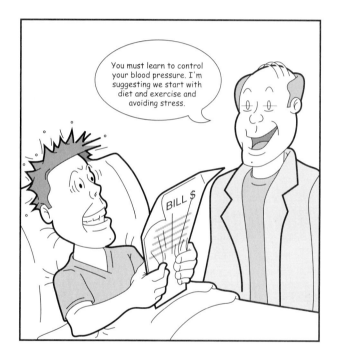

OBJECTIVES

Upon completion of this chapter you will be able to

- Define key terms related to blood pressure and thrombosis
- Relate cardiovascular physiology to pharmacological treatments
- Understand the variables that affect blood pressure
- Describe indications and pharmacological effects of various types of antihypertensive agents
- Describe indications and pharmacological effects of anticoagulants, antiplatelet agents, and thrombolytic agents

ABBREVIATIONS

BP	blood pressure	ACE	angiotensin-converting enzyme
CO	cardiac output	ICP	Intracranial pressure

PTT	Partial thromboplastin time	JNC	Joint National Committee
GP IIb/IIIa inhibitors	glycoprotein IIb/IIIa receptor inhibitors	DVT	deep vein thrombosis
CCB	calcium-channel blocker	tPA	tissue plasminogen activators
PT	prothrombin time	CNS	central nervous system
INR	international normalized ratio	CHF	congestive heart failure
		ECG	electocardiogram
TPR	total peripheral resistance	TOD	target organ disease

INTRODUCTION

Chapter 9 focused on drugs that affect the heart. This chapter will focus on regulating the pressure within the cardiovascular system. The drugs that regulate pressure within the cardiovascular system will primarily affect sympathetic tone, the diameter of the blood vessels, or the actual blood volume. In addition, this chapter will discuss agents to ensure the blood itself will flow freely through blood vessels and not be affected by intravascular blood clots. Anticoagulants will prevent vascular clots from ever forming or extending and/or breaking off to form a clot to block vital blood flow to tissues and organs. In addition, this chapter will discuss thrombolytic agents that will dissolve already existing blood clots, as well as antiplatelet agents that prevent adhesion and aggregation of platelets.

BLOOD PRESSURE

The Basics

The cardiovascular system must be pressurized in order for blood to flow throughout it and provide vital gas exchange, nutrients, immunologic defense, etc. Too much pressure can be disruptive and have serious consequences, whereas too little pressure will not allow enough perfusion to vital areas such as the brain or kidneys and can again have dire consequences.

The heart, as discussed in Chapter 9, is the pump that is connected to a roadway of blood vessels traveling throughout the body. Circulatory flow results as pressure differences are created within the system by the cardiac contraction. The vessels offer varying resistance to flow depending on their diameter or level of dilation or constriction. Just as the heart can be broken down into a right- and left-sided pump with different purposes, the circulatory system can be divided between the pulmonary vascular and systemic vascular systems. The pulmonary vascular system represents the vessels that flow through the lungs for gas exchange. The systemic vascular system comprises all the other vessels that supply all the tissues and organs with blood flow (perfusion). Each system contains arteries, arterioles (small arteries), veins, venules (small veins), and capillaries.

The Blood Vessels

A layer of endothelial cells lines each vessel within the vascular system. This layer is a passive barrier keeping cells and proteins from going into tissues; it also contains substances that control the contraction of underlying smooth muscle, such as prostacyclin (vasodilator), nitric oxide (vasodilator), and endothelin (vasoconstrictor) (see Figure 10-1). Notice that in Figure 10-1, the walls of arteries, arterioles, veins, and venules all contain smooth muscle but in different proportions. The capillaries contain no smooth muscle, since this would act as a diffusion barrier to the vital gas exchange that occurs within capillaries.

The sympathetic nervous system, discussed in Chapter 3, controls the activity of smooth muscle. Both neural and humoral (circulating within the blood) mechanisms control blood vessel contraction. Because the arterioles contain more smooth muscle and are

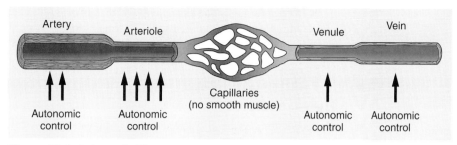

Figure 10-1 Schematic Diagram of Various Blood Vessels

under more nervous system control, they are the main resistance vessels and regulate the force against which the heart must pump, or the **afterload.** If the arterioles are vaso-constricted, this will narrow the circulatory highway, thereby increasing afterload and systemic vascular resistance. This leads to an increase in blood pressure. Conversely, vasodilation would relax the smooth muscle layers in the vessels and thereby reduce afterload and lower blood pressure. Arterioles branch into capillaries at the tissues where vital gas exchange takes place, and the blood now delivers its oxygen and picks up the waste carbon dioxide.

The systemic venules and veins then collect the deoxygenated blood from the tissue sites and return it to the right side of the heart to be pumped through the pulmonary vascular system to gain vital oxygen (inhalation) and rid the body of waste carbon dioxide (exhalation). The systemic veins and venules have a large capacity to hold blood and relatively little musculature as compared to arteries and arterioles and therefore can distend much easier without major pressure changes. The veins are therefore considered capacitance vessels; they regulate **preload.** Preload is the amount of blood returning to the heart and contained in the ventricles prior to a contraction.

Compliance is the extent to which the volume of the vascular system increases as pressure increases. More work is needed to push blood through a constricted vessel, so in that case the compliance is decreased, resulting in a greater pressure. If the compliance increases and the vessels vasodilate, the pressure will be reduced.

Thus far we have focused on the systemic vascular system; however, it is important to note that pressure must also be regulated within the pulmonary vascular system, and this will be discussed in later chapters. Finally, the kidneys play a role in regulating blood pressure in addition to their other roles of ridding the body of waste products, drug excretion, and maintaining fluid, electrolyte, and acid–base balance. This will be discussed later in this chapter.

Blood Pressure Regulation

Blood pressure is controlled by centers in the brain that respond to changes in the **baroreceptors** (pressure sensors) in the arterial system. Baroreceptor reflexes are the primary autonomic mechanism for blood pressure homeostasis. These reflexes react to input from the carotid sinus and output from parasympathetic and sympathetic nerves to maintain blood pressure control. If the baroreceptors are stretched too far, thus sensing high pressure, they send signals that will decrease sympathetic tone and thus reduce blood pressure. If the receptors sense low pressure, they will increase sympathetic tone to increase blood pressure and maintain perfusion.

A mathematical relationship describing blood pressure is helpful in understanding the various ways pharmacological control of blood pressure can be exerted. The equation is as follows:

blood pressure (BP) = cardiac output (CO) $\times$ total peripheral resistance (TPR)

LEARNING HINT

A balloon represents a good way to understand these relationships. A new balloon is very noncompliant, so it takes more pressure to inflate. If we stretch the balloon (vasodilate) it, it then becomes more compliant and takes less pressure to inflate. A good disease analogy would be an aneurysm, which is like a weak patch in a balloon. This section is too compliant, and high pressures (hypertension) could cause it to burst.

From this equation, it's simple to see that anything that increases CO or TPR will increase blood pressure and vice versa. Cardiac output, as established in Chapter 9, is directly related to heart rate and stroke volume. Therefore, anything that decreases heart rate, diminishes stroke volume, or decreases total peripheral resistance will lower blood pressure.

Hypertension

CLINICAL PEARL

Many people with hypertension are asymptomatic, yet other people with hypertension complain of a pounding in their heads. If pressure increases in your arms or legs, there is a certain "give," since the tissues are not rigid, so some of the pressure increases will dissipate. However, the skull does not allow this flexibility, and small increases in cerebral blood flow or pressure can increase the intracranial pressure (ICP) dramatically.

Hypertension can be characterized by an elevation in systolic blood pressure, diastolic blood pressure, or both. It is classified into three stages which guide therapy. There are various causes of hypertension. If no specific cause can be found for the hypertension, it is termed **essential hypertension,** and this represents the majority of patients who have hypertension.

<CONTROVERSY>

Some of the etiologic factors that may contribute to the pathophysiology of hypertension are subject to debate, and they include the following: defective baroreceptors, defective kidney response to fluid and electrolytes, excess sodium, potassium depletion, and even low calcium in the diet.

Because the disease is frequently asymptomatic, hypertension is frequently called the "silent killer." This is because hypertension is one of the leading causes of stroke, blindness, congestive heart failure, and renal disease. If hypertension goes untreated, target organ disease (TOD) can result. Target organ disease may include, for example, left ventricular hypertrophy, transient ischemic attacks, peripheral vascular disease, retinopathy, or protein in the urine. If TOD is present at the time of diagnosis, it suggests that hypertension has been present long-term but not treated adequately.

Antihypertensives work on different parts of the blood pressure equation to either decrease cardiac output or decrease total peripheral resistance (see Figure 10-2, which shows the relationship between antihypertensive agents and the blood pressure equation). By looking at Figure 10-2, you can more clearly see the potential role for combination antihypertensive therapy that uses two drugs that work on different parts of the equation.

How would you explain the importance of treating a potentially asymptomatic disease like hypertension to a newly diagnosed patient?

Before discussing the various pharmacological agents to treat hypertension, it should be noted that nonpharmacologic treatment is preferred if possible. By using lifestyle changes such as exercise, weight loss, alcohol restriction, smoking cessation, and salt restriction, patients may be able to control high blood pressure or decrease the amount of drug needed to control the disease. Unfortunately, not all patients are salt-sensitive, meaning that some patients don't benefit from salt restriction as much as others. The different mechanisms for the pathophysiology of hypertension may explain why patients respond differently to nonpharmacological treatment as well as different antihypertensives.

If the hypertension cannot be treated effectively nonpharmacologically, then initial drug therapy is individualized according to patient age, race, pathophysiology, presence of TOD, and concurrent compelling medical conditions.

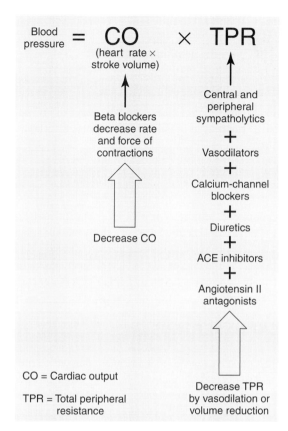

Figure 10-2 Relationship Between Antihypertensive Agents and Blood Pressure Equation

Depending on the stage of hypertension and the presence or absence of TOD, an initial decision is made to treat by lifestyle changes alone or drug therapy concurrently. By looking at Table 10-1, you can see that the higher the blood pressure, the sooner drug treatment is started, rather than waiting for lifestyle changes to work. An example of a treatment choice based on concurrent compelling medical condition would be a hypertensive patient with congestive heart failure. This patient would most likely be started on an ACE inhibitor since this drug could treat both medical conditions. If single-drug therapy is not successful, then additional drugs from a different class or a new drug from a different class are given until the right combination works. The various types of antihypertensive agents include the following: (1) central- and (2) peripheral-acting sympatholytics, (3) beta blockers, (4) diuretics, (5) ACE inhibitors, (6) angiotensin II antagonists, (7) calcium-channel blockers, and (8) vasodilators. See Table 10-1 for the classification and recommendations for initial treatment of hypertension.

Table 10-1   Recommendations for Initial Treatment of Hypertension

Blood Pressure Category	*No Target Organ Disease*	*Target Organ Disease*
High normal (130–139/85–89)	lifestyle change	drug therapy
Stage 1 (140–159/90–99)	lifestyle change	drug therapy
Stages 2 and 3 ($\geq$160/$\geq$100)	drug therapy	drug therapy

Source: The Sixth Report of the Joint National Committee on Prevention, Detection, Evaluation, and Treatment of High Blood Pressure. Arch Intern Med 1997;157:2413–2445. ©2000, Pinnacle Health System.

www.prenhall.com/colbert

The Joint National Committee (JNC)-VI on the Treatment, Prevention, Detection, Evaluation, and Treatment of High Blood Pressure is the most current reference for hypertension treatment guidelines. Check the algorithms used in selecting which antihypertensive is preferred in individual patients and why.

> CONTROVERSY

JNC-VI recommends diuretics or beta blockers for first-line antihypertensive therapy. This is because those drugs have been proven in scientific studies to decrease strokes, heart failure, and total mortality. Prescribers do not always follow those recommendations, and the choice of which antihypertensive to start individual patients on is considered controversial, despite JNC-VI recommendations.

DRUG CATEGORIES TO TREAT HYPERTENSION

CLINICAL PEARL

Clonidine can also be used to treat nicotine withdrawal for patients quitting smoking or going through opiate withdrawal. It is proposed to work by decreasing the noradrenergic hyperactivity common in those situations.

CLINICAL PEARL

Alpha blockers used for hypertension are also effective for benign prostatic hypertrophy. They work because the prostate has α receptors whose blockade results in decreased smooth muscle tone and less obstruction. Treating two diseases with one drug is like killing two birds with one stone. What a terrible saying!

From Chapter 3, you have learned that any agent that would inhibit sympathetic nerve function would result in decreased venous tone, decreased heart rate, decreased contractility of the heart, decreased cardiac output, and decreased total peripheral resistance. On this basis, it only makes sense that sympatholytics would be used as antihypertensives. Sympatholytic antihypertensives are classified by their central (the brain) or peripheral (circulating vessels) site or mechanism of action. These antihypertensive agents affect the α or β receptors.

Direct-Acting, α_2-Agonists, or Central-Acting Sympatholytics

Central-acting agents work directly on the α_2 receptors found within the CNS to decrease sympathetic outflow of activity from the CNS. α_2 receptors, when stimulated, block the release of norepinephrine. Remember that norepinephrine is an endogenous vasoconstrictor, and thus its blockage would cause vasodilation and reduce blood pressure. α_2-selective agonists such as clonidine therefore decrease centrally controlled sympathetic outflow from the brain, thus resulting in decreased cardiac output and decreased vascular resistance.

Rebound hypertension may occur when a central α_2-agonist is discontinued. This means that the blood pressure can overshoot and become higher than it was before treatment. Although commonly mentioned with this drug class, it may occur with any antihypertensive class. Another side effect to be aware of with this class and all anti-hypertensives is orthostatic hypotension. Orthostatic hypotension occurs when blood pressure drops as patients move from sitting to standing position. Patients should always rise slowly from a horizontal or sitting position to minimize dizziness that may accompany the orthostasis and lead to falls. Common types of central-acting or α_2-agonists are:

℞

- **clonidine** (Catapres)
- **guanfacine** (Tenex)

α_1-Blockers or Peripheral-Acting Sympatholytics

α_1 receptors are found mainly within the blood vessels themselves, and their stimulation causes vasoconstriction. However, α_1 blockers or antagonists block receptors in both arterioles and veins, thus causing vasodilation. α_1 blockers such as prazosin therefore decrease vascular resistance. Alpha blockers are well known for their ability to cause orthostatic hypotension, especially with the first dose. Patients should always be counseled to take their first dose at bedtime as a method to lessen first-dose hypotension. Some common α_1 blockers or peripheral-acting sympatholytics are:

R̥

- **prazosin** (Minipress)
- **terazosin** (Hytrin)
- **doxazosin** (Cardura)

Beta Blockers

β_1 receptors are found primarily within the heart, and their stimulation leads to an increase in the rate and force of contraction. Beta blockers would therefore inhibit sympathetic activity and decrease the rate and force of contraction, thus lowering blood pressure.

Beta blockers need to be cautiously used in patients with peripheral vascular disease and insulin-dependent diabetics. This is because beta blockers can exacerbate symptoms of arterial insufficiency and mask warning signs of hypoglycemia. Beta blockers can also cause bradycardia or atrioventricular conduction abnormalities. Some common beta blockers include:

R̥

- **metoprolol** (Lopressor)
- **propranolol** (Inderal)
- **atenolol** (Tenormin)

See Figure 10-3, which illustrates the sites of action of sympatholytic antihypertensive agents.

Diuretics

As discussed in Chapter 9, diuretics are used to treat edema associated with CHF as well as to treat hypertension. Diuretics lower blood volume by increasing sodium and water excretion and will therefore lower blood pressure. There are three different classes of diuretics used to treat hypertension: thiazides, loop, and potassium-sparing. Different diuretics work on different sites in the kidney. Blood pressure–lowering effects are not necessarily dose related. There can be a ceiling effect for drugs, as in the thiazide class of diuretics, where increased doses just cause more side effects and do not lower blood pressure. Thiazide diuretics are preferred over other diuretic classes in mild to moderate hypertension, as they are more effective than loop diuretics for this indication.

Loop diuretics such as furosemide (Lasix) can be used for hypertension, but they have a shorter duration of action than thiazide diuretics. Loop diuretics are also useful in the treatment of edema and acute pulmonary edema. In that situation, in addition to diuresing, they act as pulmonary vasodilators, so they will decrease the pulmonary system pressure rise found in pulmonary edema. Loop diuretics are also used in the treatment of hypercalcemia of malignancy to lower calcium levels.

Potassium-sparing diuretics such as spironolactone (Aldactone) may be administered in combination with other diuretics to prevent potassium depletion. They have a weak antihypertensive effect when used alone but can be additive with thiazide or loop diuretics. Thiazide and loop diuretics both cause potassium loss and are not potassium-sparing.

Side effects of diuretics include hypokalemia, hypomagnesemia, hyperuricemia, and hyperglycemia. Loop diuretics cause less hyperglycemia and differ from thiazides in that

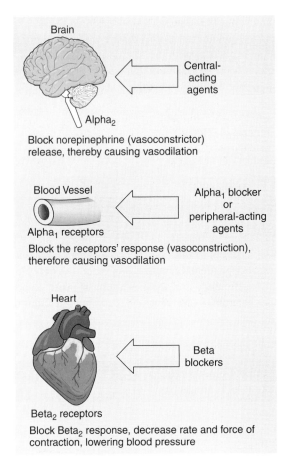

Figure 10-3 Sites of Action of Sympatholytic Antihypertensive Agents

they cause hypocalcemia, while thiazides can be calcium-sparing. Common diuretics include:

- **furosemide** (Lasix)
- **hydrochlorothiazide** (HydroDiuril)
- **spironolactone** (Aldactone)
- **amiloride** (Midamor)

STOP & REVIEW

How do diuretics differ from each other?

Angiotensin-Converting Enzyme (ACE) Inhibitors

The kidneys are involved in blood pressure regulation through the renin–angiotensin system. They release renin into the bloodstream when renal blood flow decreases. Renin acts on angiotensinogen (also known as angiotensin precursor) in the bloodstream to form angiotensin I. It is then converted to angiotensin II as it circulates through the lungs, and angiotensin II is a powerful vasoconstrictor. Angiotensin II also causes the release of the hormone aldosterone, which increases sodium and water reabsorption into the bloodstream. The increased blood volume, along with the vasoconstriction, will increase the blood pressure. ACE inhibitors decrease blood levels of angiotensin II and aldosterone by interrupting the renin–angiotensin–aldosterone system and thereby lower blood pressure. They reduce peripheral arterial resistance without affecting heart rate and cardiac output.

These drugs can have a 30% incidence of cough as a side effect. Cough can occur after anywhere from 1 week to 6 months of therapy and is more common in women than in men. Another side effect of ACE inhibitors is hyperkalemia, especially in patients with decreased renal function. They can also cause renal damage even though they are also used to protect renal function (renal sparing), and they decrease protein loss in the urine in patients with diabetes. Common ACE inhibitors include:

℞
- **benazepril** (Lotensin)
- **captopril** (Capoten)
- **enalapril** (Vasotec)

Angiotensin II Receptor Blockers

Angiotensin II antagonists inhibit angiotensin II at receptor sites on the blood vessels and therefore act differently than ACE inhibitors. They are an alternative for patients with a cough side effect from an ACE inhibitor. Representative drugs in this category include:

℞
- **losartan** (Cozaar)
- **valsartan** (Diovan)

See Figure 10-4, which shows the site and mechanism of action of diuretics, ACE inhibitors, and angiotensin II receptor blockers.

Calcium-Channel Blockers (CCBs)

CCBs produce arteriole relaxation by the same mechanisms they use to relieve angina. By blocking calcium needed for contractility, they relax vascular smooth muscle, and therefore vasodilation results. Any effects related to the drug's action on calcium in smooth muscle are unrelated to dietary calcium.

The most common side effects of CCBs are peripheral edema and dizziness. As explained in the arrhythmia section of Chapter 9, CCBs have different effects on heart rate and atrioventricular nodal conduction. This may cause side effects when used for hypertension. Common CCBs include:

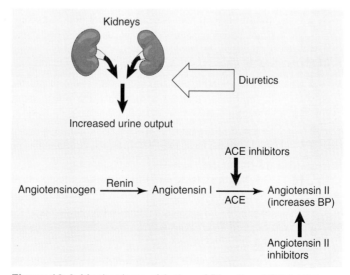

Figure 10-4 Mechanisms of Action of Diuretics, ACE Inhibitors, and Angiotension II Inhibitors

℞

- **amlodipine** (Norvasc)
- **diltiazem** (Cardizem)
- **verapamil** (Calan)

Vasodilators

Vasodilators such as hydralazine are more effective at relaxing the smooth muscle in arteries than in veins. Vasodilators are usually considered last-line for nonacute hypertension treatment.

Vasodilators can cause a reflex tachycardia and peripheral edema. For those reasons, they are frequently used in combination with a beta blocker and a diuretic. One vasodilator you may recognize by name is minoxidil. One of minoxidil's side effects is hypertrichosis, or increased hair growth. Drug manufacturers capitalize on this side effect and market minoxidil (Rogaine) for male-pattern baldness. Rogaine's vasodilator action reestablishes blood flow to the hair follicles of some individuals when applied topically. Common vasodilators include:

℞

- **hydralazine** (Apresoline)
- **minoxidil** (Loniten)

After reading about all the side effects from blood pressure medications and reading about hypertension being a silent killer, how would you explain the importance of treatment compliance with antihypertensives?

Agents for Hypertensive Emergencies/Urgencies

Although hypertensive emergency and urgency sound like the same condition by name, they are different medical conditions and are treated differently. They differ not so much by an absolute blood pressure value but by the absence or presence of neurological symptoms along with the elevated blood pressure. Physicians will do an ophthalmologic exam to detect eye changes that may be present with neurological symptoms. This can guide treatment aggressiveness and drug therapy selection.

If there is a rapid rise in blood pressure, it can become an immediately life-threatening condition requiring fast-acting treatment. Stroke or death may occur if not treated. Other times blood pressure rise may be just as high quantitatively but may have occurred more gradually and may therefore require a slower decrease. In this case, too rapid a reduction in blood pressure can be dangerous. Both oral and parenteral antihypertensive drugs are options, depending on the situation. The oral antihypertensives clonidine or captopril have been given in loading doses to achieve a fast response.

℞ **Diazoxide** (Hyperstat) is a long-acting direct-acting parenteral arteriole vasodilator. Because of the rapid reduction in blood pressure, one must monitor BP and ECG changes, as the patient may become severely hypotensive. Diazoxide increases plasma volume, so it is common to use a diuretic concurrently.

℞ **Nitroprusside sodium** (Nipride, Nitropress) is another potent agent used for minute-to-minute control of hypertension. Nipride is a potent vasodilator that dilates both venous and arterial vessels and has an immediate onset of action, within 30 to 60 seconds. Its most common side effect is too rapid a reduction in blood pressure, which as previously mentioned can be dangerous.

℞ **Nitroglycerin IV** dilates both arterioles and veins, reducing both preload and afterload. It is especially useful when hypertension occurs concurrently with myocardial ischemia. See Table 10-2, which puts all the various categories of antihypertensive agents, along with representative drugs, in one rather large table.

Table 10-2   Categories of Antihypertensive Agents with Representative Drugs

Class	Action	Generic	Brand Name
Sympatholytics (central)	decrease in sympathetic outflow from brain	guanfacine clonidine	Tenex Catapres
Sympatholytics (peripheral)	peripheral vasodilation	doxazosin prazosin terazosin	Cardura Minipress Hytrin
Beta blockers	decrease in CO	acebutolol atenolol metoprolol propranolol	Sectral Tenormin Lopressor Inderal
Diuretics	decrease in blood volume	thiazides furosemide spironolactone	Diuril Lasix Aldactone
ACE inhibitors	vasodilation	benazepril captopril enalapril	Lotensin Capoten Vasotec
Angiotensin II antagonists	vasodilation	losartan valsartan	Cozaar Diovan
Calcium-channel blockers	vasodilation	amlodipine verapamil diltiazem	Norvasc Calan Cardizem
Vasodilators	direct relaxation of smooth muscle	hydralazine minoxidil	Apresoline Loniten
Emergency/urgency hypertensives	acute vasodilation	nitroprusside diazoxide nitroglycerin IV	Nipride Hyperstat

www.prenhall.com/colbert

Hyperlipidemia is a general term for elevated serum cholesterol levels, which can increase blood pressure by clogging the arteries (arteriosclerosis). Go to the Web site to learn more about hyperlipidemia and the drugs used to treat this condition.

Treating Hypotension

The treatment of hypotension and shock will be covered in Chapter 15 on advanced cardiac life support (ACLS). These drugs are primarily vasopressor and cardiotonic agents. Vasopressor drugs increase smooth muscle tone and thus cause vasoconstriction. Cardiotonic agents stimulate the heart to increase the rate and/or force of contraction of the heart to increase blood pressure and perfusion.

THE HEMOSTATIC SYSTEM

The Clotting Process

One of the amazing things about blood is its ability to normally flow freely through blood vessels and yet to clot when the need occurs. The hemostatic system's job is to maintain fluidity of blood within the vasculature and minimize blood loss when blood leaks outside the vessels by clotting. Without the clotting mechanism, a minor cut would cause us to literally bleed to death. However, the clotting mechanism, like all physiologic mechanisms, can get out of balance owing to disease states or other factors. If a clot forms within a blood vessel or an organ cavity such as the heart, it is termed a thrombus. This intravascular clot can partially or totally occlude the blood flow, which will diminish or stop the supply to the local tissue being fed by this vessel. Lack of blood flow will lead to infarction and subsequent tissue necrosis.

The thrombus can dislodge and travel through the bloodstream. A traveling thrombus is called a **thromboembolism.** The thromboembolism will continue to move along the bloodstream until it reaches a vessel where its size matches the vessel's diameter, and it will eventually obstruct and totally occlude blood flow beyond the obstruction. This has very serious consequences, especially since many emboli may reach the lungs (pulmonary emboli) or brain (cerebral emboli) and cause serious irreversible tissue damage. The goal of anticoagulant therapy is to prevent clot formation in patients at risk and to prevent clot extension and embolization.

A thrombus can form because of local trauma to a blood vessel. This stimulates the specialized thrombocytes or platelets within the blood to bind together or aggregate, forming a sticky gelatinous mass to begin to plug the leak. Platelet aggregation also causes the release of thromboplastin, which begins a cascade of steps that are simplified as follows:

CLINICAL PEARL

An embolism is a general term for an obstruction of a blood vessel by a foreign substance. This can be fat or even a gas bubble. A thromboembolism refers specifically to a blood clot.

1. Thromboplastin forms in the presence of Vitamin K (released from aggregating platelets).
2. Prothrombin, in the presence of thromboplastin and calcium, forms thrombin.
3. Fibrinogen, in the presence of thrombin, forms fibrin, which causes the clot.

Vascular stasis or turbulent flow such as occurs in atherosclerotic disease and anything that damages the inner lining of the blood vessels can cause platelet aggregation and subsequent release of thromboplastin. Vascular clots can form in the venous or arterial system. Venous clots usually occur due to stasis, since it is a relatively low pressure/low flow system. Platelet aggregation usually occurs in the higher flow/higher pressure of the arterial systems.

Three categories of drugs are used to treat or prevent the formation of thrombi. **Anticoagulants** prevent the formation of the fibrin clot by interfering with one of the steps leading up to fibrin formation. **Antiplatelets** inhibit the aggregation and release of thromboplastin to begin the process. Finally, **thrombolytics** (fibrinolytics) actually dissolve and liquefy the fibrin of the existing clot.

Anticoagulants

Anticoagulants are distinguished as either indirect or direct thrombin inhibitors. Indirect thrombin inhibitors include warfarin, unfractionated heparin, and low molecular weight heparin. Direct thrombin inhibitors include lepirudin, argatroban, and bivalirudin. Anticoagulants inhibit steps in the clotting cascade leading to fibrin formation and *do not* dissolve existing clots. They do prevent new clots from forming as well as the extension of existing clots. They prevent mostly venous thrombosis formation. Anticoagulants are primarily used prophylactically to prevent deep venous thrombosis (DVT), prevent clots forming postoperatively after heart, valve, or vascular surgery, and decrease the risk of further clots in stroke patients. Candidates for anticoagulants may have any of the following:

- history of embolus formation
- prolonged bed rest
- coronary artery disease
- venous thrombosis
- phlebitis
- surgery with previous history for thrombosis (especially pelvic surgery)

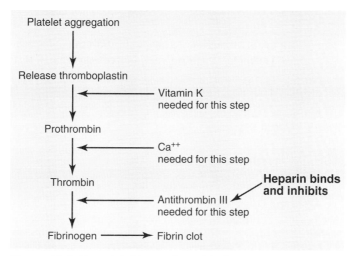

Figure 10-5 Heparin's Mechanism of Action

Heparin. Standard heparin (unfractionated) is a parenteral anticoagulant that binds with antithrombin III to inhibit the conversion by thrombin of fibrinogen to fibrin. See Figure 10-5 for an illustration of its mechanism of action.

Heparin is a naturally occurring substance in our mast cells and is broken down in the stomach, so it is only effective as an injectable medication. Low-dose subcutaneous heparin is used to prevent venous thromboembolism in immobile, bedridden patients postoperatively. IV boluses or infusions of heparin are used to treat pulmonary emboli. Heparin is also used to prevent clots in cannulas or may be included in an IV or in procedures such as hemodialysis. In arterial blood kits, needles are heparinized to prevent clotting from occurring and blocking the return of blood into the syringe.

The therapeutic goals, depending on the heparin indication, are aimed at increasing clotting time two to three times normal. The partial thromboplastin time (PTT) lab test is used to make dosage adjustments for heparin. The PTT time should be maintained at 2 to 2.5 times its normal value of 22 to 37 seconds. The PTT lab test is different from the Prothrombin Time (PT) lab test, which is used to make dosage adjustments for warfarin. The PT measures the vitamin K–dependent factors. It has been largely replaced by the more reliable International Normalized Ratio (INR), which will be discussed later with warfarin.

Heparin Side Effects. Standard heparin doesn't cross the placental barrier, has a rapid action, and is readily excreted (because the body recognizes it). However, bleeding is the most important side effect of heparin. Watch for bleeding in the mucosa (petechiae) and gums and for hematuria and GI bleeding. An antidote for excess bleeding is **protamine sulfate,** which complexes with heparin to antagonize its action.

Heparin can cause thrombocytopenia and even osteoporosis with long-term use. Heparin is contraindicated in any active bleeding or thrombocytopenia. Use of heparin with brain, eye, or spinal cord surgery can be very risky, since the slightest bleed can increase intracranial pressure greatly.

Low molecular weight heparins (LMWH) are the more modern version of heparin. These agents differ in their antithrombotic properties, pharmacokinetics, side effects, and monitoring. They are also referred to as unfractionated heparin (UFH). As suggested by the name, LMWH is smaller in weight than standard heparin. This allows LMWH to have a different antithrombotic effect that is as effective as standard heparin but may have fewer side effects and less need for monitoring.

℞

CLINICAL PEARL

Protamine, which is derived from salmon sperm, is an anticoagulant alone, but given with heparin neutralizes its effects. This reversal agent acts instantaneously and is long acting.

Representative drugs in the heparin group are:

R

- **Standard Unfractionated heparin sodium** (Calciparine)
- **Low Molecular Weight Fractionated enoxaparin** (Lovenox)

What precautions would you take if you were obtaining an arterial blood gas from someone on heparin?

Warfarin. The warfain agents are oral anticoagulants. Warfarin acts differently than heparin and works on vitamin K–dependent liver synthesis of certain clotting factors by inhibiting vitamin K, which is vital to the clotting process (See Figure 10-6 for this mechanism).

Warfarin is used to prevent blood clots in patients with various medical conditions, such as atrial fibrillation, a prosthetic mechanical heart valve, or stroke. Depending on the indication, the goal INR (international normalized ratio) may be 2 to 3 times normal or higher. Chronic warfarin therapy requires monthly lab monitoring and frequent dosage manipulations, since anything that affects clotting factors in the liver will affect the body's response to warfarin.

CLINICAL PEARL

Warfarin is an oral anticoagulant that is sometimes referred to by patients as rat poison, because the active components are similar. This drug was discovered when cattle died mysteriously after eating sweet clover. It turned out that the sweet clover was spoiled. This led to the isolation of the chemical components of the spoiled sweet clover and development of oral anticoagulants.

< CONTROVERSY >

There are legitimate questions about whether warfarin or aspirin is better and/or safer at preventing blood clots in atrial fibrillation. Consensus guidelines are published periodically to make treatment recommendations, yet they are not always followed by physicians because of this controversy.

Warfarin Interactions and Side Effects

Diet drug interactions with warfarin are important. Anything that increases vitamin K, such as yellow or green leafy vegetables can also affect warfarin response. This can be used advantageously in cases of over-anticoagulation by administering pharmacological doses of vitamin K. Patients on anticoagulants need to be monitored for bleeding gums, nose bleeds, petechiae, or blood in the urine or stools. Before surgery or certain dental procedures, war-

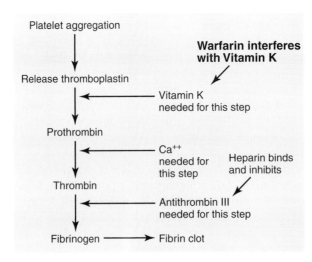

Figure 10-6 Warfarin's Mechanism of Action

farin patients may need to hold doses. Any drug has the potential to interact with warfarin on the basis of the mechanistic principles described in Chapter 1. Most, but not all, patients on warfarin are instructed not to take aspirin concurrently, since it may increase bleeding potential.

www.prenhall.com/colbert

On the Web site you will find long lists of drugs that interact with warfarin but frequently must be taken concurrently. You will also find current consensus recommendations for warfarin use and goals of therapy.

A representative drug includes:

R̥

• **warfarin** (Coumadin)

R̥ *Lepirudin.* The direct thrombin inhibitor **lepirudin** has distinct pharmacological properties relating to how it interacts with thrombin. This drug may be used in conjunction with aspirin in patients with unstable angina who are undergoing percutaneous transluminal coronary angioplasty (PTCA) or as an alternative to heparin in patients with heparin-induced thrombocytopenia. In the future it may have a role as an alternative to warfarin.

What is the difference between the PT, PTT, and INR lab tests, and why are they important to pharmacotherapy?

Antiplatelet Drugs

Antiplatelet agents inhibit the platelet phase of clotting (See Figure 10-7). Antiplatelet drugs are also called antithrombotic drugs and include aspirin. Aspirin irreversibly inhibits the enzyme prostaglandin synthetase, which is required for thromboplastin release. This means that once aspirin is taken, a platelet will be affected by aspirin's antiplatelet effects

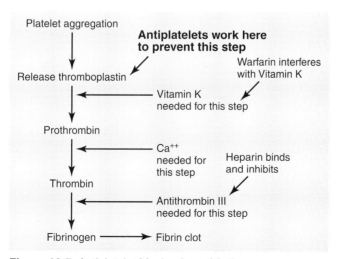

Figure 10-7 Antiplatelet Mechanism of Action

for the lifetime of that platelet. The cardioprotective effects of an aspirin a day warrant that most patients, with few exceptions, take daily low-dose aspirin. One of the controversies addressed in the consensus guidelines on the Web is whether a baby aspirin is enough or whether a full dose of aspirin is needed.

Besides aspirin, antiplatelet representative drugs include:

℞

- **dipyridamole** (Persantine)
- **ticlopidine** (Ticlid)
- **clopidogrel** (Plavix)

These drugs are usually used if patients "fail" or still have symptoms on aspirin or don't tolerate aspirin.

Glycoprotein IIb/IIIa Platelet Receptor Inhibitors
Platelet glycoprotein (GP) IIb/IIIa receptor inhibitors are a new class of drugs administered parenterally. They bind with and block GP IIb/IIIa receptors, which initiate platelet aggregation. They are used in unstable angina and myocardial infarction, and they have been used concurrently with heparin.

Representative GP IIb/IIIa platelet receptor inhibitors include:

℞

- **tirofiban** (Aggrastat)
- **eptifibatide** (Integrilin)

Thrombolytics

Thrombolytics stimulate fibrinolytic mechanisms to dissolve existing clots. Pharmacological thrombolysis occurs when plasminogen is converted to plasmin, an enzyme that digests fibrin strands. In essence, thrombolytics promote the lysis of the fibrin to a gel or liquid, thereby dissolving the existing clot. Thrombolytics are used in patients with acute myocardial infarction, because they lyse the thrombus that caused the infarction and can reduce mortality and salvage heart tissue by reperfusion. These drugs dissolve existing clots but do not affect the underlying cause of the occlusion.

There are different generations of thrombolytics, each generation striving to be better than the previous. Improvements include things like longer half-life, bolus IV administration, and fewer side effects. Bolus administration is easier and quicker, so you have a faster "door-to-needle time." This is important, since the goal is to treat myocardial infarction patients as early as possible after the onset of chest pain.

There are two main types of thrombolytics: enzymes and tissue plasminogen activators (tPAs). The enzyme thrombolytic streptokinase is derived from streptococcus and can cause antigenicity, making repeat administration not safe. Urokinase is isolated from urine or kidney cultures. The tPAs are produced commercially by DNA technology. Cost is the predominant selection criterion influencing which thrombolytic is used most often. Since thrombolytics can't differentiate between pathologic clots and hemostatic plugs, the biggest complication of thrombolytics is bleeding. Representive thrombolytics include:

LEARNING HINT

Notice that all these drugs end in "ase," which is a formal suffix denoting an enzyme.

℞

- **alteplase** (Activase) (tPA)
- **reteplase** (Retavase) (tPA)
- **urokinase** (Abbokinase) (thrombolytic enzyme)
- **streptokinase** (Streptase) (thrombolytic enzyme)

See Table 10-3 for a summary of the classes of antithrombotic agents.

Table 10-3   Classes and Representative Drugs Used for Antithrombotic Therapy

Class	Generic	Brand Name
Anticoagulant agents	heparin sodium	Calciparine
	enoxaparin	Lovenox
	warfarin sodium	Coumadin
	lepirudin	Refludan
Antiplatelet agents	aspirin	
	dipyridamole	Persantine
	ticlopidine	Ticlid
	clopidogrel	Plavix
Thrombolytic agents	alteplase	Activase
	reteplase	Retavase
	urokinase	Abbokinase
	streptokinase	Streptase
Glycoprotein IIb/IIIa platelet receptor inhibitors	tirofiban	Aggrastat
	eptifibatide	Integrilin

www.prenhall.com/colbert

Thrombolytics are a very dynamic group of drugs. On the Web site, you can see the most current drugs available. You will also see an example of a treatment algorithm.

SUMMARY

This chapter concluded a two-chapter sequence on cardiac pharmacotherapy. Antihypertensives, anticoagulants, antiplatelet agents, and thrombolytic agents have greatly influenced cardiac morbidity and mortality. The high prevalence of the conditions these drugs are used to treat indicates that you will encounter these drugs frequently in your professional practice and even in your personal life.

REVIEW QUESTIONS

1. Nonpharmacological approaches to hypertensive treatment include:
   (a) fluid restriction
   (b) salt supplementation
   (c) exercise
   (d) folic acid
   (e) vitamin C
2. Which of the following is not an antihypertensive drug class?
   (a) beta agonist
   (b) beta blocker
   (c) alpha agonist
   (d) alpha blocker
   (e) diuretic
3. Sympatholytics:
   (a) decrease venous tone
   (b) increase heart rate
   (c) increase cardiac contractility
   (d) increase total peripheral resistance
   (e) increase cerebral blood flow
4. Diuretics
   (a) can cause hyperkalemia
   (b) have dose-related antihypertensive effects

(c) are classified by where they work in the kidney

(d) should not be used with other anti-hypertensives

(e) b and c

5. ACE inhibitors:

(a) may cause a cough

(b) may cause hypokalemia

(c) increase aldosterone

(d) work the same as angiotensin II receptor blockers

(e) may cause CHF

6. Explain the mathematical equation that describes blood pressure and how it relates to antihypertensive therapy.

7. Discuss the factors that influence which antihypertensive is used in an individual.

8. Explain the steps involved in platelet aggregation and clot formation.

9. Describe three categories of drugs used to treat or prevent thrombus formation.

10. A 47-year-old male presents with mild hypertension without target organ disease (TOD). Is pharmacotherapy indicated at this point? If not, what suggestions would you make?

11. A 53-year-old female patient with past medical history of pulmonary emboli is admitted for pelvic surgery. What prophylactic pharmacotherapy may be indicated presurgery? What would be the therapeutic goal? What tests would help to confirm the effectiveness of the presurgical medications? If a pulmonary embolism did develop, what medications may now be indicated? If this patient is discharged to home, what medications may be prescribed and what precautions emphasized?

GLOSSARY

afterload   force against which the heart must pump, including tension that develops in ventricular wall during systole.

anticoagulant   drug used to prevent formation of fibrin clot.

antiplatelet   drug used to inhibit platelets' release and aggregation.

baroreceptors   homeostatic mechanism the body uses to maintain blood pressure.

compliance   flexibility of the blood vessels responding to pressure.

essential hypertension   high blood pressure with no identifiable cause.

hypertension   high blood pressure.

preload   filling pressure of the heart during diastole.

thromboembolism   a traveling thrombus that leads to obstruction and blood flow occlusion.

thrombolytic   drug used to dissolve the fibrin of an existing clot.

www.prenhall.com/colbert

Use the address above to access the free, interactive Companion Web site created specifically for this textbook. Enhance your studying by viewing videos and animations, answering practice quiz questions, and reviewing an audio glossary and much more related to Chapter 10.

CHAPTER 11

Neuromuscular, Anesthetic, Sedative, and Analgesic Agents

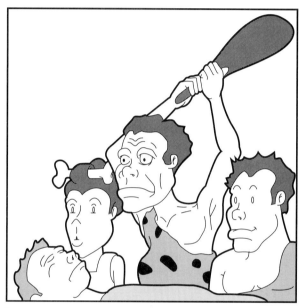

Dr. Aagh, the first anesthesiologist, demonstrating his techniques.

OBJECTIVES

Upon completion of this chapter you will be able to

- Apply the principles of nerve transmission to pharmacology of neuromuscular blocking drugs
- Describe the clinical applications of neuromuscular blocking drugs
- Discuss the mechanisms of action of medications that are hypnotic, sedative, or anxiolytic and their importance in cardiorespiratory practice
- Describe the mechanism and role for ventilatory stimulants
- Explain the pain pathway (nociceptive pathway) and the role of medications that are used as analgesics
- Discuss the role of medications used for general anesthesia and distinguish them from local anesthesia

Main contributing author Roger G. Hefflinger

ABBREVIATIONS

NSAID	nonsteroidal anti-inflammatory drugs	PCA	patient-controlled analgesia
GABA	γ-aminobutyric acid	COX	cyclooxygenase
DTs	delirium tremors	REM	rapid eye movement
Benzos	benzodiazepines	ACh	acetylcholine
CNS	central nervous system	AChE	acetylcholinesterase
MAC	minimum alveolar concentration	FDA	Food and Drug Administration
		NMBD	neuromuscular blocking drugs
		TOF	train of four
CSF	cerebrospinal fluid	NMBA	neuromuscular blocking agents

INTRODUCTION

Healthcare professionals are responsible for the safe administration of all medications utilized in the provision of patient care. There is no better example of the complete control healthcare providers have than the case of general anesthesia, or when medications are administered to cause paralysis of respiratory muscles. If a patient were not on ventilatory support in either of these circumstances, rapid death would ensue. To appreciate and understand the pharmacologic activities of these medications, it is imperative to have a thorough understanding of nervous system transmission, explained previously in Chapter 3 but to be reviewed briefly in this chapter.

Many medications covered in this chapter will somehow influence muscle contraction or patient sensorium. Drug classes in this chapter are commonly used to facilitate ventilation. In some situations, in order to achieve effective ventilation, the muscles around the airway must be relaxed. Sometimes, relaxation and sedation of the individual person alone is enough to provide sufficient muscle relaxation for the situation, although at other times complete and total respiratory paralysis is the desired outcome to reduce the work of breathing and decrease oxygen consumption. Once the patient and/or respiratory muscles are relaxed and ventilation is appropriately controlled, there is frequently a need to decrease the pain associated with invasive cardiorespiratory procedures. This is accomplished by using analgesics or local anesthesia. If the need is broader, general or surgical anesthesia is used, and the practitioner must make decisions about using intravenous or inhalational routes. There may also be a need for sedation, so sedatives, anxiolytics, and hypnotics will be discussed in this chapter. The consequences of drugs from each of these classes for blood pressure and heart rate must be considered, not just the isolated respiratory effects. In each situation a different drug and dose would be indicated.

This chapter will also discuss the role of opioid and nonopioid pain medications and their corresponding relationship to the cardiorespiratory system. For completeness and balance to the discussion of all these drugs, which potentially cause respiratory depression, this chapter will also discuss the role of ventilatory pharmacological stimulants.

NERVE TRANSMISSION

Physiology of Muscle Contraction

Agents that affect skeletal muscle contraction affect the somatic part of the peripheral nervous system. As you recall from Chapter 3, the somatic nervous system originates in the CNS and is the portion of the nervous system that is responsible for skeletal and respiratory muscle activity.

Nerve conduction occurs when ions move across cells, and electrical energy moving along the fiber results in eventual interaction at the target organ. That target organ may be another nerve junction, as in the case of the ganglia, or it may be a target organ such as muscle in the eye, arms, legs, or diaphragm. When a nerve impulse reaches the end of the fiber, it is converted into a chemical that facilitates the impulse propagation. There are a variety of types of nerve fibers as well as chemicals that help to continue the impulse. These nervous system chemicals are called neurotransmitters.

Nerve conduction only occurs when there is a precise transfer of electrolytes such as potassium and sodium, which results in cellular depolarization. Cells have a particular electrical charge at which a cell is most likely to depolarize; this is called threshold level. When electrical energy moves along the fiber and is depolarized, there is a time period when that nerve can't accept any more electrolyte transfer. This time period is called the refractory period. Once depolarization and muscle contraction occur, repolarization must now take place. All of this occurs faster than the time it takes you to read about it. The traveling of the impulse down the fiber is referred to as an **action potential.**

The nerve junction with skeletal muscles is referred to as the motor end plate. This is where the binding sites for acetylcholine are located. When these receptors are stimulated, they will become activated, and acetylcholine will be released into the synapse and allow for calcium influx. Depolarization of the muscle fiber occurs when calcium is released. Calcium is required for the contractile proteins actin and myosin to interact, resulting in muscle contraction (see Figure 11-1, which illustrates this process).

Different tissues specialize in conduction of different impulses. In Chapter 9, we talked about cardiac muscle and its action potential and refractory periods. In that case, the different action potential and refractory period were what maintained a proper balance between the stimulation of the cardiac muscle and the contraction of the heart as an effective pump. In this case, the same can be said about the proper balance of skeletal muscle contraction and relaxation.

From this discussion, you can see that several things can happen at the neuromuscular junction. Cholinergic agonists can stimulate more acetylcholine (ACh) and thus facilitate muscle contraction. Conversely, agents can be given to decrease levels of ACh or block its action and thus result in neuromuscular blockade, which inhibits muscle contraction.

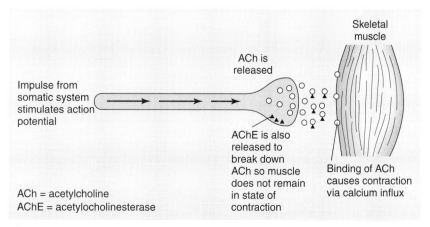

Figure 11-1 Nervous Transmission and Muscle Contraction

Acetylcholinesterase (AChE)

Acetylcholinesterase (AChE) breaks down acetylcholine, ending the contraction, or else we would be in a constant state of contraction. AChE is the enzyme that inactivates acetylcholine to relax the muscle, end the contraction, and result in a resting state. When AChE is inhibited, there is increased acetylcholine available at the muscle end plate. Drugs can stimulate muscles by stopping the breakdown of ACh by the AChE enzyme. This makes impulse transmission easier and makes the duration of action of acetylcholine longer. For this reason, cholinesterase inhibitors are considered cholinergic stimulants.

Neuromuscular Blocking Drugs

Neuromuscular blocking agents have several indications pre- and postoperatively and in the emergency and critical care departments. One of the factors that has influenced neuromuscular blockade use over the years has been the method of ventilation available. The more the patient "fought the ventilator," the more likely pharmacologic paralysis was needed. Depending on what mechanical ventilation mode is in vogue, future neuromuscular blockade use may or may not increase in intensive care settings for patients on ventilators. For example, when pressure-controlled inverse ratio ventilation is used, heavier sedation and paralysis may be needed.

By paralyzing chest wall muscles, practitioners can alleviate problems associated with the patient being out of place with the ventilator. Depending on the situation, bolus doses for short-term or infusions for longer use are used. It's unusual to need these drugs for longer than 72 hours. Neuromuscular blocking agents (NMBAs) are beneficial in ventilation therapy because they (1) reduce spontaneous breathing, (2) prevent movement that can dislodge chest tubes, (3) reduce oxygen consumption in patients with poor cardiopulmonary function, and (4) improve patient synchrony, thereby reducing the pressure needed for mechanical ventilation. NMBAs are also used to facilitate endotracheal intubation as a one-time dose.

Now that we've talked in generalities about NMBA uses, let's get specific about the pharmacology of different types of neuromuscular blockers. We will then pick up again with some clinical applications. Neuromuscular blockers can be classified as **nondepolarizing** or **depolarizing agents,** and we will discuss them according to this classification.

Nondepolarizing Agents

Nondepolarizing agents are competitive antagonists and bind to the receptor sites that acetylcholine would occupy. If a binding site is occupied by a nondepolarizing neuro-

Table 11-1   Neuromuscular Blocking Agents

Generic	*Trade*
Depolarizing neuromuscular blocking agents	
succinylcholine	Anectine
Nondepolarizing neuromuscular blocking agents	
pancuronium	Pavulon
vecuronium	Norcuron
atracurium	Tracrium
rocuronium	Zemuron
rapacuronium	Raplon
mivacurium	Mivacron
cisatracurium	Nimbex
doxacurium	Nuromax

muscular blocking agent, acetylcholine can't stimulate the muscle, and muscle paralysis results. The drugs are called nondepolarizing because they prevent the motor endplate from depolarizing. These drugs are competitive antagonists, which means their effect can be reversed if more acetycholine is available to compete at the receptor site.

Nondepolarizing agents are nonselective in cholinergic receptor stimulation, which means they will bind with other cholinergic sites that stimulate parasympathetic responses, as in the heart. This is what causes side effects such as hypotension and tachycardia, and one factor that influences selection of NMBAs.

Nondepolarizing agents can be reversed. This is useful in situations of toxicity or side effects. The antidote for a nondepolarizer's neuromuscular blockade would be to increase ACh levels at receptor sites. Neuromuscular blocking action ceases when the drug's plasma concentrations decline via metabolism or the effect is reversed by cholinesterase inhibitors. These inhibitors inhibit the enzyme acetylcholinesterase, which breaks down acetylcholine. More acetylcholine is then available to compete with the neuromuscular blocker. During the reversal situation, it's important to recover spontaneous ventilation and neuromuscular transmission before the artificial ventilation is discontinued. Examples of nondepolarizing agents include pancuronium, rocuronium, and rapacuronium, to name a few. Examples of agents that reverse neuromuscular blockade or cholinesterase inhibitors include **neostigmine** and **pyridostigmine**.

What respiratory intervention is needed for patients on a nondepolarizing agent?

Depolarizing Agents

Depolarizing agents are agonists that actually bind to the ACh receptor sites and initiate a massive depolarization of the muscle, which then sends it into a prolonged refractory period. Muscle twitching (fasciculation) takes place, followed by complete muscle paralysis. This is different from nondepolarizing agents, which don't cause the initial muscle fasciculations and go straight to muscle paralysis.

Depolarizing neuromuscular blocking agents such as succinylcholine bind with cholinergic receptors and start depolarization by causing total body muscle contraction, followed by muscle paralysis. This lasts until the binding of the receptor by the depolarizing agent ends, or the drug is inactivated by the enzyme pseudocholinesterase. Cholinesterase inhibitors can't reverse the effects of depolarizing neuromuscular blocking agents the way they can for nondepolarizing agents. Since depolarizing agents have a short duration of action, this is not a problem clinically, except in those rare patients who have a genetic deficiency of the pseudocholinesterase enzyme. In those cases, paralysis can last for hours.

Neuromuscular blockers may have drug interactions with inhalation anesthetics, antibiotics, and other drugs, so they require close monitoring and dosing. Neuromuscular blockade is monitored clinically and subjectively by patient movement (or lack thereof) and objectively by nerve stimulation with a peripheral nerve stimulator.

www.prenhall.com/colbert

To learn more about monitoring neuromuscular blockers via a peripheral nerve stimulator and a specific monitoring technique called the train of four (TOF), go to the Web.

CLINICAL PEARL

To fasciculate or not to fasciculate? Fasciculations may increase gastric pressure and put a patient at risk for gastric reflux, which could lead to aspiration.

CLINICAL PEARL

Even anesthesia in the dentist's office requires strict monitoring. A 17-year-old undergoing dental surgery was given succinylcholine and had to be resuscitated and ventilated after finding out the hard way that she had a genetic deficiency of the pseudocholinesterase enzyme. There is a lab test available to identify whether this deficiency is present and may therefore result in this adverse effect of succinylcholine.

Neuromuscular blocking agents are classified not only by the type of block produced (either depolarizing or nondepolarizing), but also by chemical structure, side effects, duration of action, and onset of action. See Table 11-2 for a comparison of neuromuscular blocking agents.

NMBD Selection Factors

Before administering a drug, it's important to know which patients should or should not receive a drug and which patients might be at risk. The ideal NMBA is one that is not influenced by the liver or renal dysfunction common in acutely ill patients and one that doesn't have the vagolytic activity that increases heart rate or releases histamine to cause hypotension or reflex tachycardia. It's also important to know what other drugs the patient is on to avoid drug interactions. Neuromuscular blocking drugs may have drug interactions with inhalation anesthetics, antibiotics, and other drugs.

All patients that receive NMBAs should receive sedatives or anxiolytics and analgesics first to decrease awareness and anxiety and to relieve pain. Patients on NMBAs and mechanical ventilation will frequently also require blood thinning to decrease their risk of having a blood clot secondary to immobility. Since concurrent use of these drugs with NMBAs is necessary, drug interactions are always a potential and need to be monitored for.

Resistance has been reported with nondepolarizing NMBAs. How would you know whether this was occurring?

Usually once paralysis is no longer needed, patients regain muscle function spontaneously with NMBA discontinuation. This is assessed clinically by patient ability to open the eyes wide, protrude the tongue, grip a hand, lift the head, or cough on demand. If reversal needs to be done, acetylcholinesterase inhibitors are used.

As previously mentioned, the NMBDs differ in some of their pharmacological properties. The FDA defines NMBDs by their onset and duration of action. Ultrashort-duration NMBAs respond in a minute or less, rapid or short in between 1 and 3 minutes, intermediate from 2 to 4 minutes, and long or slow in 4 minutes or longer. The duration of ultrashort NMBAs is less than 8 minutes; short, from 15 to 25 minutes; intermediate, from 20 to 50 minutes; and long, more than 50 minutes.

The following is a brief summation of available NMBAs.

R̥ ***succinylcholine (Anectine), the Only Depolarizing Agent.*** With various neuromuscular blocking drugs on the market, there is a need to compare and contrast them

Table 11-2 Comparison of Neuromuscular Blocking Agents

Category	Drug	Onset (min)	Duration (min)	Cardiovascular Effects
Ultrashort duration	succinylcholine	1–1.5	7–12	++
Short duration	rapacuronium	1–1.5	15–25	+++
	mivacurium	3–5	15–25	++
Intermediate duration	atracurium	3–4	35–45	++
	cisatracurium	4–6	40–50	0
	rocuronium	1.5–3	30–40	+
	vecuronium	3–4	35–45	0
Long duration	doxacurium	5–7	90–120	0
	pancuronium	3–5	90–120	+++

The numbers listed here are approximate and may vary depending on patient characteristics.

and to define their roles. We will first start with a review of succinylcholine, the single depolarizing agent and long the gold standard drug for quick action for intubation. This drug has been used for more than 50 years. Its rapid onset and short duration of action make it a popular drug.

It can be used as a bolus or infusion, and it works quickly at the vocal cords, which makes for good intubating conditions and rapid recovery. Unfortunately, it has cardiovascular effects such as dysrhythmias and pulmonary edema, increases intraocular, intragastric, and intracranial pressure, and has been associated with hyperkalemia and myoglobinemia.

Patients with genetic muscle weakness disorders are prone to hyperkalemia when given succinylcholine, inhalation anesthetics, or the combination. Hyperkalemia can also occur with succinylcholine in patients with burns, polio, or Guillain-Barré Syndrome, so it should not be used for such patients.

Succinylcholine has also been associated with malignant hyperthermia, which is characterized by spasm of the jaw muscles, skeletal muscle damage, hyperthermia, rapid breathing, and death if not treated properly. It is commonly associated with metabolic and respiratory acidosis.

℞ **pancuronium (Pavulon).** Pancuronium has a higher incidence of residual neuromuscular block postoperatively than other agents, probably owing to its duration of action. This could cause a patient to be at risk for pulmonary complications. Patients with renal failure have longer recovery times with pancuronium.

℞ **mivacurium (Mivacron).** This drug has a short duration of action and midrange onset. Rapid recovery from this drug is due to rapid metabolism. At higher doses, mivacurium has a faster onset without prolonging muscle recovery. The limitation is with the side effect of histamine release, which is dose related.

℞ **rocuronium (Zemuron).** Rocuronium has a faster onset of action and controllable duration of action relative to other intermediate-duration drugs. It has neutral cardiac side effects and is available in a liquid dosage form, which may allow for faster administration. It rarely causes histamine release. It may interact with theopylline, resulting in a need for increased rocuronium doses.

℞ **cisatracurium (Nimbex).** This drug is a chemical isomer of atracurium that is less likely to cause histamine release. It has a longer duration of action that atracurium and does not depend on liver or renal elimination but rather is broken down in the bloodstream.

℞ **rapacuronium (Raplon).** It is faster in onset than rocuronium and leads to a quicker recovery. At higher doses it causes histamine release. This drug may have direct arterial vasodilating effects and calcium channel–blocking effects. It causes blood-pressure lowering—an average of 10–15 mm Hg. Rapacuronium has an active metabolite that is cleared by the kidney and is 2.5 times as potent. It is not used as a continuous infusion, and doses are repeated no more than two to three times. Bronchospasm has been reported, unrelated to histamine release.

℞ **atracurium (Tracrium).** Atracurium requires no dosage change in patients with renal or liver impairment. It has a metabolite that can cause seizures. It produces histamine release and probably shouldn't be used in unstable ICU patients.

℞ **vecuronium (Norcuron).** Vecuronium is very similar to rocuronium. It has a neutral cardiac side-effect profile with no histamine release. It requires reconstitution prior to administration.

℞ **doxacurium (Nuromax).** Doxacurium has no active metabolites, which results in a faster recovery time.

SKELETAL MUSCLE RELAXANTS

In many situations, relaxation rather than paralysis of the muscle is needed. For example, someone experiencing painful back spasms or that ever-typical "pulled muscle" would benefit from a muscle relaxant. Skeletal muscle relaxants relieve musculoskeletal pain or spasm. They are used to treat spasticity in patients with multiple sclerosis, spinal cord injuries, or in stroke patients. These medications are occasionally used as an adjunct to pain control, which will be discussed later.

Skeletal muscle relaxants can be divided into two classes: central- and peripheral-acting. Unlike the neuromuscular blocking agents, central-acting relaxants do not block the motor end plate junction but are thought to act directly on the CNS to decrease muscular tone by interfering with overstimulated reflex nerve pathways in the spinal cord. These drugs are frequently used in acute and chronic back pain.

Peripheral muscle relaxants work on the muscles themselves. Peripheral muscle relaxants such as dantrolene (Dantrium) decrease the force of skeletal muscle contraction by stopping the release of calcium. This results in less actin and myosin linkage and decreased force of contraction, since calcium is a necessary part of that mechanism. Since its major effect is directly on muscle rather than on the brain, dantrolene causes fewer CNS side effects than centrally acting agents. Examples of common muscle relaxants are listed in Table 11-3.

Table 11-3   Common Muscle Relaxants

Generic	Trade (type)
methocarbamol	Robaxin (central)
cyclobenzaprine	Flexeril (central)
orphenadrine	Norflex (central)
chlorzoxazone	Parafon Forte (central)
dantrolene	Dantrium (peripheral or direct-acting)

SEDATIVE/HYPNOTICS/ANXIOLYTICS

Terminology

A drug that reduces CNS arousal is a **sedative.** Any medication that induces sleep is a **hypnotic.** Any medication that reduces the symptoms of anxiety is an **anxiolytic.** Some drug classes, such as benzodiazepines, may have all of these characteristics and be categorized as all three. Differences among sedatives, hypnotics, and anxiolytics are in reality minor and may be dose related.

Sedatives are often needed with analgesics to improve tolerance of endotracheal tubes, facilitate acceptance of mechanical ventilation, suppress spontaneous ventilation, and prevent self-extubation. It's preferable to adjust the ventilator to patient tolerance rather than to sedate the patient to match the ventilator, but this may not always be possible. One of the biggest challenges is to measure sedation in patients. Different modes of ventilation require different amounts of sedation. Sometimes sedation allows avoidance of neuromuscular blocking agents.

Tolerance and addiction are real possibilities with these drug classes. Depending on the drug indication, some of these drugs are only used for the short term to avoid this potential. With indications such as chronic anxiety, long-term use is the reality. What we refer to as sleeping pills or hypnotics, regardless of the drug class they belong to, are only meant to be used for a maximum of one or two consecutive weeks at a time. With longer-term use, hypnotics can change the characteristics of a normal sleep cycle and alter rapid eye movement (REM), sleep quality, and sleep quantity.

Benzodiazepines

Benzodiazepines are by far the most common drug class with sedative, hypnotic, and anxiolytic pharmacological effects. Benzodiazepines work by enhancing the inhibitory effect on the receptor for the neurotransmitter γ-aminobutyric acid (GABA) within the brain. Benzodiazepines can cause respiratory effects such as loss of airway reflexes at high doses and decreased tidal volume at lower doses. The duration of action influences the extent of hypnotic hangover felt in the morning. One of the common short-acting sedative benzodiazepines is midazolam (Versed). See Table 11-4 for more examples of the benzodiazepines.

If it were three o'clock in the morning and you couldn't get back to sleep, would you want to use the same sleeping pill as the one you had taken right before bedtime? Why or why not?

Barbiturates

Barbiturates are some of the oldest drugs around and have been used for ages to treat seizure, sleep, and anxiety disorders. Barbiturates work differently than benzodiazepines to block the excitatory impulse and decrease the level of arousal in the CNS. Like benzodiazepines, the barbiturates differ in their onset of action and duration of action. The primary side effect—drowsiness—is a natural extension of their desired actions. Patients using these drugs for seizure treatment fortunately get tolerant to this side effect. In overdose situations, barbiturates cause respiratory depression, CNS depression, cardiovascular collapse, coma, and death. For this reason, barbiturates, even though they are a time-honored drug class, are not used as frequently as benzodiazepines.

Cocktails

A variety of drugs are used in surgical and office procedure arenas to decrease the patient's level of consciousness and produce a retrograde amnesia so the patient won't remember the negative aspects of the procedure. Sometimes these drug combinations are referred to as "cocktails." Individual prescribers frequently develop their own combination or recipe of drugs they feel comfortable with to decrease patient consciousness. Two such examples are

CLINICAL PEARL
Benzodiazepines are also used for effects other than sedative, hypnotic, and anxiolytic. Status epilepticus is treated with intravenous diazepam. Symptoms of alcohol withdrawal and delirium tremens (DTs) are prevented by giving benzodiazepines. One of the short-acting agents, midazolam (Versed), is used as an adjunct to anesthesia. There is a drug available that is an antagonist to GABA receptors and that can be used in benzodiazepine overdoses; it is called **flumazenil** (Romazicon).

CLINICAL PEARL
Analgesic and sedative tapering on withdrawal of mechanical ventilation is not well defined. Usually, daily attempts at dose reduction are effective at decreasing the duration of unneeded drug administration. As mechanical ventilation is reduced, so should sedatives and analgesics be.

℞

Table 11-4 Common Benzodiazepines

Generic	Trade
alprazolam	Xanax
chlordiazepoxide	Librium
diazepam	Valium
midazolam	Versed

morphine given in combination with diazepam or meperidene given with droperidol. The desired endpoint is to make a patient comfortable yet still able to respond to commands such as "lift your arm" or "open your eyes."

ANESTHETICS

General versus Local

The term anesthesia refers to the inability to perceive sensations. The route and the type of agent administered will depend upon the individual patient situation. **Local anesthesia** refers to the administration of an agent that will act locally to stop the transmission of sensations from that area. **General anesthesia** refers to the induction of a total anesthetic state in which the patient will not respond to any stimuli. General anesthesia is reserved for surgical procedures in which the normal stresses placed on the patient are substantial.

General Anesthesia

Important anesthesia terms are induction, maintenance, and termination. Induction relates to the time it takes to create the appropriate level of anesthesia. Maintenance relates to the continuation of the anesthetized state. Termination refers to the time it takes for a patient to recover from the anesthesia. Pharmacologic and patient characteristics of each agent will determine and influence each of these components of anesthesia.

One of the most influential factors determining which anesthetic medication a patient will receive or whether the person is even a candidate for anesthesia is the medical condition of the patient. Age, organ function, and disease being treated—all influence the selection process. Elderly people tend to have decreased liver, kidney, lung, and immune function, as well as a lower serum albumin concentration. All of these contribute to the altered efficacy, elimination, accumulation, and potential toxicities of the anesthetic agents. Likewise, neonatal patients may have a reduced ability to clear medications, and this may result in drug accumulation and toxicity.

Drug allergy or sensitivity also impacts which route and type of anesthetic medication will be administered. Patients who have experienced an adverse effect from a particular type of anesthetic or analgesic in the past are more likely to have that same adverse event the next time they receive the medication. These adverse reactions may range from a mild gastrointestinal discomfort after receiving an opioid analgesic or a dysphoric reaction (unpleasant CNS sensations) with inhaled nitrous oxide all the way to a severe cardiovascular collapse following the administration of inhaled general anesthetic medications.

Drug factors also influence the type of anesthetic used. The characteristics of the drug molecule are going to determine whether it may be administered by an enteral, intravenous, intramuscular, or inhaled route. Onset of action will be critical for each of these routes, as well as the duration of medication action.

Stages of Anesthesia

The depth of anesthesia can be categorized as stages 1 through 4. Stage 1 is analgesia, with the patient retaining consciousness without experiencing pain. Stage 1 anesthesia is sometimes called "conscious sedation" and is frequently used for outpatient endoscopies, colonoscopies, and minor procedures. Stage 2 anesthesia is the level representing a loss of consciousness. During Stage 2, the patient may have a number of reflexes activated that result in coughing, increased salivation, increase in cardiovascular output, and increase in blood pressure. Stage 3 anesthesia is surgical anesthesia and progresses to a state of complete respiratory depression. During Stage 3, there is a loss of the blink reflex and loss of eye movement, and respiratory depression soon ensues. Stage 4 is complete loss of respiratory drive, and there may be a loss of cardiovascular tone. As you can see, there is a fine line between the desired level of anesthesia and the level that produces adverse effects.

As the level of anesthesia progresses, there are some characteristic responses that can be anticipated. Can you think of any medication that may be administered as a "preanesthetic" that can decrease the complications of general anesthesia?

Specific General Anesthetics

You can administer medications to create a state of surgical anesthesia. These medications are administered by the inhaled route or by the intravenous route. General anesthesia has four characteristics: unconsciousness, analgesia, muscle relaxation, and depression of reflexes. Undesirable characteristics that can occur with anesthesia relate to cardiovascular hemodynamics.

Inhaled general anesthetics work by binding to a protein-binding site in the neurons of the CNS. The interaction of the anesthetics and the neurons results in a decrease in the neuronal firing rate. Inhaled anesthetics are a diverse group of compounds that exist in a gaseous state. The medications must pass through the alveoli, diffuse through the blood stream, cross the blood–brain barrier, and then diffuse into the CNS. Characteristics of the individual compounds will determine the ease with which they pass through membranes. It is nearly impossible to determine the actual concentration of the medication in the CNS, so inhaled anesthetic medications are discussed and compared by using a concept called minimum alveolar concentration (MAC). MAC is a number that correlates to the minimum inhaled drug concentration that results in 50 percent of patients failing to move in response to surgical incision. You have to feel bad for the other fifty, who do move, but remember that they usually have no memory of this event.

The desired CNS actions of inhaled anesthetics are useful for surgery. However, as the chemicals are distributing throughout the body, they come in contact with all organ systems. Side effects of inhaled anesthetics include cardiovascular complications such as reductions in blood pressure, increase in peripheral tissue blood flow, decrease in vessel and cardiac response to sympathetic nervous system activity, and alteration of cardiac conduction. Respiratory complications include reduction in the ventilatory response to falling O_2 levels, decrease in depth of respiration, increase or decrease in rate of respiration, and alteration of the ventilatory response to rising CO_2 levels.

Muscle complications may include increased sensitivity of motor end plates to the actions of neuromuscular blocking agents, relaxation of skeletal muscles, or, rarely, development of **malignant hyperthermia.** Malignant hyperthermia is a condition in which there is sustained skeletal muscle contraction that if untreated results in muscle breakdown, and potential renal impairment. See Table 11-5, which lists common inhaled anesthetics.

Table 11-5   Inhaled Anesthetics

Generic	Trade
nitrous oxide	
halothane	Fluothane
methoxyflurane	Penthrane
enflurane	Ethrane
isoflurane	Forane

Intravenous anesthetics are commonly used as adjuncts to inhaled anesthesia or as the primary agent for maintaining a state of anesthesia. IV induction agents rapidly induce unconsciousness in a predictable way. These medications are generally classified as rapid-acting barbiturates (thiopental), rapid-acting benzodiazepines (midazolam), or as miscellaneous agents. These medications when administered by the intravenous route cross into the CNS and cause a global reduction in neuronal activity. This may be done by the inhibition of pre- and postsynaptic neuronal interactions (barbiturates), alterations of electrolyte channels (barbiturates and benzodiazepines), or by an unknown global cerebral suppression (propofol). Importantly, they blunt the stress response to laryngoscopy and intubation.

They also induce a short-lived global amnesia. Complications of barbiturates have included respiratory depression, suppression of cardiac conduction, and severe reductions in arterial blood pressure. Because of these complications, the short-acting benzodiazepines have become the preferred agents in the acute setting. Midazolam (Versed) is an ultrashort-acting benzodiazepine. This medication is used to induce an amnesia state in major and minor surgical procedures.

Propofol (Diprivan) is a lipid-soluble medication that can be administered intravenously to induce and maintain general anesthesia. Propofol is chemically unrelated to barbiturates, benzodiazepines, and inhaled anesthetics, and its exact mechanism of action is unknown. Propofol comes in a lipid emulsion containing soybean oil that can occasionally cause an elevation of serum triglycerides. This intravenous anesthetic is used frequently in the ICU setting to assist with anesthesia and sedation of the ventilated patient. It can be discontinued with a rapid taper and allows for earlier extubation. Some of these drugs can be used for maintenance of general anesthesia alone or in combination with inhalational anesthetics.

Ketamine (Ketalor) is used clinically intravenously as an analgesic and sedative at lower doses and an anesthetic at high doses. It can be used in nonintubated patients but has been reported to be associated with aspiration and ventilatory compromise. Ketamine (Ketalor) is a bronchodilator also, but it can increase respiratory secretions.

See Table 11-6 for a list of common IV anesthetics.

Local Anesthetics

Many circumstances in medicine do not require administration of general anesthesia. Local anesthesia relates to the administration of a medication that will make a specific region of the body insensitive to pain without loss of consciousness. The most common situation for local anesthesia is when a potentially painful procedure is required. Suturing, removing moles, and taking skin biopsies are examples of times when administration of a topical local anesthetic is appropriate.

For certain procedures, such as a bronchoscopy or an intubation, local anesthethics help deaden the gag reflex that can cause the patient discomfort or, worse yet, an aspiration of vomitus into the lungs. Another situation in which local anesthetics may be administered is

CLINICAL PEARL
Propofol infusions shouldn't be suddenly interrupted, because rapid awakening can be hard on the patient. This drug also causes a green discoloration of the urine.

CLINICAL PEARL:
Another case when local anesthetics may be administered is when a local block is desired in a particular anatomic site. Regional spinal anesthesia is frequently used in surgical situations. Epidural anesthesia refers to the injection of the analgesic medication into the dural tissue, as in the case of obstetrical Caesarian section birth. Intrathecal anesthesia results with the direct injection of the medication into the CSF. These local blocks can be accomplished with narcotic analgesics or with local anesthetic medications.

Table 11-6 IV Anesthetics

Type	Generic	Trade
Barbiturates	**thiopental**	Pentothal
	methohexital	Brevital
Miscellaneous	**propofol**	Diprivan
	ketamine	Ketalar
Benzodiazepine	**midazolam**	Versed

Table 11-7 Common Local Anesthetics

Type	Generic	Trade	Duration (hours)
Esters	**procaine**	Novocaine	0.5–1.5
	benzocaine	Anbesol	0.5–1.5
	tetracaine	Pontocaine	1.25–3
Amides	**lidocaine**	Xylocaine	0.5–1
	mepivacaine	Carbocaine	0.5–1.5
	bupivacaine	Marcaine	2–4

CLINICAL PEARL

A common application of local anesthetics is topical lidocaine applied when inserting an arterial line.

in joint injuries that may require a joint space injection. Torn rotator cuffs and sprained fingers are frequently injected in athletes. Local anesthetics can also be topically placed on mucous membranes for surface anesthesia to decrease pain and discomfort. Local anesthetics are found in hemorrhoidal cream preparations and in topical sprays that may be used for sunburn or even sore throats. The most commonly known drug with local anesthetic properties is cocaine. It also has therapeutic pharmacological applications for ophthalmic anesthesia used topically.

STOP & REVIEW

The last time you went to the dentist and had a cavity fixed, or better yet, a root canal, what types of local anesthetics did you receive?

CLINICAL PEARL

A lidocaine spray is often used prior to a bronchoscopy procedure to reduce the gag reflex and aid in comfort. Once the area is numb (no gag reflex or sensation with tongue depressor), adding more lidocaine will not numb it further. Rather, it will just be systemically absorbed.

Local anesthetics work by binding to a membrane site that when stimulated results in an inability of the neuron to depolarize. This action is related to the closing of the sodium channels that propagate the action potential. Adverse effects of local anesthetics are primarily related to a skin sensitivity to the structure of the medications. "Caine" anesthetic medications can be divided chemically into amide and ester types. If a patient has had an adverse reaction to an amide type anesthetic, there is a high probability of a cross-reaction to any other structurally related products. Examples of the amide-type anesthetics include lidocaine (Xylocaine), bupivacaine (Marcaine), and mepivacaine (Carbocaine). The second type of local anesthetics is known as esters. These medications include cocaine, benzocaine (Anbesol), and procaine (Novocain). See Table 11-7, which describes local anesthetics.

VENTILATORY STIMULANTS

So far, we've talked mostly about depressing the respiratory system. However, there are times when we need to stimulate the ventilatory drive with **ventilatory stimulants.** A drug that causes nervous system arousal and increases the rate and depth of ventilation is technically classified as an **analeptic** but is more commonly referred to as a ventilatory stimulant. These drugs act on the respiratory center in the medulla to increase the rate and depth of ventilation. Drugs that are useful as ventilatory stimulants also stimulate the CNS, although not all CNS stimulants are useful as ventilatory stimulants.

Drugs used clinically for these effects include doxapram (Dopram), caffeine, theophylline, protriptyline (Vivactyl), and medroxyprogesterone (Depo-Provera). In reality, these drugs are used infrequently for this indication and are not practical for reversing CNS depression. It only makes sense that by stimulating respiration, breathing becomes more work and requires more oxygen, which may exacerbate tissue hypoxia.

℞

Table 11-8 Ventilatory Stimulants

medroxyprogesterone	obesity hypoventilation syndrome
protriptyline	daytime symptoms of obstructive sleep apnea
doxapram	post-anesthesia for drug-induced respiratory depression
caffeine	apnea of prematurity

Ventilatory stimulants are used to treat sleep apnea, postanesthesia respiratory depression, acute hypercapnea in chronic pulmonary patients, patients who need to be weaned from ventilators, and apnea of prematurity.

Caffeine is well known as a CNS stimulant but less known as a xanthine that can increase the ventilatory drive, similar to theophylline. One of the differences for this indication between caffeine and theophylline is the potency and duration of action. By increasing responsiveness of the medullary respiratory center to carbon dioxide levels and hypoxia, these drugs increase ventilatory rate and depth. Side effects of the stimulants include nausea, vomiting, nervousness, insomnia, tremors, and even convulsions.

Medroxyprogesterone is a progesterone hormone that stimulates alveolar ventilation and increases the body's ventilatory response to hypercapnea and hypoxia. Since it increases the sensitivity of the medullary respiratory centers to respond to hypercapnea and hypoxia, it is most useful for obstructive sleep apnea. It can cause nervousness, nausea, male impotence, and alopecia.

Protriptyline is an antidepressant used for sleep apnea, although its mechanism is not that of a ventilatory stimulant. Rather, it suppresses REM sleep, which is the sleep period most associated with loss of upper airway muscle tone. It also increases muscle tone of the upper airways. It doesn't directly affect arterial carbon dioxide tension. See Table 11-8 for a list of ventilatory stimulants.

ANALGESIA

Principles of Analgesia

Analgesia refers to the reduction in the sensation of pain. Anything that decreases the patient's perception of pain or pain intensity is an analgesic. The physiologic consequence of stress response caused by pain can be tachycardia, increased oxygen consumption, and immunosuppression. One of the roles of analgesics is to minimize physiologic results of pain by decreasing pulmonary complications. Almost all ICU patients are in pain, whether it's due to an endotracheal tube, postoperative discomfort, trauma, or inability to position oneself comfortably.

Pain can certainly impair ventilatory function if the pain is located in the abdominal thoracic region. If you have ever damaged your ribs, you became "painfully aware" of your breathing process and even more aware of your cough reflex. Postoperative abdominal and/or thoracic patients must be encouraged to breathe deeply or the pain may lead to hypoventilation and poor cough effort. This in turn can lead to atelectasis (lung collapse), pneumonia, or even the need for mechanical ventilation.

Analgesics include drugs that relax a patient or decrease patient pain perception, as well as drugs or devices that interrupt nerve transmission. This section will focus on pharmacologic analgesic treatment. The principles that guide the use of analgesic medications are similar to those that guide other medications and include medication class, mechanism of action, side effects, patient tolerability, cost, and route of administration. Frequently medications from different classes are combined for synergistic effects.

Analgesics work on neurotransmitters and different locations in the pain pathway. Morphine-like drugs target opioid-binding sites. Steroidal and nonsteroidal anti-inflammatory agents inhibit the formation of pain-producing cytokines that start the pain impulse. Other drugs, such as some of the antidepressants, increase levels of the regulatory neurotransmitters norepinephrine and serotonin, and still other drugs, such as some of those used for seizures, slow the nerve impulses for pain.

The Pain Response

The specialty organ system that is responsible for dealing with painful noxious stimuli is the nociceptive nervous system. It is also worthwhile to consider that pain is a normal protective response that helps to warn the organ system (you!) of any potential or real damage.

Pain receptors are referred to as nociceptors. There are four different types of receptors that we will discuss briefly, although in reality there are probably dozens of different types and subtypes of nociceptors that can start an impulse. These four are stretch, temperature, pressure, and chemical receptors. Types of receptors differ in location and tissue density.

The stretch receptors, located in joints, for example, fire before there is damage and serve in a protective role. The temperature receptors have their highest density in the hands, lips, and mouth. They help warn us if we grab or try to eat something outside of our temperature tolerance. The deep pressure receptors have no pharmacologic interventions yet, but stay tuned to the Web site as developments occur. The chemical receptors regulate the inflammatory and healing responses. When tissue damage has taken place, chemicals such as prostaglandins are released as a natural response to damaged tissue by the arachidonic acid cascade.

Once impulses from pain receptors reach the brain, there are hundreds, if not millions, of innervations in the cerebral cortex that allow for the psychological, behavioral, and physical responses to the impulse. Psychological activity in response to pain is usually an increase in arousal and awareness. Behavioral and physical responses include increased heart rate and blood pressure, increased motor activity (attempts to get away from the painful stimuli), and vocalization (usually cursing in acute pain and moaning and groaning in chronic pain).

www.prenhall.com/colbert

There is more to the story of "pain," but it would make this chapter too long and a "pain to read." Therefore, concepts such as totality of pain, reflex responses to pain, and endorphin and serotonin pathways are discussed on the Web.

What are some physical symptoms you can look for in a patient who may not be able to verbalize their level of pain (e.g., ICU ventilated patients)?

Analgesics

This section will focus on pharmacologic modalities that have analgesic properties. The principles that govern the use of analgesic medications include medication type, mechanisms of action, side effects, patient tolerability, and cost. Routes of administration become important and may include oral, intravenous, intramuscular, or direct infusion of medications into the cerebrospinal fluid space (intrathecal administration).

Also important is whether or not a local analgesic can be administered (intra-articular administration or local anesthetic injections), contrasting with a major surgical procedure that may require a general anesthetic. Frequently multiple medications from different classes are used for synergistic analgesia. All patient factors and medication factors need to be taken into account to determine the ideal analgesic regimen.

Outcomes Assessment Analgesic Therapy

No two people report pain in the same way. Because of this, it becomes very difficult to quantify such a subjective perception. The best way to quantitate the pain response is to let the patient rate their pain on a visual analog scale or a verbal number scale. If time allows a more thorough discussion with the patient, a few simple questions may start to reveal contributing factors to the patient's pain response. Occasionally the acronym PQRST is used to help with the pain assessment. **P**alliative information relates to what relieves the pain. **Q**uality relates to a description of the pain (such as sharp, acute, penetrating versus dull, aching, or sickening pain qualities). **R**adiation helps to identify where the pain starts and where it goes—frequently internal pain may present with a characteristic radiating pattern; the heart-attack patient who presents with neck, shoulder, and jaw pain illustrates this example. **S**everity relates to the perceived intensity of the pain; the analog scales help to quantify the severity assessment. **T** translates into the time course of pain. This may be time of day, time of month, time of year, or any relationship to an event that may exacerbate the pain response.

Specific Analgesics

Analgesics exert their mechanisms of action by targeting a number of different locations and neurotransmitters within the nociceptive pathway. These medications may target opioid-binding sites, causing the opioid receptors' inhibition of the pain impulse (morphine-like drugs), or they may inhibit the formation of the pain production cytokines that start the pain impulse (steroids and nonsteroidal anti-inflammatory agents). Other medications that are used in pain situations may act to increase the regulatory neurotransmitters norepinephrine and serotonin or slow the nerve impulse propagation.

Opioids

CLINICAL PEARL

Remember from Chapter 9 that the opioid morphine is beneficial also for its ability to decrease preload and afterload, which helps patients with pulmonary edema, congestive heart failure, and myocardial infarction.

One of the first analgesic medications to be used was heroin, obtained from the poppy seed. Within the juice of the poppy seed are a number of opiate congeners that have been shown to have analgesic properties as well as many of the unwanted CNS side effects. Morphine sulfate is the best known of this class of medications. The term opioid refers to any natural or synthetic chemical that can bind to an opioid receptor and exert an action. Opioids differ in their potency, onset of action, duration of action, chemical structure, available routes of administration, side effects, abuse potential, and cost. See Table 11-9 for a list of the opioid analgesics.

The opioids that cross quickly into the CNS and produce rapid analgesia and euphoric effects are the agents more likely to be abused by patients with addictive personalities. It should be noted that in acute pain situations, where the source of the pain is very well defined, there is a very low probability of patients demonstrating drug-seeking behavior or progressing to opioid addiction. However, in the chronic pain situation, where the source of pain is not well defined, patients will frequently present with drug-seeking behavior and chemical dependency.

The Food and Drug Administration heavily regulates manufacture, distribution, and sale of opioid analgesics. The scheduling of controlled drugs is based upon the potency and

Table 11-9   Opioid Analgesics

Generic	Trade	Onset (min)
morphine sulfate	many	15–60
hydromorphone	Dilaudid	15–30
oxymorphone	Numorphan	5–10
oxycodone	Roxicodone	15–30
oxycodone in combinations	Tylox Percodan Percocet	15–30
hydrocodone	many	15–60
codeine	many	10–30
levorphanol	Levo-Dromoran	60
butorphanol	Stadol	10–15
methadone	Dolophine	30–60
propoxyphene	Darvon	30–60
meperidine	Demerol	15–30
fentanyl	Sublimaze, Duragesic	5–10

℞

potential for abuse of the various chemicals. See Table 11-10 for drug schedules and their regulations.

The route of administration of opioid analgesics will depend upon the severity of the pain situation. If a patient is in mild to moderate pain, oral administration of opioids is appropriate. If the patient is not controlled on oral regimens, intramuscular or intravenous medications may be administered. A self-administration technique is patient-controlled analgesia (PCA). This allows the prescriber to determine the medication, continuous infusion rates, and bolus doses. However, the patient can self-dose the medication to an appropriate level of analgesia by pressing a button that is connected to the PCA infusion device. PCA infusion devices have decreased patients' pain and suffering while minimizing nursing and prescriber time in the acute pain settings.

An additional option for the management of pain is to directly infuse opioids into the CNS. This may be done in the acute situation, such as delivering a baby, with epidural administration. In a more prolonged surgery, a drug may be directly infused into the intrathecal space to produce a local analgesia. In the circumstance of malignant pain,

Table 11-10   Drug Schedules

Schedule	Criteria	Examples
I	no medical use— high addiction potential	heroin
II	medical use— high addiction potential	cocaine, opioids, amphetamines
III	medical use— moderate potential for dependence	codeine
IV	medical use— low abuse potential	benzodiazepines

catheters placed intrathecally or epidurally may be connected to continuous infusion pumps. In each of these situations, the goal is to provide optimal analgesia while minimizing the central side effects.

Opioid analgesics exert similar side effects. They differ slightly in their ability to cause side effects such as respiratory depression or constipation. It is important to note that patients who have not had opioids in their systems (opioid-naive patients) will be more likely to have side effects. Patients who are not opioid naive are much more tolerant to larger doses and side effects. One of the most serious side effects is respiratory depression. Administration of opioid analgesics causes a central depression of the brainstem's ability to sense CO_2. This can result in a decrease in respiratory rate, tidal volume, minute ventilation, and the CO_2 response-curve slope. The peak respiratory depression effect will correspond with the route of administration and the peak in CNS concentration of the opioids. As an example, the peak actions following IV morphine will be in 8–10 minutes. See Table 11-11 for a list of opioid analgesic side effects.

CLINICAL PEARL

All opiates produce equivalent respiratory depression in equipotent doses. Regular use of opiates can cause tolerance to respiratory depression.

Opioid Antagonists

Opioid antagonists such as **naloxone** reverse the CNS and ventilatory depression that can be caused by opioids. The antagonism they cause at the opioid receptor can be as soon as five minutes after administration. Since naloxone administration in the absence of opioids is not harmful, naloxone administration is frequently used in cases where narcotic overdose is suspected but unknown. It will not reverse CNS and ventilatory depression from other causes.

Steroid Anti-inflammatory Agents

In any situation in which there is a destruction of tissue, the arachidonic acid cascade will be activated. The end products of this cascade include leukotrienes that act as inflammatory mediators as well as prostaglandins, which are potent simulators of the chemical nociceptors. Corticosteroid anti-inflammatory medications act to inhibit the arachidonic acid cascade, resulting in decreased production of leukotrienes and prostaglandins.

Corticosteroids for pain may be administered by a number of routes. Systemic routes include enteral administration of oral tablets or solutions, or parenteral administration of intravenous or intramuscular injections. Short-term systemic administration of corticosteroids is occasionally very helpful in controlling the pain response. However, long-term

Table 11-11 Opioid Analgesic Side Effects

System or Area of Concern	Side Effect
Major concerns	respiratory depression, apnea circulatory depression, shock respiratory arrest, cardiac arrest
CNS	light-headedness dizziness, syncope seizures dysphoria, hallucinations
Respiratory	depression, decrease rate, and depth of breathing
Cardiovascular	reduction in venous and arterial pressures
Skin	histamine release resulting in blood vessel dilation, flushing sweating, pruritus
GI, nauseant	inhibition of peristaltic waves, leading to constipation

side effects of systemic corticosteroids, including peptic ulcer disease, bone demineralization, alteration of blood glucose, and muscle atrophy, limit their use.

Corticosteroids are utilized by local injections into painful joints for analgesic/anti-inflammatory action. Corticosteroid joint injections are limited by the amount of fluid that can be injected into the space. Naturally, a large shoulder joint will require a larger volume than a small finger joint. One of the complications of joint injections is that they mask the damage at the joint. If an injured athlete does not want to take time off from the sport to allow the injury to heal, they may receive a joint injection that will mask the pain, which may result in further injury to the joint.

Nonsteroidal Anti-inflammatory Agents

One of the most commonly used classes of analgesic medications is the nonsteroidal anti-inflammatory drugs (NSAIDs). NSAIDs are considered the drugs of choice in situations of tissue destruction pain. Any circumstance that has caused a disruption of the tissues will respond to NSAID therapy. NSAIDs exert their mechanism of action by inhibiting the enzyme system known as cyclooxygenase. This enzyme system causes the production of thromboxanes, prostacyclins, and prostaglandins. NSAIDs can be used for acute pain, chronic pain, malignant pain, osteoarthritis pain, arthritis pain, migraine headache, regular headache, and gout pain. See Table 11-12 for a list of nonsteroidal anti-inflammatory medications.

Side effects of NSAIDs are primarily an extension of the desired action. Inhibition of prostaglandin production can result in a decrease in the protective effects of prostaglandins on the GI tract. This may present acutely with gastritis, irritation, and intestinal discomfort, or chronically it may contribute to peptic ulcer disease. CNS effects include dizziness and drowsiness, but to a much lesser degree than with the opioid-type medications. NSAIDs may also alter renal function and can contribute to renal dysfunction in patients with underlying tenuous renal perfusion. NSAIDs are also metabolized extensively in the liver, and these medications can occasionally cause toxicities to the liver cells.

Analgesic Synergy

It should become apparent that there is a pharmacologic rationale for the administration of analgesics from different classes to better control the pain. Remember from Chapter 1 that the concept of synergy relates to the phenomenon best illustrated with a numeric example: $1 + 1 = 3$. When you use two medications, the analgesia is better than the sum of the two agents separately. A significant number of combination products are commercially available. Acetaminophen (an analgesic but not anti-inflammatory) is combined with codeine to

℞

Table 11-12   Common Nonsteroidal Anti-Inflammatory Medications

Generic	Brand Name
aspirin	Bayer, et al.
ibuprofen	Motrin, et al.
ketoprofen	Orudis, et al.
naproxen HCl	Naprosyn, et al.
naproxen sodium	Anaprox, et al.
indomethacin	Indocin, et al.
sulindac	Clinoril
piroxicam	Feldene
ketorolac	Toradol

create the product line known as Tylenol with codeine. It is also combined with a number of different strengths of hydrocodone to form the product lines Vicoden, Anexia, and Lortab. Aspirin is combined with codeine to form Empirin, while aspirin plus the potent opioid oxycodone is known as Percodan. Not to be outdone, Ibuprofen has been added to hydrocodone to form the product Vicoprofen! All of these medications have been shown to be more effective than either medication by itself in improving pain scores. See Table 11-13 for suggested pain severity dosing regimens.

℞

Adjuncts to Analgesics

A number of other medications have been utilized as adjunctive analgesics. Phenothiazine antiemetic medications have been administered to decrease the nausea and vomiting associated with the pain response. These medications include **prochlorperazine** (Compazine) and **promethazine** (Phenergan).

In patients with chronic pain, it is known that they have a functional decrease in circulating levels of the neurotransmitters serotonin and noerepinephrine. Tricyclic antidepressant (TCA) medications have been shown effective in improving pain response scores. These medications act by blocking the pre-synaptic uptake of catecholamines released into the synaptic cleft. This results in an increase in serotonin and norepinephrine that then decreases the release of the pain-propagating neurotransmitter substance P. See Table 11-14 for common antidepressant medications.

In the treatment of depression, there has been a recent emphasis on putting patients on selective serotonin reuptake inhibitors (SSRIs). This has largely taken place because of their lower side effect profiles and greater safety profile in an overdose setting. However, in pain situations, the selective SSRIs are NOT more effective than the older TCA types of medications. This is probably because the TCAs also block the reuptake of norepinephrine, which also regulates the pain transmission process. SSRIs however, only affect the serotonin-related aspects of pain transmission.

Table 11-13 Suggested Pain Dosing Regimens

Mild Pain	*Moderate Pain*	*Severe Pain*
APAP 500 mg q 4 hr	tramadol (Ultram) 50 mg 2 tabs q 4 hr	ketorolac (Toradol) 30–60 mg IM, 15–30 mg IV
ASA 650 mg QID	ketorolac (Toradol) 10 mg q 6 hr	hydrocodone/APAP (Lorcet) 10/650 1-2 q 4–6 hr
ibuprofen 600 mg QID	hydrocodone 5/500 1–2 q 4–6 hr	hydrocodone/APAP (Norco) 10/325 1–2 q 4–6 hr
propoxyphene/APAP 100/500 1–2 q 4–6 hr	APAP 300/COD 30 mg 1–2 q 4–6 hr	oxycodone/APAP (Tylox) 5/500 1–2 q 3–4 hr
tramadol (Ultram) 50 mg TID	APAP-300/COD 60 mg 1–2 q 4–6 hr	oxycodone/ASA (Percodan) 5/325 1–2 q 4–6 hr
hydrocodone 2.5/500 1–2 q 4–6 hr	hydrocodone 7.5/500 1–2 q 4–6 hr	morphine 30–60 mg TID levorphanol (Levo-Dromoran)
APAP 300/COD 15 mg 1–2 q 4–6 hr		2 mg 1–2 q 6–8 hr methadone (Dolophine)
		20 mg q 12 hr meperidine (Demerol)
		50 mg 4–6 tabs q 6 hr hydromorphone (Dilaudid)
		2 mg 1–2 q 4–6 hr

Abbreviations: APAP (acetaminophen); ASA (aspirin); COD (codeine)

Table 11-14 Common Antidepressant Medications

Category	Generic	Trade
Tricyclic antidepressants (TCAs)	**amitriptyline**	Elavil
	imipramine	Tofranil
	doxepin	Sinequan
	nortriptyline	Pamelor
	desipramine	Norpramin
Selective serotonin reuptake inhibitors (SSRIs)	**fluoxetine**	Prozac
	paroxetine	Paxil
	sertraline	Zoloft

Tricyclic antidepressants have a characteristic side effect profile that may affect a patient's tolerance. Drowsiness and confusion are the first side effects. These will go away if the dose is started low and titrated upward on a weekly basis. Dry mouth, urinary retention, hot dry skin, and constipation are the other anticipated side effects of this class of medications.

Neuropathic pain is characterized by a well-defined nerve pathway involvement. This pain is generally described as sharp and piercing, or a constant burning along a specific nerve root. A good example of neuropathic pain is post-herpetic neuralgia, which may become quite debilitating in patients following a herpes zoster infection. Neuropathic pain also presents in diabetic patients and HIV patients, and occasionally following injuries. The medications that work well in this circumstance are some of the antiseizure medications. These medications act by decreasing the membrane depolarization and somehow decreasing the intensity of pain. Carbamazepine (Tegretol), **divalproex sodium** (Depakote), and **gabapentin** (Neurontin) have all been shown to be helpful in select nerve pain situations.

SUMMARY

In this chapter, we have learned about the role of neuromuscular function blocking agents before surgery, in intubations, with mechanical ventilation, and in specialized cases postoperatively. We have learned that these drugs can have consequences on blood pressure and heart rate and not just isolated respiratory effects. Since analgesia must accompany neuromuscular relaxation, and pain can impair ventilation, other broad classifications of drugs were also reviewed. In addition, anesthesia agents were reviewed, with attention paid to the impact on the respiratory system.

REVIEW QUESTIONS

1. Neuromuscular blocking agents are classified by:
   (a) duration of action
   (b) the type of block produced
   (c) route they are administered
   (d) all of the above

2. The terms induction, maintenance, and termination are relevant to:
   (a) local anesthesia
   (b) sedative/hypnotics
   (c) general anesthesia
   (d) anxiolytics

3. Inhaled anesthetics may adversely affect:
   (a) cardiovascular function
   (b) respiratory function
   (c) muscular function
   (d) all of the above

4. Match the NMBA to its duration of action:
   pancuronium   short
   succinylcholine   intermediate
   rapacuronium   long
   vecuronium   ultra short

5. Match the drug with its pharmacological class:

ibuprofen	anxiolytic
morphine	NSAID
Valium	opioid

6. Explain some of the principles that guide the use of analgesics.

7. Describe some of the different neurotransmitters involved in the pain pathway and why they are important to cardiorespiratory pharmacotherapy.

8. What are some of the side effects of opioid analgesics?

9. What is the role of concurrent analgesic use with NMBAs?

10. Describe the characteristics of an ideal drug used to facilitate endotracheal intubation.

11. What are some methods of monitoring efficacy of neuromuscular blocking agents?

12. What pharmacological effects does the benzodiazepine class have?

13. A vehicular accident patient with massive chest injuries requires emergency intubation. What pharmacological agent would be indicated? Once intubated, the patient is difficult to ventilate because he is combative, and in addition, the physician wants to depress spontaneous ventilation to assist in healing the chest trauma. What pharmacological agents would be indicated?

GLOSSARY

action potential   change in membrane voltage when the membrane is excited.

analeptic   drug that stimulates the CNS.

analgesic   an agent that relieves pain.

anxiolytic   a drug that reduces anxiety.

depolarizing agent   an agent causing skeletal muscle paralysis by persistent depolarization of the neuromuscular end plate.

general anesthesia   state of deep sleep with no response to stimulation.

hypnotic   a drug that induces sleep.

local anesthesia   condition that results when sensory transmission from a local area of the body to the CNS is blocked.

malignant hyperthermia   increase in temperature to 42°C or higher; this can be a lethal complication of anesthetics.

nondepolarizing agent   an agent causing skeletal muscle paralysis by blockade of the nicotinic end plate.

opioid   class of drugs that mimic actions of opiates, which are drugs derived from opium.

sedative   a drug that produces sedation.

ventilatory stimulant   a drug that acts on the respiratory center in the medulla to increase the rate and depth of ventilation.

www.prenhall.com/colbert

Use the address above to access the free, interactive Companion Web site created specifically for this textbook. Enhance your studying by viewing videos and animations, answering practice quiz questions, and reviewing an audio glossary and much more related to Chapter 11.

CHAPTER 12

Therapeutic Medical Gases

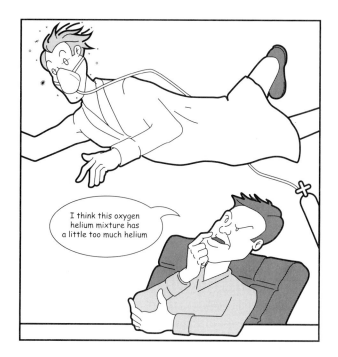

OBJECTIVES

Upon completion of the chapter you will be able to

- Identify the indications for oxygen, helium, carbon dioxide, and nitric oxide therapy
- List and describe the function of oxygen delivery devices
- Describe the effects of oxygen, helium, carbon dioxide, and nitric oxide therapy
- List the hazards of oxygen, helium, carbon dioxide, and nitric oxide therapy
- Describe the monitoring and assessment of oxygen, helium, carbon dioxide, and nitric oxide therapy

ABBREVIATIONS

ABG	arterial blood gas	CO_2	carbon dioxide
ARDS	acute respiratory distress syndrome	COPD	chronic obstructive pulmonary disease
CHF	congestive heart failure	CPAP	continuous positive airway pressure
CO	carbon monoxide		

EDRF	endothelium-derived relaxing factor	PEEP	positive end expiratory pressure
FIO_2	fraction of inspired oxygen	ROP	retinopathy of prematurity
He	helium	SaO_2	arterial blood gas measurement of the saturation of oxygen on the hemoglobin molecule
INO	inhaled nitric oxide		
MI	myocardial infarction		
NO	nitric oxide		
NO_2	nitric dioxide	SpO_2	measure of hemoglobin saturation via a pulse oximety
$PaCO_2$	blood gas measurement of pressure of carbon dioxide within the arterial system	USP	United States Pharmacopoeia
		V/Q	the relationship of alveolar ventilation (V) to capillary perfusion (Q)
PaO_2	blood gas measurement of the pressure of oxygen within the arterial system		

INTRODUCTION

℞ Therapeutic gases are indeed drugs because they exert a physiologic effect upon the body. **Oxygen** is listed in the United States Pharmacopoeia (**USP**), and **oxygen therapy** is used extensively in both the hospital and home setting. The transport and delivery of oxygen to our body's tissue is vital for life. Without adequate oxygen delivery to tissues, we would suffer irreversible brain damage in 4 to 6 minutes. However, too much oxygen can also be dangerous and have serious consequences by disrupting normal tissue function, possibly leading to oxygen toxicity.

Oxygen therapy can be administered with relative ease. However, many misconceptions and the fact that it is easy to administer can lead to situations where oxygen therapy is taken for granted and is not used rationally and properly. Working through this chapter will give you the knowledge to decide "when" and "how" to properly administer oxygen therapy to your patients. In addition, this chapter will focus on gases mixed with oxygen to achieve certain desired physiologic effects. These gases include helium, carbon dioxide, and nitric oxide.

www.prenhall.com/colbert

To learn some fun and interesting historical and chemical facts about oxygen, visit the Web site.

OXYGEN THERAPY

Physiologic Background

One of the most basic human functions in maintaining life is the extraction of oxygen from the atmosphere and its delivery via the bloodstream to cells and tissues to be used for such functions as energy, growth, and repair. We obtain the oxygen from our atmosphere and deliver it to the blood stream by the processes of **ventilation** and **respiration.** Ventilation is

LEARNING HINT

Think of hemoglobin as a bus and the oxygen molecules as kids who can get on and off the bus. Hemoglobin (the bus) has an affinity for (wants to pick up) oxygen (kids) at the lungs. When oxygen-rich hemoglobin reaches the tissues, the oxygen molecules are released to the tissues and carbon dioxide is picked up to return to the lungs for exhalation. This learning hint bus analogy will be used throughout this chapter.

LEARNING HINT

Whenever someone draws and analyzes an arterial blood gas for oxygen levels, they are measuring the amount of oxygen dissolved in the blood, NOT the amount on the hemoglobin molecule. This value is called the partial pressure of arterial oxygen or PaO_2 value. You can think of this value representing kids running around outside the bus waiting to get in. If there are a lot of kids running around outside the bus (high PaO_2) then the bus is probably too full to fit any more in (saturated); if there aren't many kids around (low PaO_2), then the bus is probably not very full.

simply the process of breathing in and out or carrying the oxygen-rich atmosphere from outside the body down to the millions of thin-walled alveoli within the lungs. Respiration is the process of gas exchange at the alveolar capillary membrane, where oxygen is transferred from the alveoli into the bloodstream and the waste product carbon dioxide is transferred into the alveoli to be exhaled. Respiration occurs via diffusion of gases from areas of high concentration to areas of low concentration. In essence, the fundamental purpose of the respiratory system is to supply oxygen to the individual tissue cells and to remove their gaseous waste product, carbon dioxide. Disruption or impairment of either the ventilation or the respiration process will impair oxygenation of the blood. See Figure 12-1 for the process of respiration at the alveolar–capillary membrane.

Once oxygen is transported across the alveoli into the bloodstream, it must be carried to the tissues via the hemoglobin molecule, found within the red blood. **Hemoglobin** has an affinity to bind with oxygen in a reversible manner and thus can combine with oxygen at the alveoli and then release it to the tissues.

This basic background can now be used as a foundation to explain the indications for oxygen therapy.

Hypoxemia

The terms **hypoxemia** and **hypoxia,** while sounding similar, are two related but different clinical terms. We will first discuss the term hypoxemia. Hypoxemia is defined as low levels of oxygen in the blood and can be verified by measuring an arterial blood gas (**ABG**), which shows the partial pressure of oxygen dissolved in the blood (PaO_2). Normal PaO_2 values range between 80 and 100 mm Hg. A PaO_2 of less than 80 mm Hg indicates hypoxemia. See Table 12-1 for a classification of the types of hypoxemia according to the PaO_2 value.

The earth's atmosphere contains approximately 21% oxygen, which provides ample oxygen for a healthy person to survive. However, several conditions can cause hypoxemia, which may require supplemental oxygen. These conditions fall under the following four categories:

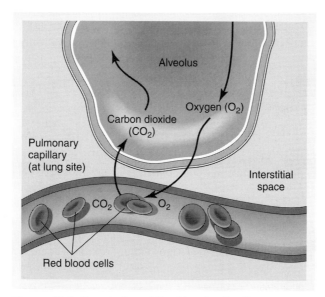

Figure 12-1 Respiration at the Alveolar Capillary Membrane

Table 12-1 Classification of Hypoxemia

Type	PaO₂
Hyperoxemia	greater than 100 mm Hg
No hypoxemia (normoxemia)	80–100 mm Hg
Mild hypoxemia	60–79 mm Hg
Moderate hypoxemia	40–59 mm Hg
Severe hypoxemia	less than 40 mm Hg

Note: The PaO_2 normally decreases with age, and a general rule is that for every year of age over 60, subtract 1 mm Hg from the normal range limits. For example, a 75-year-old patient would have 65 to 85 mm Hg as their adjusted normal range.

1. Low levels of atmospheric oxygen. An example would be high altitudes, where the low barometric pressure allows only low oxygen tensions to be available.
2. Alveolar hypoventilation. Anything that interferes with the transport of oxygen to the alveoli, thereby decreasing ventilation, may cause hypoxemia. Ventilatory depression due to narcotic overdoses, COPD, neuromuscular disease, chest trauma, or pain are some examples.
3. Ventilation-to-perfusion (**V/Q**) mismatching: Any process that impairs the balance between ventilation reaching the alveolus and perfusion to the surrounding capillary may lead to hypoxemia. For example, lung diseases such as emphysema, interstitial pulmonary fibrosis, lung cancer, and pneumonia all create conditions that impair the ventilation process (decreasing V) by either destroying the integrity of the alveolus or impairing diffusion by causing secretion barriers. In addition, cardiac diseases that affect the cardiac output, such as CHF or MI, or that interfere with capillary perfusion, such as pulmonary emboli, will alter the perfusion (Q) of the capillary and thus lead to a V/Q mismatch.
4. Right-to-left shunt. This occurs when the blood leaving the right heart either bypasses a portion of the pulmonary circulation or flows by nonfunctional alveoli. This blood will enter the left heart unoxygenated and therefore lower the overall PaO_2. Right-to-left shunting examples include cardiogenic pulmonary edema, acute respiratory distress syndrome (ARDS), and atelectasis, where the alveolus is totally nonfunctional because of collapse or being completely filled with fliud.

CLINICAL PEARL
Oxygen therapy will help under conditions 1 to 3, but not 4, because in the last case the oxygen never gets to the nonventilated alveolus. The right-to-left shunt requires positive end-expiratory pressure (PEEP) or continuous positive airway pressure (CPAP) in addition to oxygen therapy to reestablish ventilation to these nonfunctional units.

Why do mountain climbers need supplemental oxygen, and why do airplane cabins need to be pressurized?

Clinical Manifestations of Hypoxemia

The clinical manifestations of hypoxemia relate to the body's attempt to combat and compensate for the hypoxemic condition. The following is a list of these responses:

- Tachycardia and systemic hypertension. The tachycardia is an attempt to speed up oxygen delivery, and hypertension is a result of the increased heart rate. If the heart is weakened by disease, bradycardia and hypotension may result.
- Tachypnea. The increased respiratory rate is an attempt to get more oxygen into the blood. The depth will probably also increase, resulting in hyperventilation, as evidenced by a decrease in $PaCO_2$.
- Pulmonary hypertension. Constriction of pulmonary capillaries allows slower blood flow and therefore more oxygen to be loaded onto the hemoglobin at the lungs.

- Cerebral and coronary vasodilatation. This leads to increased blood flow to the vital areas of the heart and brain.
- Cyanosis, diaphoresis, and pallor. These may all be present.
- Restlessness, agitation, and confusion. Not enough oxygen to the brain causes these.
- Secondary polycythemia. With chronic hypoxemia, as in COPD, or in the case of individuals living at high altitudes, the body will stimulate the production of more RBCs and therefore have higher hemoglobin levels.

Hypoxia

Whereas hypoxemia is easy to assess with a blood gas, it doesn't necessarily mean that you have hypoxia. Hypoxia means low levels of oxygen to the tissue. A patient could have low levels of oxygen in the blood (hypoxemia) but not necessarily have low levels reaching the tissues (hypoxia), because the body will have compensated with tachycardia, pulmonary vasoconstriction, or polycythemia. Conversely, a patient could have hypoxia but not have hypoxemia. For example, a patient may have normal or high PaO_2 (no hypoxemia), yet the hemoglobin may be defective, or the tissues may not be able to utilize the oxygen, leading to hypoxia. Of course, you could have situations where both hypoxemia and hypoxia occur at the same time. Let's review some specific types of hypoxia.

Hypoxemic Hypoxia. Sounds like a redundant term? Basically, this is hypoxia caused by anything that interferes with the ability of oxygen to get to the alveoli or diffuse across them. Some examples of causes include atmospheres with insufficient oxygen, such as mountain climbers contend with; airway obstructions that do not let oxygen pass; fluid in the alveoli, which would act as a barrier to diffusion; and any situation that would lead to hypoventilation, such as muscle weakness/disease, brain injuries, or drug overdoses that suppress the respiratory system. Hypoxemia will always be present in these situations, since an adequate oxygen supply never reaches the alveoli.

Anemic Hypoxia. This is anything that interferes with the hemoglobin's oxygen-carrying capacity. For example, anemic patients or patients with dysfunctional hemoglobin, as in carbon monoxide poisoning or sickle cell anemia, may not be able to carry sufficient oxygen to the tissues. Hypoxemia may or may not be present in these patients, because they may have normal amounts of dissolved oxygen (PaO_2) but be unable to properly load it onto the hemoglobin molecule.

Stagnant or Circulatory Hypoxia. Anything that interferes with the circulatory system's ability to transport oxygen causes stagnant hypoxia. Examples include decreased cardiac output, cardiogenic shock, hypovolemia, and any cardiovascular instability, such as congestive heart failure. In these cases, hypoxia will almost always be present.

Histotoxic Hypoxia. Here we have an inability of the tissue to utilize available oxygen, no matter how much is presented. Cyanide poisoning is the classic example. It is rarely accompanied by hypoxemia, but it is deadly.

Demand Hypoxia. In hypermetabolic states, the tissue demand for oxygen may exceed the supply. Fever and strenuous exercise are examples of demand hypoxia where hypoxemia will be present.

As you can see, when you assess a patient for hypoxia you need to look at more than just the PaO_2. You must also look at the oxygen saturation of the hemoglobin (**SaO_2**), the amount and type of hemoglobin, and the cardiovascular status.

Contrast hypoxemia and hypoxia in terms of definition and clinical assessment.

CLINICAL PEARL

Not all patients have a PaO₂ of 80–100 mm Hg as their normal range. Premature infants and chronically hypoxemic COPD patients may have lower limits of acceptability.

CLINICAL PEARL

Cyanosis is a bluish discoloration of the skin. This bluish color comes from excessive amounts of deoxygenated hemoglobin (a lot of blue buses). Be careful, though; if a patient has low hemoglobin levels (anemia), they may not show signs of cyanosis, because in essence they don't have enough hemoglobin to effect a color change in the blood. Nevertheless, they are probably still suffering from hypoxia and still need supplemental oxygen.

CLINICAL PEARL

The ultimate goal is to treat the underlying cause of the hypoxia, whether it is hypoxemia that will respond to oxygen therapy or anemia or cardiovascular instability that may need additional treatments in addition to oxygen therapy.

CLINICAL PEARL

Medical oxygen is regulated by the FDA and must be 99% pure. It can be stored as a compressed gas in cylinders or as stored liquid oxygen that is converted to a gas before being delivered to a patient. Oxygen cylinders and oxygen piping systems are color-coded green in the United States; however, white is the international color for oxygen.

www.prenhall.com/colbert

The oxygen–hemoglobin dissociation curve shows the relationship between how many kids are outside the bus (PaO₂ we get from blood gases) to how many are inside it (the saturation of hemoglobin, or SaO₂). Visit the Web site to view an animation that explains this curve and why it is important to us. You may want to view this more than once.

Goals of Oxygen Therapy

The three major goals for oxygen therapy are to (1) treat hypoxemia, (2) decrease the work of breathing, and (3) decrease myocardial work.

Treating Hypoxemia. The following guidelines are used for assessing hypoxemia in adults, children, or infants who are breathing room air at rest. If the patient's ABG shows either a PaO₂ of less than 60 mm Hg or a saturation (SaO₂) of less than 90%, or if pulse oximetry is used and a reading of less than 90% (**SpO₂**) is obtained, you can document that your patient needs oxygen therapy.

Decrease the Work of Breathing. A patient who is having a difficult time breathing consumes a lot of oxygen in order to survive. The body increases the work of the respiratory muscles by increasing the rate and depth of breathing in order to bring in more oxygen. A clinical assessment of the patient in respiratory distress and in need of oxygen therapy may find an increase in the rate and depth of breathing, accessory muscle use, and cyanosis.

Decrease Myocardial Work. The heart is the major organ that pumps the blood containing oxygen to the tissues of the body. When there is a decrease in the blood's oxygen levels, the heart attempts to correct this situation by increasing its pumping action and rate. This action also produces an increased need for oxygen for the heart's muscles, because of its increased workload. This can lead to arrhythmias or heart failure. Therefore, oxygen therapy should be started to assist the heart with this increased work, so that it may safely provide more oxygen to the tissues.

Oxygen Administration Devices

Before discussing particular devices for oxygen therapy, it is important to talk about the idea of **fractional inspired oxygen** or **FIO₂**. Our atmosphere consists of approximately 21 parts in 100 oxygen, or 21%; therefore, the FIO₂ of room air is .21. When supplemental oxygen is delivered to the patient, we increase the FIO₂ in order to provide more oxygen to the body for gas exchange. You can deliver from 22% up to 100% oxygen, depending upon the type of device used. Successful oxygen therapy depends upon choosing the right type of device and the proper FIO₂.

www.prenhall.com/colbert

Oxygen therapy that can deliver 100% oxygen at increased atmospheric pressures is called hyperbaric oxygen therapy. Hyperbaric oxygen is used to treat carbon monoxide poisoning, thermal burns, decompression sickness, air embolism, and anaerobic infections. Go the Web to learn more about this therapy.

Low-Flow Oxygen Devices

After assessing your patient and determining that oxygen therapy is needed, the next step is to decide what device will provide the amount of oxygen needed for this patient. **Low-flow oxygen systems** provide only a portion of the total amount of gas the patient is breathing. For example, while a portion of what the patient is breathing is coming from the oxygen device, the rest must be added from room air. Common low-flow oxygen devices include the **nasal cannula, simple mask,** and **nonrebreathing mask.**

Nasal Cannula. One of the most commonly used low-flow oxygen therapy devices is the nasal cannula. The small-bore flexible plastic tubing has two short extensions that insert into the nostrils and direct the oxygen into the nasal cavity. It is well tolerated by most patients and has advantages over a mask for comfort of eating or speaking. The major disadvantage is that, as with all low-flow oxygen devices, as the patient increases the rate and/or depth of breathing in a crisis situation, they will pull in more room air but the oxygen delivered will remain fixed, so the FIO_2 will drop because of air dilution. The nasal cannula is frequently used for low FIO_2s for long-term oxygen therapy with COPD patients to treat hypoxemia and in cardiac intensive care to decrease myocardial work (see Figure 12-2, which shows a nasal cannula).

Simple Mask. A simple mask is a low-flow oxygen device that fits over the patient's nose and mouth and acts as a reservoir for the next breath. The FIO_2 varies with this device because of a number of factors, including a poor sealing system, variable tidal volumes and breathing rates, and low gas flows. This mask can deliver an FIO_2 between .35 and .50, depending on the patient's ventilation rate and depth. A simple mask is generally used for emergencies and short-term therapies, which require a moderate FIO_2 (see Figure 12-3).

Nonrebreathing Mask. A nonrebreathing mask is designed to fit over the patient's nose and mouth as the simple oxygen mask does; however, a 500 to 1000 ml plastic bag is added to the mask, and it acts as an oxygen reservoir for the next breath. This mask has a series of one-way valves that permit the reservoir bag to fill only with pure oxygen, the exhaled gases being vented outside the mask. This reservoir of 100% oxygen and the exhalation valves on the mask force the patient to take the next breath from the reservoir bag, providing higher FIO_2s, in the range of 50% to 70%.

CONTROVERSY

In many textbooks, the range for the nonrebreathing mask is given as 70% to 100%, but studies have shown that owing to removal of one valve for safety and difficulty in obtaining a perfect seal, the percentage of oxygen delivered to the patient is lowered.

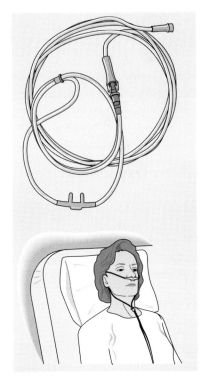

Figure 12-2 Nasal Cannula

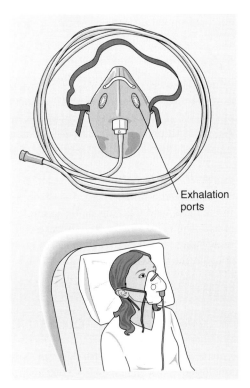

Exhalation ports

Figure 12-3 Simple Mask

It is very important to note that the flow to the reservoir bag must be enough that the bag does not deflate more than one third when the patient inhales. If the flow rate is too low, the patient could suffocate, especially if the mask has a tight seal; if not, the delivered FIO_2 will be decreased if the patient has to breathe around the mask (see Figure 12-4).

If a patient on a low-flow device such as 2 liters/min nasal cannula suddenly experiences respiratory distress and increases their rate and depth of ventilation, what happens to the FIO_2 reaching the lungs?

www.prenhall.com/colbert

Go to the Web site to view videos concerning low-flow oxygen therapy devices.

High-Flow Oxygen Systems

High-flow oxygen systems provide enough gas flow to meet all of the patient's ventilatory demands regardless of what their demands are and thus prevents dilution of the set FIO_2. High-flow systems deliver a precise FIO_2 that doesn't change with a patient's ventilation rate, their breathing pattern, or the depth of their breathing, so high-flow systems are advantageous when a closer monitoring of a patient's oxygenation status is needed. Types of high-flow systems include the **jet mixing mask** and **large-volume nebulizers.**

Jet Mixing Mask. A jet mixing mask (also referred to as a venti mask) is an example of a high-flow device that delivers a total high flow by mixing oxygen with room air. This mask uses the Bernoulli principle to take pure oxygen from the flow meter and mix it with

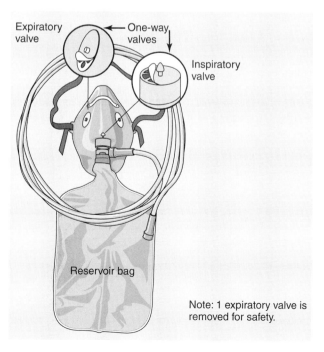

Figure 12-4 Nonrebreathing Mask

Expiratory valve

One-way valves

Inspiratory valve

Reservoir bag

Note: 1 expiratory valve is removed for safety.

a certain proportion of room air and then deliver oxygen concentrations ranging from 24% to 50% to the patient. Every percentage of oxygen has its own ratio of air to oxygen. The most common proportions are listed in Table 12-2.

Large-Volume Nebulizers. A large-volume nebulizer is another example of a high-flow system and is typically used for a patient who requires a precise nonchanging FIO_2 coupled with high moisture levels in aerosol form, for retained secretions, or for a patient whose body's natural humidification system is impaired or bypassed. This device works on the same principle as the jet mixing mask but also provides **bland** (nonmedicated) **aerosol therapy.** The large-volume nebulizer can be connected to a variety of devices, including an aerosol mask, a face tent for patients with facial burns or who cannot tolerate a mask, a **T-**piece or Briggs adapter for intubated patients, or a tracheostomy mask (collar) for patients with a tracheostomy (see Figure 12-5).

Monitoring Oxygen Therapy

Patients on oxygen therapy should have the following monitored:

- Sensorium. The patient should think more clearly and become less restless and agitated because of more oxygen being delivered to the brain.
- Dyspnea. Shortness of breath should improve, and the patient's accessory muscle use should decrease.
- Color. Cyanosis may improve and should be monitored via the skin and nail beds.
- Vital signs. Vital signs should return toward normal.
- PaO_2 value. The PaO_2 obtained from an ABG should rise toward acceptable limits for that particular patient.
- Pulse oximetry. The amount of hemoglobin saturated with oxygen (SaO_2) should show improved values with the proper use of oxygen therapy. A value of 95% to 98% is considered normal, but most physicians will accept a reading of 90% to 92%.

Give four positive clinical signs that oxygen therapy is effective.

Hazards of Oxygen Therapy

Oxygen is considered a drug, and if proper delivery of this drug is not monitored, some problems could occur that might be harmful. Some of the hazards of oxygen therapy include:

- **Oxygen toxicity** is a serious condition that may occur if too much oxygen is delivered for too long, and it could possibly lead to death. If a normal person breathes 100% oxygen for longer than 12 to 24 hours, he or she will show early signs of oxygen toxicity, which include a sore throat, dyspnea, cough, and substernal discomfort.

Table 12-2 Common Oxygen Percentages and Air-to-Oxygen Ratios

Oxygen (%)	Approximate Air : Oxygen Ratio
24	25 : 1
28	10 : 1
30	8 : 1
35	5 : 1
40	3 : 1
60	1 : 1

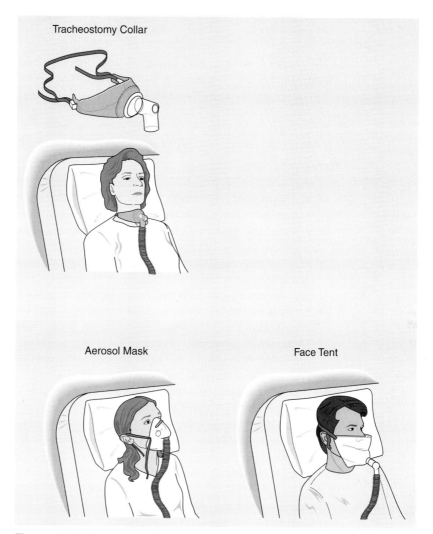

Tracheostomy Collar

Aerosol Mask

Face Tent

Figure 12-5 Bland Aerosol Devices

If oxygen is continued, then nausea, vomiting, diffuse infiltrates, atelectasis, and eventually ARDS may develop. This is because too much oxygen in this person's system causes the formation of **free radicals** or oxidants, which are charged particles that disrupt tissue formation.

• **Oxygen-induced hypoventilation** is a problem that may occur in patients who suffer from chronic obstructive pulmonary disease (COPD). These patients may have chronic retention of carbon dioxide ($PaCO_2$), which depresses the respiratory centers in the brain, which usually control the stimulus to breathe. When they are depressed, the patient's stimulus to breathe is controlled by the **peripheral chemoreceptors,** which respond to arterial oxygen tension (PaO_2) of less than 60 mm Hg. This is known as the **hypoxic drive** mechanism. Administering high oxygen concentrations to these patients may lead to a decrease in the rate and depth of their breathing. A general rule of thumb when applying oxygen therapy to a COPD patient who has *chronic* hypoxemia is to maintain their PaO_2 in the 50 to 60 mm Hg range.

⟨ CONTROVERSY ⟩

The "hypoxic drive theory" has come under question and it is theorized that the oxygen-induced hypoventilation may be caused by hypoxic pulmonary vasoconstriction that occurs in chronic COPD patients. This compensatory vasoconstriction shunts blood to better ventilated regions of the lungs. Relieving the vasoconstriction with high oxygen levels may increase the blood flow to poorly or nonventilated regions of the lungs and thus increase shunting and increase arterial carbon dioxide levels.

- **Retinopathy of prematurity (ROP),** formerly called **retrolental fibroplasia,** is caused by both prematurity and high PaO_2 levels in premature infants, which causes vasospasm to occur in the retinal area, leading to the formation of fibrous scar tissue behind the lens of the eye (retrolental fibroplasia), causing vision impairment or blindness.
- **Absorptive atelectasis** can occur when high concentrations of oxygen wash out the inert nitrogen in the lungs. With subsequent absorption of oxygen into the circulatory system, the lower pressures in the airways become subatmospheric and lead to atelectasis.
- **Environmental hazards** can occur because oxygen promotes combustion, causing a fire to burn hotter and faster. This is why oxygen is used in welding to increase the temperature. Therefore, if a facility is not a smoke-free environment, a "No Smoking—Oxygen in Use" sign must be posted, and the danger of fire must also be emphasized in the home care setting. Because of the large use of oxygen in the hospital, all healthcare personnel should know where all oxygen shut-off valves and fire extinguishers are located as well as how to use them.

While these hazards may be present, oxygen therapy should not be withheld from patients in critical need. For example, patients may require 100% oxygen to survive a cardiopulmonary arrest or carbon monoxide poisoning, and the resulting possible hazards are less ominous than the resulting death if high levels of oxygen are withheld.

In summary, the oxygen amount in the blood tension (PaO_2) and the length of exposure will determine if a toxic response is likely. Generally speaking, an FIO_2 of less than 50% should not result in a meaningful amount of toxic response in adults. The best advice when administering oxygen therapy is to follow this general rule: **Administer oxygen at the lowest possible FIO_2 to get the desired PaO_2 or SaO_2.**

CARBON DIOXIDE

Introduction

Carbon dioxide (CO_2) is a by-product of cellular metabolism that must be excreted via the respiratory and renal systems at a homeostatic rate to maintain the body pH within an acceptable limit. CO_2 exerts powerful effects on the respiratory, circulatory, and central nervous systems and has limited therapeutic uses because of these effects.

Physiologic Effects

The central chemoreceptors, located in the medullary centers, control ventilation according to the levels of CO_2 within the blood. High levels of CO_2 will activate the medullary centers to increase ventilation in order to rid the body of the excess CO_2. Therefore, inhaled carbon dioxide is a potent respiratory stimulant; it will rapidly increase the rate and depth of ventilation.

With rising CO_2 levels, the circulatory response is to increase perfusion to vital areas to deliver more oxygen and excrete the high level of CO_2 that could become toxic to the tissues. Therefore, the major circulatory effects of inhaled carbon dioxide include cerebral vasodilation, coronary vasodilation, tachycardia, and increased blood pressure.

Inhaled carbon dioxide is also a powerful CNS depressant. Inhalation of small percentages of carbon dioxide may produce mental confusion, and with higher doses, seizures and unconsciousness can result.

Patients who have respiratory acidosis are often confused and complain of a headache. Can you see the correlation of the increased CO_2 to these symptoms?

Indications for Carbon Dioxide Therapy

Inhaling CO_2 to elevate $PaCO_2$ levels has limited uses because of the adverse effects. The current therapeutic indications for carbon dioxide therapy include the following:

- Respiratory stimulant and increased cerebral perfusion agent—to reverse anesthetic gas–induced respiratory depression.
- Treatment for singulation (commonly called hiccups)—one of the many home cures for hiccups is to breathe into a paper bag. This makes physiologic sense, since hiccups occur when an irritated phrenic nerve sends erratic impulses to the diaphragm. Inhalation of low concentrations of carbon dioxide hyperstimulates the respiratory center, which overrides the spasmodic impulses to the diaphragm that produce the hiccups, thereby restoring normal breathing.
- Improved retinal blood flow—some ophthalmologists use carbon dioxide therapy to vasodilate the retinal vessels to enhance perfusion when it is inadequate.

CLINICAL PEARL

O_2/CO_2 cylinders are colored green/gray in the United States, with the majority green representing the majority gas oxygen. The FDA purity standard for carbon dioxide is 99.9%.

Carbon Dioxide Administration

Carbon dioxide does not support life and therefore must be combined with oxygen. CO_2/O_2 mixtures are usually either 5% CO_2 and 95% O_2 or 10% CO_2 and 90% O_2. Patients breathe these mixtures through a well-fitting nonrebreathing mask for 5- to 10-minute treatments. The patient must be continuously monitored for adverse effects such as nausea, vomiting, dizziness, headaches, palpitations, muscle tremors, high blood pressure, and confusion. Carbon dioxide therapy is contraindicated for patients who are chronic retainers of CO_2, because additional carbon dioxide will further exacerbate their condition.

HELIUM THERAPY

Introduction

Helium is an odorless and tasteless gas that is very light and low in density. This is why helium balloons float so well and inhaled helium allows the vocal cords to vibrate much easier and give a high-pitched cartoon character-like sound to the voice. Helium is also physiologically inert and poorly soluble in water and therefore will not react within the body.

Indications for Helium Therapy

Like CO_2, helium does not support life, and the practice of inhaling helium to cause vocal distortion is dangerous. Helium, like carbon dioxide, must be mixed with oxygen to form a **heliox** mixture. This mixture has been demonstrated to be effective in treating patients with upper airway obstructions. The airway obstruction enhances the rough turbulent flow already present in the larger airways. The low-density helium/oxygen mixture favors a smoother, more laminar flow through the airways, thus reducing the airway resistance and

CLINICAL PEARL

Helium is an excellent heat conductor and can be used during laser airway surgery to absorb the heat from the laser beam, thereby lessening the surrounding tissue damage within the airway. Breathing helium/oxygen diving mixtures minimizes the risk of oxygen toxicity and decompression sickness (the bends). Helium is also used in certain pulmonary function tests.

work of breathing and allowing more flow beyond the obstruction. Helium/oxygen mixtures are less useful in lower airway obstruction, where flow is laminar and independent of gas density.

Administration of Helium/Oxygen

The helium/oxygen mixture is compressed in cylinders color-coded brown (helium) and green (oxygen), with a percentage mixture of either 80% He and 20% O_2 or 70% He and 30% O_2. Helium/oxygen is administered via a well-fitting nonrebreathing mask or through patient artificial airways.

www.prenhall.com/colbert

Because of helium's lighter density, oxygen flowmeters will read inaccurate flows. There is a way to calculate the true flow of an oxygen/helium mixture flowing through an oxygen flowmeter, though, and the Web site will show you how it is done.

Hazard of Helium/Oxygen Therapy

Although it's not a true hazard, the patient should still be told that their voice will be changed temporarily to a higher pitch and will return to normal shortly after the therapy. It has been suggested that breathing helium/oxygen mixtures may affect the cough mechanism, because an effective cough requires turbulent flow in the larger airways to generate the explosive pressure. However, this will only be a temporary diminishment of cough effectiveness; it will return within minutes after the treatment, when the helium is cleared from within the airways.

What is the main indication for heliox therapy?

NITRIC OXIDE THERAPY

Introduction

Certain conditions and disease states can lead to increased pulmonary hypertension. This increase in pulmonary vascular resistance not only puts a strain on the heart but can cause damage and leakage of the pulmonary capillaries, which would greatly impair gas exchange capabilities. All blood vessels have a single cell layer that lines their inner lumen; this is referred to as the endothelial layer or endothelium. The capillary vessels contain only an endothelium layer and are void of the smooth muscle and collagen layers that the veins and arteries contain. In the early 1980s it was discovered that the endothelium produces a chemical substance that is a very potent vasodilator and can reduce pulmonary vascular resistance. This chemical was originally termed **endothelium-derived relaxing factor (EDRF)** but was later shown to be equivalent to **nitric oxide (NO).**

LEARNING HINT

Do not confuse nitric oxide (NO)—the potent inhaled vasodilator—with nitrous oxide (N_2O), the anesthetic gas commonly referred to as laughing gas.

Physiology of Nitric Oxide

Nitric oxide binds to the enzyme guanyl cyclase and increases levels and stability of cGMP, which causes vasodilation within blood vessels. However, nitric oxide is rapidly metabolized on contact with blood and reacts with hemoglobin to form methemoglobin. In essence, contact with blood destroys nitric oxide's vasodilation effects. Although this may seem like a disadvantage, it is actually advantageous in treating pulmonary hypertension. Inhaled nitric oxide (**INO**) diffuses across the alveoli and *first* comes in contact with the endothelium layer of the capillaries and pulmonary arterioles, producing vasodilation and decreasing pulmonary vascular resistance. Further diffusion of nitric oxide now causes it to enter the bloodstream and neutralizes its effect so that it does not cause systemic vasodilation. Therefore, INO is a selective pulmonary vasodilator.

INO can only travel to well-ventilated alveoli, so it will improve the ventilation/perfusion ratio and thus oxygenation by redistributing capillary blood to well-ventilated lung units, causing enhanced gas exchange. In addition, the decreased pulmonary vascular resistance reduces the stress on the right heart, which is pumping into the pulmonary vascular bed. Table 12-3 summarizes the beneficial effects of INO.

<u>CLINICAL PEARL</u>
Nitric oxide is not exclusively a vascular smooth muscle relaxant but also relaxes bronchial smooth muscle, so it is a bronchodilator and may have potential future use.

INO Administration and Dosage

Nitric oxide combined with oxygen is rapidly oxidized into toxic substances; therefore it is combined with inert nitrogen in compressed gas cylinders. It is generally provided through the inspiratory line of the ventilator, and continuous monitoring for NO and **nitrogen dioxide (NO$_2$)** levels should be performed. Many studies have demonstrated that inhaled nitric oxide seems to be relatively effective and safe at doses between 2 and 80 parts per million (ppm), although a specific dosage has not been approved by the FDA. Please refer to the Web site for references and updates for more specific and current information.

Therapeutic Indications for Inhalation of Nitric Oxide

INO has been shown to be effective in treating patients with increased pulmonary vascular resistance secondary to severe pulmonary hypertension. Inhalation of nitric oxide has proven beneficial for the following conditions:

- Acute respiratory distress syndrome (ARDS)
- Infant respiratory distress syndrome (IRDS)
- Persistent pulmonary hypertension of the neonate (PPHN)
- Other conditions that cause pulmonary hypertension

Monitoring of Nitric Oxide Therapy

Although studies have suggested that short-term, low-dose inhalation of nitric oxide is a relatively safe procedure, continuous monitoring of the NO should be maintained to ensure

Table 12-3 Beneficial Effects of INO

Lowers pulmonary hypertension
Reduces pulmonary vascular resistance with no change in systemic vascular resistance
Enhances right-heart function
Improves arterial oxygenation by enhancing ventilation/perfusion ratio

remaining within the prescribed dose. In addition, the toxic metabolites of nitric oxide when combined with oxygen (NO_2, NO_3), along with methemoglobin levels, should be monitored. Premature infants may be more prone to higher methemoglobin levels than adults during nitric oxide therapy.

SUMMARY

Medical gases are indicated for a variety of clinical conditions. Oxygen therapy is one of the most frequently prescribed drugs in medicine and is delivered via a host of devices. The major goals of oxygen therapy include treating hypoxemia, decreasing the work of breathing, and decreasing myocardial work.

In addition to oxygen therapy, other medical gases are used, including helium, carbon dioxide, and nitric oxide therapy. The low-density helium is mixed with oxygen to primarily treat airway obstruction. Carbon dioxide has many side effects that limit its use, but it can be used as a respiratory stimulant, to treat hiccups, and to improve retinal blood flow. Inhaled nitric oxide is used to lower pulmonary hypertension, which also serves to enhance right-heart function.

REVIEW QUESTIONS

1. Hypoxemia is
   (a) low levels of tissue oxygen
   (b) low levels of arterial oxygen
   (c) low levels of hemoglobin
   (d) low levels of red blood cells
2. Which of the following are clinical manifestations of hypoxemia?
   I. tachycardia
   II. cerebral vasodilation
   III. tachypnea
   IV. pulmonary hypotension
   (a) all
   (b) I and III
   (c) I, II, and II
   (d) II and IV
3. Which of the following medical gases need(s) to be mixed with oxygen before delivering to a patient?
   (a) carbon dioxide
   (b) argon
   (c) helium
   (d) a & c
4. Inhaled nitric oxide (INO) will:
   (a) increase pulmonary hypertension
   (b) increase systemic vascular resistance

(c) decrease pulmonary hypertension
(d) decrease arterial oxygenation

5. Classify the following PaO_2s:
   100 mm Hg _____
   55 mm Hg _____
   39 mm Hg _____
   45 mm Hg _____
   125 mm Hg _____
6. Classify the type of hypoxia:
   Low hemoglobin levels _____
   CNS drug overdose _____
   Severe hypotension _____
   Fever _____
7. List and explain the three major goals of oxygen therapy.
8. Explain how a patient could have hypoxemia but not hypoxia.
9. Contrast low-flow and high-flow oxygen delivery devices.
10. Give three positive clinical responses expected with effective oxygen therapy.
11. Explain why carbon dioxide therapy is very dosage dependent.
12. List the indication for heliox therapy and what properties of helium make it useful for this purpose.

CASE STUDY

A 68-year-old woman in congestive heart failure has a PaO$_2$ of 41 mm Hg. Pharmacological treatment of the CHF is begun. She has tachycardia and tachypnea and is showing signs of acrocyanosis. What oxygen therapy recommendations would you make at this time?

How would you monitor the treatment's effectiveness?

What would be your response to an order that read, "Simple oxygen mask at 2 liters per minute"?

GLOSSARY

absorptive atelectasis   a hazard of breathing high concentrations of oxygen, which can wash out the inert nitrogen within the lungs and lead to collapse of lung tissue when the oxygen is absorbed into the bloodstream.

anemic hypoxia   hypoxia due to low levels of hemoglobin or dysfunctional hemoglobin.

bland aerosol therapy   nonmedicated aerosol therapy.

cyanosis   bluish discoloration of the skin.

demand hypoxia   hypoxia as a result of a hypermetabolic state.

free radicals   charged particles or oxidants that are formed with excess oxygen; they can disrupt tissue function.

heliox   mixture of oxygen and helium gas.

hemoglobin   molecule that transports oxygen by binding with it in a reversible manner.

high-flow oxygen systems   oxygen delivery devices that provide the patient's total ventilatory requirement.

histotoxic hypoxia   hypoxia as a result of the tissue's inability to utilize oxygen for metabolism.

hyperoxemia   higher-than-normal oxygen levels within the blood.

hypoxemia   low levels of oxygen in the blood.

hypoxemic hypoxia   hypoxia caused by impairment of oxygen delivery to the alveoli.

hypoxia   low levels of oxygen at the tissues.

hypoxic drive   the ventilatory drive when it is stimulated by the peripherial chemoreceptors' response to low levels of oxygen in the blood.

jet mixing mask   a high-flow oxygen mask that utilizes the Bernoulli principle to mix oxygen and room air to deliver a precise FIO$_2$.

large-volume nebulizers   nebulizers that can deliver oxygen and aerosol particles.

low-flow oxygen systems   oxygen delivery devices that provide only a portion of the patient's ventilatory requirement.

nasal cannula   a common low-flow oxygen device inserted into the nostrils.

nonrebreathing mask   an oxygen mask with a reservoir and valves to increase the amount of delivered oxygen or FIO$_2$.

oxygen-induced hypoventilation   hypoventilation caused by excessive oxygen blunting the hypoxic drive in sensitive patients.

oxygen therapy   the delivery of oxygen for therapeutic value.

oxygen toxicity   serious condition that can occur if excess oxygen is delivered.

peripheral chemoreceptors receptors in the carotid and aortic bodies that respond to low levels of oxygen.

polycythemia higher-than-normal levels of hemoglobin.

respiration process of gas exchange of oxygen and carbon dioxide.

simple mask low-flow oxygen mask.

stagnant hypoxia hypoxia due to an impairment in the circulatory system's ability to transport oxygen.

ventilation the movement of gas into and out of the respiratory system.

www.prenhall.com/colbert

Use the address above to access the free, interactive Companion Web site created specifically for this textbook. Enhance your studying by viewing videos and animations, answering practice quiz questions, and reviewing an audio glossary and much more related to Chapter 12.

COPD: The Pharmacological Treatment of Asthma, Chronic Bronchitis, and Emphysema

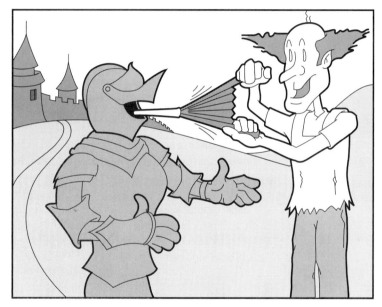

The first bronchodilator, administered by a medieval physician

OBJECTIVES

Upon completion of this chapter you will be able to

- Explain the pathophysiology of chronic obstructive pulmonary disease (COPD)
- Distinguish among the various forms of COPD
- Develop a pharmacologic regimen for asthma, chronic bronchitis, and emphysema
- Develop a monitoring and educational plan for asthma, chronic bronchitis, and emphysema

ABBREVIATIONS

ATS	American Thoracic Society	FTND	Fagerstrom test for nicotine
COPD	chronic obstructive pulmonary disease		dependence
		MDI	metered-dose inhaler

Main contributing author Carla Frye

NAEPP2	National Asthma Education and Prevention Program, Second Expert Panel	$PaCO_2$	arterial partial pressure of carbon dioxide
NRT	nicotine replacement therapy	PaO_2	arterial partial pressure of oxygen
PEFR	peak expiratory flow rate	CNS	central nervous system
NIH	National Institutes of Health	FEV_1	forced expiratory volume in 1 second
BTS	British Thoracic Society		
FVC	forced vital capacity	α_1-AT	alpha one antitrypsin
AHCPR	Agency for Health Care Policy and Research	GERD	gastroesophageal reflux disease
IgE	immunoglobulin E	ICU	intensive care unit

INTRODUCTION

Chronic obstructive pulmonary disease (COPD) is a global term used to describe abnormal pulmonary conditions associated with cough, sputum production, dyspnea, airflow obstruction, and impaired gas exchange. It is the fourth leading cause of death in the United States. Specific COPD conditions such as **emphysema, asthma,** and **chronic bronchitis** are delineated on the basis of clinical, anatomic, or physiologic criteria and can coexist, making diagnosis very difficult. See Table 13-1, which gives definitions for the various COPD states.

These overlapping disease states can sometimes lead to a "state" of confusion because of the many common features complicating their diagnosis. In addition, drug therapies for each condition overlap; this can also be confusing when developing a therapeutic plan for an individual patient. Therefore it is very important to start this discussion with an understanding of how these disease entities are defined and how they can be differentiated.

Patients with asthma, chronic bronchitis, or emphysema all share features of airway obstruction, and their treatment modalities will have similar goals. Asthma is distinguished by having reversible airway narrowing and airway hyperreactivity; it is most commonly

Table 13-1   Definitions of COPD Disease States

Disease	*Description*
Asthma	A chronic inflammatory disorder of the airways in which many cells and cellular elements play a role, in particular mast cells, eosinophils, T lymphocytes, neutrophils, and epithelial cells. In susceptible individuals, this inflammation causes recurrent episodes of wheezing, breathlessness, chest tightness, and cough, particularly at night and in the early morning. These episodes are usually associated with widespread but variable airflow obstruction that is often reversible either spontaneously or with treatment. The inflammation also causes an associated increase in the existing bronchial hyperresponsiveness to a variety of stimuli.
Chronic Bronchitis	Usually defined in clinical terms as the presence of productive cough during 3 months of the year for 2 consecutive years, provided that other causes of chronic sputum production such as tuberculosis and bronchiectasis are excluded. Airway hyperreactivity may be present.
Emphysema	A pathologic diagnosis marked by destruction of alveolar walls, with resultant loss of elastic recoil in the lung. Dyspnea on exertion is the predominant clinical feature, and airway hyperreactivity may also be present.

characterized as an inflammatory process. Patients with emphysema or chronic bronchitis, on the other hand, *may* have airway hyperreactivity.

Emphysema is characterized physiologically as the permanent, abnormal enlargement of airway spaces and destruction of the alveolar wall. Chronic bronchitis is associated with a productive cough, enlargement of mucous glands, and hypertrophy of the airway smooth muscle. Although asthma, emphysema, and chronic bronchitis can all be termed "chronic obstructive pulmonary disease," asthma is distinguished from the other two by the presence of inflammation with the participation of complex cellular and chemical mediators, as described in Chapter 7. For the purposes of our discussion, we will generally refer to chronic bronchitis and emphysema as COPD and discuss asthma as a separate disease entity.

ASTHMA

Background

Asthma is a chronic illness that affects 14 to 15 million people in the United States; as many as 4.8 million of these are children. Asthma is the most common chronic disease of childhood and younger adults, with about 80% of cases developing in people younger than 45 years of age. The incidence of asthma in the United States has increased by 66% since 1980, making the understanding of how to treat this prevalent disease a priority.

Differential Diagnosis

Wheezing is the most prominent clinical feature, especially in the early morning and after exposure to cold air or exercise. As already mentioned, COPD patients (bronchitis and emphysema) can present with many of the same symptoms, as can patients with chronic cough, hyperventilation syndromes, congestive heart failure, pulmonary embolism, gastroesophageal reflux disease (GERD), allergies, Sjogren's syndrome, and others. Asthma medication is effective in some of these diseases, but not in all. Therefore it is important to have the correct diagnosis for effective pharmacotherapy. If you are uncertain that your patient has been evaluated fully for these other diseases, or if their response to appropriate asthma medication is not optimal, refer them back to their physician for further evaluation and workup.

Table 13-2 lists the differential diagnostic markers for COPD and asthma. No one marker is conclusive, so the entire clinical picture must be assessed for correct diagnosis and treatment.

Explain this clinical statement: "All that wheezes is not asthma."

Asthmatic attack prevention and treatment focuses on the inflammatory components of the disease, and patients treated for asthma should exhibit most of the inflammatory diagnostic markers, such as episodic attacks related to irritant or allergen exposure, variable peak expiratory flow rate (PEFR), eosinophilia, and improvement on corticosteroids.

Asthma Symptoms

The most common symptoms of asthma include wheezing, shortness of breath, cough, and chest tightness. The degree of wheezing is often used as a major criterion for judging the severity of the asthmatic episode. Cough, while generally the most common asthmatic

Table 13-2   Diagnostic Markers to Differentiate COPD and Asthma

Diagnostic Markers	*COPD*	*Asthma*
Age	patient typically over 40	asthma typically presents at an early age
Smoking history	smokers and ex-smokers	no direct correlation between smoking and asthma
Dyspnea	shortness of breath, especially upon exertion	episodic attacks, especially upon exposure to allergen/irritant/exercise
Cough	productive cough, typically in the morning	cough typically in the evening
Triggers (allergens, exercise, temperature, humidity, etc.)	none usually identified for attacks	exposure leads to attacks
Spirometry	FEV_1/FVC ratio $\leq$ 70%	FEV_1/FVC ratio low during attacks only
Daily variation in peak expiratory flow rate (PEFR)	little	morning dip and day-to-day variability
Effect of corticosteroid trial	inconclusive (<20% of patients are successful)	improvement
Eosinophilia	no	maybe
Chest X-ray	overinflation	overinflation during attacks

symptom, is also the third most common presenting symptom in the ambulatory care setting. When a patient presents with cough, a thorough history, identification of triggers, and pulmonary function testing will make the diagnosis of asthma more clear.

The patient's history can be very helpful, as many asthmatic patients will have a family history of allergies. Usually, the patient or their parents will be able to identify exposures or circumstances that trigger the patient's symptoms. Asthma is a chronic disease, not an episodic one, even though certain disease triggers may wax and wane. Therefore, patients and their caregivers need to understand the chronic nature of the underlying inflammatory process. Patients will need to understand how to identify and control their exposure to environmental allergens or other types of triggers.

Persons with asthma develop bronchospasm on exposure to specific sensitizing substances usually described as "triggers." Common triggers include allergens, inhalants, viruses, cold air, and exercise. Although it may seem strange to have this discussion on preventive measures in a pharmacology text, the authors believe that *preventing the use of medications* is in fact an important pharmacologic intervention and mindset.

Allergies. Seasonal, indoor, and outdoor allergen exposure can lead to asthma symptoms. One of the most common allergens is the domestic dust mite, which is found throughout our households and businesses. It is difficult to limit exposure to this allergen, but the World Health Organization recommends frequent washing of bed linens and blankets in hot water, encasing pillows and mattresses in airtight covers, and removal of carpets, especially in bedrooms. The use of vinyl, leather, or plain wooden furniture is encouraged over fabric-upholstered furniture. Tobacco smoke should be avoided; parents and patients should not smoke. Allergies to animal fur should be identified, and, if found, animals should be removed from the home or at least from the sleeping area. Cockroach allergen is another very common triggering substance for asthma. Houses and work areas should be cleaned thoroughly and often. An appropriate pesticide should be used regularly, but not while the patient is nearby. Many patients will also experience triggers from outdoor pollens and both outdoor and indoor molds. To avoid exposure to the outdoor triggers, patients should spend most of their time inside, with windows and doors closed when pollen and mold counts are highest. To avoid exposure to indoor molds, dampness in the home should be reduced, and damp areas should be regularly cleaned and disinfected. Air conditioning will help to reduce both types of exposure. Patients may also want to consider specific immunotherapy ("allergy shots") if exposure cannot be controlled.

www.prenhall.com/colbert

To learn more about asthma triggers and preventing or minimizing the exposure to both indoor and outdoor allergens/pollutants, go to the Web site, where you will find a detailed discussion.

Exercise. Patients who experience asthma symptoms upon exposure to cold or exercise should not completely avoid these conditions. Many patients will have no problems with bronchospasm except after exercise. Symptoms can be prevented through the use of a long- or short-acting bronchodilator inhaled before exposure to cold air or strenuous exercise.

Gastroesophageal Reflux. Gastroesophageal reflux disease (GERD) has long been recognized in association with wheezing and asthma symptoms. The reflux of acidic stomach contents into the esophagus is thought to initiate a reflex bronchoconstriction.

Infections. Upper respiratory viral infections can provoke asthma attacks and, as with exposure to allergens, some viruses and bacteria increase airway responsiveness and hyperreactivity. This may occur because of damage to the respiratory epithelium and airway inflammation. It isn't very easy to avoid respiratory viral infections, but asthmatics should be aware of good handwashing techniques and other ways to reduce viral transmission. If patients develop an upper respiratory tract infection or sinus infection, they should closely monitor their peak flow rates and begin appropriate bronchodilator and/or anti-inflammatory therapy as soon as indicated. Viral upper respiratory tract infections are a major precipitant of acute asthma. The most common cause of exacerbations in both children and adults is the common rhinovirus.

Irritants. Irritants are likely to stimulate receptors along the respiratory tract and include things such as perfumes, detergents, smoke, strong smells, dust, and air pollution. Inhalation of irritants can trigger bronchospasm. The general mechanisms are not known, but it is presumed that these irritants cause epithelial damage and inflammation in the airway mucosa. If patients identify any of these substances as triggers, they should try to minimize their exposure to them, or when exposure is unavoidable, they should begin treatment with appropriate bronchodilator therapy.

CLINICAL PEARL
Emotion and stress can also be precipitating factors in some patients.

STOP
& REVIEW

What type of assessment would you perform for indoor air pollution in a home or office?

Asthma Treatment Goals

The Global Initiative for Asthma defines the goal of asthma therapy as helping patients prevent most attacks, stay free of troublesome night and day symptoms, and keep physically active. Achieving control of asthma requires selection of appropriate medications, stopping of asthma attacks, identification and avoidance of triggers that make asthma worse, education of patients to manage their condition, and the monitoring and modifying of asthma care for effective long-term control. Drug therapy must be selected carefully, monitored closely, and optimized for the individual patient. This requires extensive patient education and close cooperation among all healthcare providers.

The National Asthma Education and Prevention Program, Second Expert Panel (NAEPP2) recommends that the following goals be targeted for each patient:

1. Maintain normal activity levels (including exercise and other physical activity)
2. Maintain (near) "normal" pulmonary function
3. Prevent chronic and troublesome symptoms (e.g., coughing or breathlessness in the night, in the early morning, or after exertion)
4. Prevent recurrent exacerbations of asthma and minimize the need for emergency department visits or hospitalizations
5. Provide optimal pharmacotherapy with minimal or no adverse effects
6. Meet patients' and families' expectations of satisfaction with asthma care

Levels of Asthma

The clinical course of asthma is usually divided into three levels of disease, classified as mild, moderate, or severe, that also determine pharmacological interventions (see Table 13-3). Mild asthma is defined as causing self-limited and brief symptom episodes that may occur up to twice a week. The National Institutes of Health (NIH) further break down mild asthma into the mild intermittent and mild persistent categories. The mild persistent category has mild symptoms greater than or equal to two times a week, whereas the mild intermittent symptoms occur less than two times a week. Patients in both categories will have normal pulmonary function between episodes. Patients with mild asthma may control it with medication on an as-needed basis but need to understand how to avoid allergic triggers of their disease.

Moderate asthma has daily symptoms, with exacerbations (flare-ups) of the disease affecting daily activity. In addition, nighttime asthma symptoms are more frequent. In moderate asthma, pulmonary function does not always return to normal on its own, and patients may require therapy with inhaled or oral corticosteroids. The duration of therapy will depend on the clinical course.

Asthma is considered severe if symptoms are continuous, with frequent exacerbations and more nighttime symptoms. The patient's pulmonary activity is persistently abnormal, and the patient needs fairly regular use of inhaled bronchodilators. Patients in this category may have life-threatening episodes of bronchoconstriction and will usually require prolonged therapy with oral corticosteroids at doses of up to 60 to 80 mg per day of prednisone. Additional therapy needs may include a mast-cell stabilizer such as cromolyn, or a methylxanthine derivative.

www.prenhall.com/colbert

The Global Initiative for Asthma recommends that you ask your patients certain questions when monitoring asthma care. Go to the Web site for more information on this subject.

Table 13-3   Assessment of the Three Levels of Asthma

Factor	*Mild*	*Moderate*	*Severe*
Symptom frequency	1–2 times/week	3–5 times/week	daily
Nighttime symptoms	<2 times/week	2–5 times/week	almost nightly
Activity limitation	brief (<1/2 hour)	mild to moderate	substantial
School or work	rarely affected	performance affected	poor performance
Corticosteroid bursts/year	0 or 1	2 or 3	>3
PEFR/FEV$_1$	≥80% of best	60%–80% of best	<60% of best
Drug used to relieve symptoms	<daily	2–3 times/day	>3 times/day

Asthma Medications

The NAEPP2 report groups asthma medications into two general categories: (1) agents for **long-term control,** used to achieve and maintain control of persistent asthma, and (2) **quick-relief** medications, used to provide rapid relief in treating asthma symptoms and exacerbations. Quick-relief medications include short-acting β_2 bronchodilators and inhaled anticholinergics. See Table 13-4, which presents a glossary of quick-relief asthma medications.

Table 13-4   Glossary of Quick-Relief Asthma Medications

Medication	*Generic Name*	*Mechanism of Action*	*Side Effects (risk for serious adverse effects)*	*Long-Term Effect*	*Quick-Relief Effect*
Short-acting β_2-agonists	albuterol bitolterol isoetharine metaproterenol pirbuterol terbutaline	Bronchodilator	Inhaled β_2-agonists have fewer, and less significant, side effects than tablets or syrups.	+/−	+++
			Tablet or syrup β_2-agonists may cause cardiovascular stimulation, skeletal muscle tremor, headache, and irritability.	+/−	++
Anticholinergics	ipratropium bromide	Bronchodilator	Minimal mouth dryness or bad taste in mouth.	0	++
Short-acting theophylline aminophylline		Bronchodilator	Nausea, vomiting. At higher serum concentrations: seizures, tachycardia, and arrhythmias: theophylline monitoring may be required.	+/−	+
Epinephrine/ adrenaline injection		Bronchodilator	Similar, but more significant effects than β_2-agonists. Generally not used in adults for asthma treatment.	Not recommended for long-term treatment	In general, not recommended for treating asthma attacks if β_2-agonists are available

CLINICAL PEARL

Remember that inhaled corticosteroids should always be administered with a hand-held spacer. Use of spacers reduces the risk of oropharyngeal candidiasis (aka thrush), which often develops when the aerosol particles are deposited in the mouth. Also, remember to rinse mouth.

The most effective agents for long-term control are those with anti-inflammatory properties, such as inhaled/systemic corticosteroids and mast-cell stabilizers and mediator release inhibitors (cromolyn and nedocromil). The leukotriene modifiers (zileuton, zafirlukast, and montelukast) are also effective in persistent asthma but have no place in the treatment of acute asthma. These agents can help prevent acute exacerbations with regular use and are also thought to be helpful as adjuncts to oral corticosteroid therapy. Long-acting β_2 bronchodilators can also be used as long-term preventive medications. Finally, methylxanthines are classified as long-term control medications but are rarely used, owing to their side effects and minimal bronchodilation. See Table 13-5, which compares the long-term asthma control medications.

Asthma Management

Interest in asthma management increased dramatically in the 1990s, and this led to the development and update of asthma treatment guidelines and consensus statements. The first formal guidelines were published in 1989 to provide some uniformity in the treatment of asthma in children. Several international sets of guidelines were developed in an attempt to consolidate regionally specific guidelines into a set that could be widely used by all healthcare practitioners. The NAEPP2 developed a stepwise treatment algorithm for managing asthma in adults and children older than 5 years (Figure 13-1).

A key to the treatment algorithm is to remember which agents are for long-term, preventive care and which are the quick-relief medications. Quick-relief medications are used to treat acute symptoms and exacerbations in patients with intermittent and persistent asthma. The higher levels of therapy should be initiated to achieve control in persistent asthma, and once control is achieved, therapy should be stepped down to the lowest level needed to control symptoms. Remember that quick-relief medications can also be used to prevent symptoms. For example, the patient with exercise- or cold-induced asthma should use a quick-relief medication 15 to 30 minutes before a triggering event. Patients should track and report their use of inhaled β_2-agonists, as this may indicate the need for additional long-term medications or may signal an acute exacerbation.

Mild, persistent asthma should not be controlled by the episodic administration of quick-relief agents. Patients with this level of asthma should be treated with an agent that provides long-term symptom control, such as low-dose inhaled corticosteroids or a mast-cell inhibitor. Montelukast and zafirlukast may be used in patients as young as 6 years of age, and all leukotriene inhibitors are effective in adults and the elderly for long-term symptom control.

$\langle$ CONTROVERSY $\rangle$

Sustained-release theophylline has also been used in this category of patients for many years, but its utility has been questioned more recently as the agent has many side effects.

STOP
& REVIEW

In lay terms, how would you explain when to use quick-relief versus when to use long-term control medication to a patient?

Management of Acute Asthma Exacerbations

The NAEPP2 guidelines recommend that all patients have a written action plan to enhance awareness and monitoring of asthma. We have included a sample monitoring plan in Figure 13-2; it utilizes personal peak flow meter measurements and symptom recognition to assist the patient.

Table 13-5   Glossary of Long-Term Asthma Control Medications

Medication	Generic Name	Mechanism of Action	Side Effects (risk for serious adverse effects)	Long-Term Effect	Quick-Relief Effect
Corticosteroids	Inhaled beclomethasone budesonide flunisolide fluticasone triamcinolone	Anti-inflammatory agent	Inhaled corticosteroids have few known adverse effects. Use of spacers and mouth washing after inhalation help prevent oral candidiasis. Doses above 1 mg a day may be associated with skin thinning, easy bruising, and adrenal suppression.	+++	0 helps prevent late phase attack
	Tablets or syrups prednisolone prednisone methylprednisolone hydrocortisone dexamethasone cortisone		Tablet or syrup corticosteroids used long term may lead to osteoporosis, arterial hypertension, diabetes, cataracts, hypothalamic–pituitary–adrenal axis suppression, obesity, skin thinning, or muscle weakness	++	++ (over hours)
Cromolyn sodium		Anti-inflammatory agent	Minimal side effects. Cough may occur upon inhalation.	+	0
Nedocromil		Anti-inflammatory agent	None known	+	0
Long-acting β_2-agonists	Inhaled salmeterol	Bronchodilator	Inhaled β_2-agonists have fewer, and less significant, side effects than tablets.	++	NOT to be used to treat attacks
	sustained-release tablets terbutaline		Tablet β_2-agonists may cause cardiovascular stimulation, anxiety, heartburn, skeletal muscle tremor, headache, or hypokalemia.	+/−	
Sustained-release theophylline aminophylline		Bronchodilator with uncertain anti-inflammatory effect	Nausea and vomiting are most common. Serious effects occurring at higher serum concentrations include seizures, tachycardia, and arrhythmias. Theophylline monitoring is often required.	+	++

Treatment (Preferred treatments in bold print)

	Long-Term Control	Quick Relief	Education
Step 1: Mild Intermittent	*No daily medication is needed*	❖ Short-acting bronchodilator: **inhaled β$_2$-agonists** as needed for symptoms ❖ Intensity of treatment depends on severity of exacerbation ❖ Use of short-acting inhaled β$_2$-agonist on a daily basis, or increasing use, indicates the need for additional long-term control therapy	❖ Teach basic facts about asthma ❖ Teach inhaler spacer or holding chamber technique ❖ Discuss roles of medications ❖ Develop self-management plan ❖ Develop action plan for when and how to take rescue actions, especially for patients with a history of severe exacerbations ❖ Discuss appropriate environmental control measures to avoid exposures to known allergens and irritants
Step 2: Mild Persistent	*Once Daily Medication* ❖ **Anti-inflammatory:** either **inhaled corticosteroid** (low dosages) or **cromolyn** or **nedocromil** (children usually begin with a trial of cromolyn or nedocromil) ❖ Sustained-release theophylline to serum concentrations of 5–15 μ g/ml is an alternative but not preferred therapy. Zafirlukast, zileuton or montelukast may also be considered, although their position in therapy is not fully established.	❖ Short-acting bronchodilator: **inhaled β$_2$-agonists** as needed for symptoms ❖ Intensity of treatment depends on severity of exacerbation ❖ Use of short-acting inhaled β$_2$-agonist on a daily basis, or increasing use, indicates the need for additional long-term control therapy	Step 1 actions plus: ❖ Teach self-monitoring ❖ Refer to group education if available ❖ Review and update self-management plan
Step 3: Moderate Persistent	*Daily Medications* EITHER ❖ **Anti-inflammatory: inhaled corticosteroid (medium dosage)** OR ❖ **Inhaled corticosteroid (low-medium dosage)** and add a long-acting bronchodilator, especially for nighttime symptoms: either **long-acting inhaled β$_2$-agonist,** sustained-release theophylline, or long-acting β$_2$-agonist tablets IF NEEDED ❖ Anti-inflammatory: **inhaled corticosteroid (medium dosage)** AND ❖ **Long-acting bronchodilator,** especially for nighttime symptoms; either **long-acting inhaled β$_2$-agonist,** sustained-release theophylline, or long-acting inhaled β$_2$-agonist tablets	❖ Short-acting bronchodilator: **inhaled β$_2$-agonists** as needed for symptoms ❖ Intensity of treatment depends on severity of exacerbation ❖ Use of short-acting inhaled β$_2$-agonist on a daily basis, or increasing use, indicates the need for additional long-term control therapy	Step 1 actions plus: ❖ Teach self-monitoring ❖ Refer to group education if available ❖ Review and update self-management plan
Step 4: Severe Persistent	*Daily Medications* ❖ **Anti-inflammatory: inhaled corticosteroid (high dosage)** AND ❖ Long-acting bronchodilator: either **long-acting inhaled β$_2$-agonist,** sustained-release theophylline, or long-acting β$_2$-agonist tablets AND ❖ Corticosteroid tablets or syrup long term (2 mg/kg/day, generally do not exceed 60 mg per day)	❖ Short-acting bronchodilator: **inhaled β$_2$-agonists** as needed for symptoms ❖ Intensity of treatment depends on severity of exacerbation ❖ Use of short-acting inhaled β$_2$-agonist on a daily basis, or increasing use, indicates the need for additional long-term control therapy.	Step 2 and 3 actions plus: ❖ Individualized education and counseling

1. Review treatment every 3 to 6 months. If control is sustained for at least 3 months, a gradual stepwise reduction in treatment may be possible.
2. If control is not achieved, consider a step up, but first review the patient's medication technique, compliance, and environment control (avoidance of triggers).

Figure 13-1 Stepwise Approach for Managing Asthma in Adults and Children Older than 5 Years

Source: Modified from the NAEPP2

What happens when your patients become too sick to follow their action plan and need hospitalization? The NAEPP2-recommended algorithm for emergent asthma exacerbations is shown in Figure 13-3. Patients with mild or moderate exacerbations (pulmonary function >50% of predicted) can be treated with a metered-dose inhaler (MDI) or nebulized β$_2$-agonists administered three times during the first hour in the emergency department. Patients with more severe exacerbations (pulmonary function <50% predicted) should be

	Asthma Action Plan for _____
Addressograph here	Physician: _____ Date: _____
	Provider name and phone number: _____
	_____

Green Zone (Optimal) Peak flow = _____	**Yellow Zone (Caution)** Peak flow = _____	**Red Zone (Alert)** Peak flow = _____
No Symptoms Able to do daily activities with little difficulty	Coughing Sleep disturbed by symptoms Short of breath/wheezing Difficulty doing normal daily activities	Symptoms are worse even while resting Very short of breath Trouble walking or talking Unable to do normal daily activities
Peak Flow reading (80% – 100% of personal best)	Peak Flow Reading: (50% – 80% of personal best)	Peak Flow Reading: (Less than 50% of personal best)
☐ Review trigger control ☐ Take quick-relief medications _____ _____ as needed	☐ Rest ☐ Increase dosage of: _____	☐ Call your physician ☐ Add or increase your oral steroid: _____
☐ Before exercise or exposure to other triggers, take: _____ ☐ Annual flu vaccination	☐ Continue other **green** zone medications ☐ Add: _____ _____	☐ Continue other **green** and **yellow** zone medications ☐ Special notes: _____ _____

Figure 13-2 Sample Action Plan Management of Asthma

treated with nebulized medications, as they are probably not able to breathe deeply enough and may be too agitated over the event to benefit from the MDI. Supplemental oxygen is indicated if the patient is hypoxemic.

If symptoms persist beyond the initial treatment, systemic corticosteroids are indicated, and anticholinergic agents may be used if the prescriber considers the symptoms to be severe. Inhaled corticosteroids act much too slowly to be used in these situations and should be considered only as long-term preventive agents and to help in possible subsequent late-phase reactions. All patients whose symptoms are severe enough to require treatment in the emergency department should receive a course of oral corticosteroids.

If patients are not recovered after the initial emergency department therapy, they may require admission to the hospital. These patients should continue to receive treatment with frequent inhaled β_2-agonists plus inhaled anticholinergics and systemic corticosteroids.

If symptoms persist and the patient requires intensive care therapy, intravenous aminophylline is usually considered and may be effective. The patient in the intensive care unit should also continue to receive β_2-agonist therapy via the subcutaneous, intramuscular, inhaled, or intravenous route. They may also receive intravenous **magnesium** and aggressive therapy with oxygen. In general, patients may be discharged from the hospital when their pulmonary function returns to 70% of their predicted normal or more.

CLINICAL PEARL

Magnesium is a weak bronchodilator, and there are case reports of magnesium preventing respiratory failure in patients presenting with severe asthma exacerbations.

℞

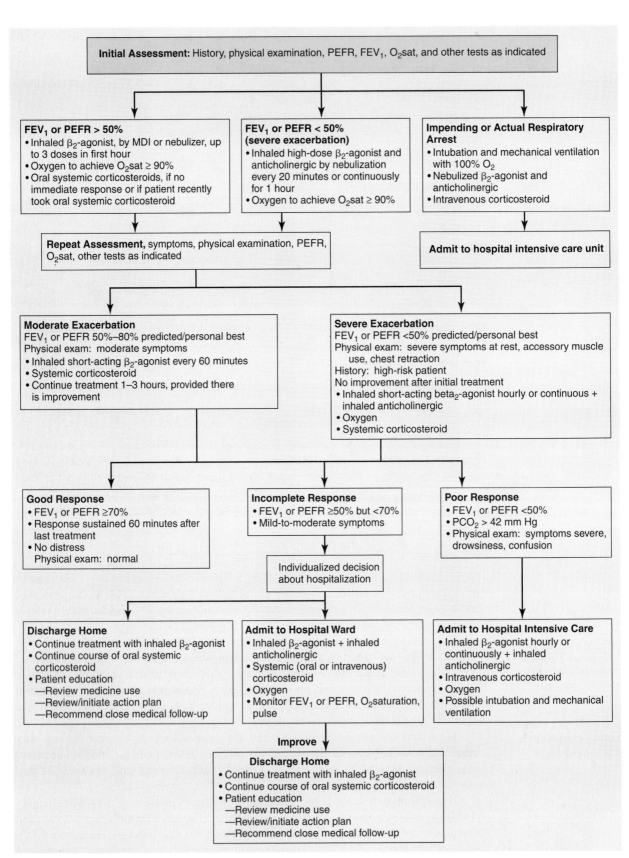

Initial Assessment: History, physical examination, PEFR, FEV$_1$, O$_2$sat, and other tests as indicated

FEV$_1$ or PEFR > 50%
- Inhaled β$_2$-agonist, by MDI or nebulizer, up to 3 doses in first hour
- Oxygen to achieve O$_2$sat ≥ 90%
- Oral systemic corticosteroids, if no immediate response or if patient recently took oral systemic corticosteroid

FEV$_1$ or PEFR < 50% (severe exacerbation)
- Inhaled high-dose β$_2$-agonist and anticholinergic by nebulization every 20 minutes or continuously for 1 hour
- Oxygen to achieve O$_2$sat ≥ 90%

Impending or Actual Respiratory Arrest
- Intubation and mechanical ventilation with 100% O$_2$
- Nebulized β$_2$-agonist and anticholinergic
- Intravenous corticosteroid

Repeat Assessment, symptoms, physical examination, PEFR, O$_2$sat, other tests as indicated

Admit to hospital intensive care unit

Moderate Exacerbation
FEV$_1$ or PEFR 50%–80% predicted/personal best
Physical exam: moderate symptoms
- Inhaled short-acting β$_2$-agonist every 60 minutes
- Systemic corticosteroid
- Continue treatment 1–3 hours, provided there is improvement

Severe Exacerbation
FEV$_1$ or PEFR <50% predicted/personal best
Physical exam: severe symptoms at rest, accessory muscle use, chest retraction
History: high-risk patient
No improvement after initial treatment
- Inhaled short-acting beta$_2$-agonist hourly or continuous + inhaled anticholinergic
- Oxygen
- Systemic corticosteroid

Good Response
- FEV$_1$ or PEFR ≥70%
- Response sustained 60 minutes after last treatment
- No distress
Physical exam: normal

Incomplete Response
- FEV$_1$ or PEFR ≥50% but <70%
- Mild-to-moderate symptoms

Poor Response
- FEV$_1$ or PEFR <50%
- PCO$_2$ > 42 mm Hg
- Physical exam: symptoms severe, drowsiness, confusion

Individualized decision about hospitalization

Discharge Home
- Continue treatment with inhaled β$_2$-agonist
- Continue course of oral systemic corticosteroid
- Patient education
  —Review medicine use
  —Review/initiate action plan
  —Recommend close medical follow-up

Admit to Hospital Ward
- Inhaled β$_2$-agonist + inhaled anticholinergic
- Systemic (oral or intravenous) corticosteroid
- Oxygen
- Monitor FEV$_1$ or PEFR, O$_2$saturation, pulse

Admit to Hospital Intensive Care
- Inhaled β$_2$-agonist hourly or continuously + inhaled anticholinergic
- Intravenous corticosteroid
- Oxygen
- Possible intubation and mechanical ventilation

Improve

Discharge Home
- Continue treatment with inhaled β$_2$-agonist
- Continue course of oral systemic corticosteroid
- Patient education
  —Review medicine use
  —Review/initiate action plan
  —Recommend close medical follow-up

Figure 13-3 Management of Acute Asthma Exacerbations
Source: Modified from the NAEPP2

A patient in acute respiratory distress with a respiratory rate of 34 should receive what type of inhaled medication? What would be the best delivery device—a MDI? Or a spontaneous nebulized treatment?

www.prenhall.com/colbert

In Chapter 1, you learned that there are differences in pharmacokinetics and pharmacodynamics in pediatrics and geriatrics. Go to the Web site for more specific information on pediatric and geriatric asthma treatment considerations.

COPD

Background

COPD is a major cause of disability in adults and is estimated to have direct economic costs in excess of $14 billion annually and indirect economic costs (lost earnings, etc.) of over $9 billion in the United States. COPD-related hospitalization is on the increase, having risen by 25% from 1992 through 1995. Men and women have similar mortality rates with COPD before the age of 55, but the rate for men rises thereafter, doubling by age 70. The death rate for COPD and related conditions has been increasing since 1966 (up by 71%), while the death rates from heart and cerebral vascular conditions have declined. The increased death rate for COPD is thought to be due to several things, including the fact that more people are living longer—the increases in death rates are most significant in the elderly who have continued to smoke cigarettes. Since we have seen a decrease in smoking frequency these past 30 years, it is believed that the COPD death rate will also decrease in the coming decades.

Etiology

The primary etiology for COPD is exposure to tobacco smoke. Smokers have higher death rates from both chronic bronchitis and emphysema. Smokers have more lung-function abnormalities, show more respiratory symptoms, and experience all forms of COPD at a much higher rate than nonsmokers. Age of starting, total pack-years, and current smoking status are predictive of COPD mortality. Passive smoking (the exposure of nonsmokers to cigarette smoke) also seems to increase the risk of COPD-related disease. Children of parents who smoke have a higher prevalence of respiratory symptoms than children of nonsmokers. Exposure to smoke at an early age may impair the attainment of maximal lung function in adult life. Air pollution, asthma, atopy, and nonspecific airway hyperresponsiveness may all play a role in the development of COPD.

CLINICAL PEARL
Men have a higher incidence of COPD than women do, and Caucasians have a higher incidence.

Emphysema. In the past, it was customary to divide persons with COPD into two categories, those with emphysema (the "pink puffer") and those with chronic bronchitis (the "blue bloater"). However, most persons with COPD have features of both of these diseases. We are going to keep the distinctions, partially to help you categorize when to use certain therapies, so we'll begin with the description and treatment of emphysema.

About two million persons in the United States are estimated to have emphysema. Of these, 60,000 to 100,000 have alpha$_1$-antitrypsin (α_1-AT) deficiency as their underlying etiology. The syndrome of α_1-AT deficiency disease is perceived by most clinicians as being rare, but the reality is that most patients with α_1-AT deficiency go undiagnosed and are treated simply as people with emphysema. Manifestations of severe α_1-AT deficiency involve the lungs, the liver, and the skin, and the major clinical feature is emphysema. The disorder is caused by a decreased level of α_1-AT to below a so-called protective value of 80 mg/dL. Normal serum levels of α_1-AT are 150 to 350 mg/dL. α_1-AT is a glycoprotein found in extracellular and intracellular fluid. It is essential in the protection of the lung against naturally occurring proteases that have the ability to break down the elastin and macromolecules in lung tissue. Low concentrations of α_1-AT cause the release of the neutrophil elastase, which causes lung connective tissue digestion and alveolar destruction.

CLINICAL PEARL

Most persons with α_1-AT deficiency are Caucasians of northern European descent.

Clinical Presentation The primary clinical features distinguishing emphysema from asthma and bronchitis are dyspnea on exertion and nonproductive cough. Emphysemic patients tend to have the "pink puffer" appearance, breathing with all of their accessory muscles. They exhale through "pursed" lips to maintain airway pressure and prevent airway collapse, but maintain a pink skin color. The work of breathing for the severely emphysemic patient is much like running a marathon. They must continually work to maintain airway pressure in their abnormally large airspaces and must maintain a rapid respiratory rate. Weight loss is typical with severe emphysema. Think how much weight you'd lose if you ran a marathon each day!

Chronic Bronchitis.

Chronic bronchitis has a prevalence of about 54.3 cases per 1,000 persons in the United States, and cigarette smoking is the major causative factor in up to 90% of cases. Patients with chronic bronchitis have an increase in size and number of the mucus-secreting glands, narrowing and inflammation of the small airways, obstruction of airways caused by narrowing and mucus hypersecretion, and bacterial colonization of the airways. Acute episodes are usually brought on by a respiratory tract infection. The usual clinical presentation of chronic bronchitis begins with morning cough productive of sputum. The patient may report a decline in exercise tolerance, although he or she may not have appreciated this decline until questioned. Wheezes may be present, and an increase in the anteroposterior diameter of the chest (the classic "barrel chest") may be present in both emphysema and chronic bronchitis. The patient who has predominantly chronic bronchitis symptoms may undergo repeated episodes of respiratory failure and frequently develop right-sided congestive heart failure.

Respiratory infections trigger acute exacerbations in the COPD patient, especially in the elderly patient with chronic bronchitis. Patients present with hypersecretion of mucus and then, owing to their decreased removal of bronchial secretions by ciliary activity, are far more likely to develop pneumonia and significant lung damage from the infection.

LEARNING HINT

Chronic progressive breathlessness occurs often in COPD, whereas asthmatic patients usually have a more episodic occurrence of these symptoms. COPD is not caused by inflammation and thus does not usually respond to a trial of inhaled or oral corticosteroids. Asthma occurs in all age groups, but COPD is usually a disease of older patients.

Clinical Presentation Wheezing and prolonged forced expiratory time strongly suggest airflow obstruction. If this is accompanied by decreased breath sounds, it is likely that the patient has at least moderately severe disease. Most patients with COPD will be short of breath, especially with any exertion, and usually have a productive morning cough. It is unlikely that the patient will be able to identify triggers that make their disease worsen. They may have cyanosis and suffer from morning headaches, which can suggest nighttime hypercapnia. Some patients will experience weight loss, which can also be a prominent symptom associated with bronchogenic carcinoma. Many COPD patients will have a somewhat characteristic physical appearance, with a hyperinflated barrel chest, wheezing on forced expiration, and subcutaneous fat wasting on their extremities and lower torso, and they may adopt positions that relieve their dyspnea. Their accessory respiratory muscles of the neck and shoulder girdle may be in full use, and they may exhale through pursed lips to maintain alveolar inflation.

Smoking history is the most important initial screening the clinician can perform, as it can help to clinically distinguish COPD from asthma. A 70-pack-year history of smoking or greater has been described as a specific finding suggestive of COPD. Pack-year history is calculated by multiplying the number of packs smoked per day by the number of years smoked.

In patients with COPD, spirometry will be diagnostic if the FEV_1/FVC ratio drops below 70%. Unlike with asthma, this should be a fairly consistent finding and will not improve between acute attacks. The sputum produced should be examined for pathogenic bacteria. Generally, a Gram stain will show a mixture of organisms and macrophages. The most frequent pathogens are *Streptococcus pneumoniae* and *Haemophilus influenzae,* although many other organisms can be cultured.

Table 13-6 describes some of the ways that chronic bronchitis differs from emphysema in clinical presentation. Much of the therapy of these diseases is aimed at symptom control, so delineating which disease the patient has is not really necessary. However, since the two terms are in common usage, you might want to review Table 13-6 so that you will have a good understanding of the patient's presentation when they are described as having emphysema or chronic bronchitis. Of the two clinical diagnoses, emphysema is the more disabling.

Table 13-6 Clinical Features of the Two Major Types of COPD

Feature	Emphysema	Chronic Bronchitis
Sputum	minimal	copious
Cor pulmonale	rare	common
Weight	marked weight loss, cachectic appearance	obesity common
Smoking history	common	common
Chest X-ray findings	hyperinflation	increased markings
Hematocrit	normal	may be increased
Blood gases	normal or slightly low PaO_2 normal pH or mild respiratory acidosis normal or slightly high $PaCO_2$	low PaO_2 respiratory acidosis elevated $PaCO_2$
Respiratory failure	rare until end stage	repeated episodes
Pulmonary function tests	decreased FEV_1 decreased FVC greatly increased residual volume	decreased FEV_1 decreased FVC increased residual volume
Dyspnea	relatively early	relatively late

PREVENTION: THE KEY TO TREATMENT OF COPD

Smoking Cessation

All patients who smoke need to be regularly encouraged to stop. Cigarette smoking kills nearly 440,000 Americans each year and debilitates nearly one half of all long-term smokers. Tobacco dependence is a powerful addiction and one that is extremely difficult to break. Tobacco relapse rates are high, and most successful quitters have made at least five attempts to stop before achieving that goal. Therefore, all healthcare providers must continually offer help and support to patients who are willing to try to stop smoking. Some patients will be successful with over-the-counter methods, but most will require encouragement and counseling from addiction specialists.

Many therapies are available to help smokers to quit. Healthcare providers should help patients identify what therapies will best suit them. They should be given written instructions on the use of the option selected. The dose and duration of therapy should be individualized. Patients should be contacted frequently and/or return to the office for encouragement and motivation and to monitor their use of the therapies chosen. The patient should be encouraged to enter a formalized smoking cessation program, and the healthcare provider should be aware of what programs are available in the community and how the patient can enter one. Finally, the healthcare provider needs to congratulate the patient on success.

Smoking Cessation Therapies

Pharmacologic therapy is an extremely important adjunct to the behavioral intervention, addictive-disorder counseling, and relapse-prevention treatment necessary to help the smoker stop. When choosing the appropriate therapy, the clinician needs to consider what the patient wants, whether they have had any adverse reactions to any of the therapies, whether the side effects are tolerable, whether the medication is effective, and how addicted the patient is to nicotine.

It is important to somehow quantify the patient's addiction to nicotine. The Fagerstrom Test for Nicotine Dependence (FTND; see Figure 13-4) is a good tool to help you do this. A score of 6 or higher on the FTND indicates a high level of nicotine dependence. Patients in this category will have difficulty overcoming the initial withdrawal symptoms of nicotine and will benefit the most from pharmacotherapy to aid cessation. Even a person with a lower score may benefit from nicotine replacement therapy or **bupropion** (Zyban) to aid in cessation. The patient's preference will also have a great deal to do with which drug therapy (if any) is chosen. The best pharmacotherapy will not be successful until the patient has

Questions and Possible Answers	Score
How soon after you wake up do you smoke your first cigarette?	
≤ 5 minutes	3
6 – 30 minutes	2
31 – 60 minutes	1
≥ 60 minutes	0
Do you find it difficult to refrain from smoking in places where it is forbidden (e.g., in church, at work, in the library, in a cinema)?	
Yes	1
No	0
What cigarette would you hate most to give up?	
The first in the morning	1
Any other	0
How many cigarettes per day do you smoke?	
≤ 10	0
11 – 20	1
21 – 30	2
≥ 31	3
Do you smoke more frequently during the first hours after waking than the rest of the day?	
Yes	1
No	0
Do you smoke if you are so ill that you are in bed most of the day?	
Yes	1
No	0

Figure 13-4 The Fagerstrom Test for Nicotine Dependence

truly decided to quit. Pharmacotherapy alone is rarely a means to successful cessation in the nicotine-addicted patient. Patients should be encouraged to seek educational and behavioral modification therapy for smoking cessation and to use pharmacotherapy as an aid to these programs.

Nicotine replacement therapy (NRT) works for many patients, because it can be adjusted to substitute partially for the nicotine the patient inhales through smoking cigarettes. In general, you will adjust the NRT to deliver less nicotine than received through smoking, but enough will be given to decrease the intensity of nicotine withdrawal symptoms. Even though nicotine is still being ingested, the carcinogens that would be delivered through smoking are not. Additionally, NRT gives more consistent blood levels of nicotine than smoking a cigarette, therefore decreasing the craving that occurs when the smoker's blood levels of nicotine drop between cigarettes. Currently, there are four methods of NRT: the patch, nicotine gum, nicotine nasal spray, and the nicotine oral inhaler. Table 13-7 gives some detail about these dosage forms.

Bupropion (Zyban) is the only FDA-approved non-NRT treatment for nicotine addiction. This agent is also used for the treatment of depression, under the brand name Wellbutrin. We do not know how this medication treats nicotine addiction, but it is speculated that the drug's adrenergic activity plays some role in easing nicotine withdrawal.

CLINICAL PEARL

Patients who use nicotine replacement therapy need to be cautioned about proper disposal of the "used" dosage forms. The patches, gum, and sprays all contain enough residual nicotine to be toxic to children and pets. It is also important that patients have completely stopped smoking before starting NRT.

Table 13-7   Nicotine Replacement Therapies and Bupropion

Dosage Form	Dosing	Adverse Effects	Rx or OTC?	Cautions
Nicotrol Patch (for patients smoking >10 cigarettes a day)	15 mg/day for 6 weeks	skin irritation, insomnia	OTC	avoid if pregnant and have heart disease
Nicoderm CQ (21, 14, 7 mg/24 hr)	<10 cigarettes/day: 14 mg/24 hr for 16–24 hr/day × 6 weeks, then one 7 mg/24 hr for 16–24 hr/day × 2 weeks >10 cigarettes/day: 21 mg/24 hr for 16–24 hr/day × 6 weeks, then 14 mg/24 hr for 16–24 hr/day × 2 weeks, then one 7 mg/24 hr for 16–24 hr/day × 2 weeks	skin irritation, insomnia	OTC	avoid if pregnant and have heart disease
Habitrol (21, 14, 7 mg/24 hr)	Healthy patients: 21 mg/day for 4–8 wks, then 14 mg/day for 2–4 wks, then 7 mg/day for 2–4 wks Patients who smoke <10 cigarettes/day, or who weigh less than 100 lbs, or who have heart disease: 14 mg/day for 4–8 wks, then 7 mg/day for 2–4 wks	skin irritation, insomnia	Rx	avoid if pregnant, use low dose if patient has heart disease
Prostep (22 or 11 mg/24 hr)	Patients > 100 lbs: 22 mg/day for 4–8 wks, then 11 mg/day for 2–4 wks Patients < 100 lbs: 11 mg/day for 4–8 wks	skin irritation, insomnia	Rx	avoid if pregnant or has heart disease

(continued)

Table 13-7   (*continued*)

Dosage Form	Dosing	Adverse Effects	Rx or OTC?	Cautions
Nicorette gum (2 and 4 mg) **Nicorette Mint gum** (2 and 4 mg)	2 mg (4 mg for highly dependent patients who request it, or for those who failed the 2 mg), chewed and held between the cheek and gum intermittently over 30 min every 1–2 hrs for 6 wks, then every 2–4 hrs for 3 wks, then every 4–8 hrs for 3 wks; do not exceed 30 pieces/day	mouth irritation, sore jaw, dyspepsia, nausea, hiccups	OTC	avoid in denture wearers, pregnancy, heart disease
Nicotrol NS nasal spray 10 mg/ml	1–2 one-mg doses (each dose is two 0.5-mg sprays, one in each nostril) per hour initially, increased as needed. Do not exceed 5 doses/hr or 40 doses/day. Full dose for up to 8 wks, then taper dose over 4–6 wks.	rhinitis, sore throat, sneezing, coughing	Rx	avoid in rhinitis, common cold symptoms, pregnancy, heart disease
Nicotrol oral inhaler (10-mg nicotine cartridges, 4 mg delivered)	Cartridge must be inserted into mouthpiece and activated. Initial use is 6–16 cartridges/day. Patient controls depth and frequency of inhalation.	dyspepsia, coughing, mouth irritation, and burning	Rx	avoid in COPD, asthma pregnancy and heart disease
Zyban (bupropion)	Start 2 weeks before quitting cigarettes; begin with 150 mg/day × 3 days. If needed, increase to 150 mg twice daily; use for 7–12 weeks.	headache, insomnia, and dry mouth	Rx	several possible drug interactions—avoid in seizure disorders, bulimia, anorexia, CNS disorders, or alcoholism

Bupropion has several drug interactions and some significant side effects, so patients must be carefully screened before beginning this therapy.

Vaccinations

Pneumococcal vaccine is recommended for all COPD patients, with revaccination every 6 years. The available vaccines incorporate the antigens of 23 species that are responsible for 90 percent of the pneumococcal pneumonia occurring in the United States. Mild redness and pain at the injection site are the only common adverse reactions to the vaccine, which is given as a single intramuscular injection.

Influenza vaccines are essential for all COPD patients. Chemoprophylaxis with amantadine or similar agents should be considered in unimmunized patients who are at risk for contracting influenza, or for whom there is an inadequate amount of time for the immunization to become effective, or in patients for whom the vaccine is contraindicated. The annual influenza vaccine is recommended for all COPD patients who are not allergic to eggs.

What are some key COPD prevention methods?

COPD TREATMENT GOALS

Drugs Used to Treat COPD

β_2-agonists and Anticholinergics.
Pharmacotherapy of COPD is very similar to that of asthma, but certain differences need to emphasized. β_2-agonists will produce less bronchodilation in COPD than in asthma. As a group, COPD patients are older than asthmatic patients and will probably be less tolerant of the sympathomimetic effects (tremor, nervousness, palpitations, etc.) of the β_2-agonists. Anticholinergics may be more effective than β_2-agonists at controlling symptoms, and the side-effect profile may be less troublesome for the older COPD population. However, anticholinergic drugs have a slower onset and longer duration than β_2-agonists and will need to be used on a regular basis, not "as needed." The use of a combination product containing both albuterol and ipratropium (e.g., Combivent) in the same MDI may help the patient by simplifying therapy. Table 13-8 summarizes the pharmacologic properties of the inhaled bronchodilators used in COPD.

Theophylline.
Theophylline at one time was probably the most common agent used in this patient population. However, its potent toxicities have caused it to fall from favor. The agent is still of value for the management of both asthma and COPD in patients who are less compliant or not capable of using a MDI effectively. Theophylline and other xanthine derivatives help to improve respiratory muscle function, stimulate the respiratory center, and enhance activities of daily living in patients who are severely limited by their COPD and who also have cardiac disease or cor pulmonale. Careful dosing is required, and blood levels of the drug must be monitored regularly, especially when any other medication is started or the patient has coexisting diseases.

Anti-inflammatory Drugs.
In sharp contrast to the therapy of asthma, anti-inflammatory drugs are of far less benefit in COPD patients. Cromolyn and nedocromil have

Table 13-8   Pharmacologic Properties of Inhaled Bronchodilators for COPD

Drug	Dose/puff (mg)	β_1 Activity	β_2 Activity	Anticholinergic Effect	Time to Onset (min)	Peak Effect (min)	Duration (min)
Albuterol (Proventil, Ventolin, various generics)	.09	+	+ + + +	0	5–15	60–90	240–360
Bitolterol mesylate (Tornalate)	.37	+	+ + + +	0	5–10	60–90	300–480
Isoetharine HCl (Bronkometer)	.34	+ +	+ +	0	3–5	5–20	60–150
Isoproterenol (Isuprel Mistometer, Medihaler-Iso)	.08	+ + +	+ + +	0	3–5	5–10	60–90
Metaproterenol sulfate (Alupent, Metaprel)	.65	+	+ + +	0	5–15	10–60	60–180
Pirbuterol acetate (Maxair)	.20	+	+ + +	0	5–10	30–60	180–240
Salmeterol (Serevent)	.021	+	+ + + +	0	10–30	120–360	>720
Terbutaline sulfate (Brethaire)	.20	+	+ + + +	0	5–30	60–120	180–360
Ipratropium bromide (Atrovent)	.018	0	0	+ + + +	5–30	60–120	240–480
Ipratropium and albuterol (Combivent)	.09/.018	+	+ + + +	+ + + +	5–15	60–120	240–480

no established use unless the patient has coexisting airway hyperreactivity. Corticosteroids may be of benefit, but usually only oral corticosteroid therapy has been shown to help. Since the COPD patient population is typically older than the asthma population, it is important to remember the side effects of oral corticosteroid use. Complications such as skin damage, cataracts, diabetes, osteoporosis, gastric ulceration, and secondary infection are more likely to occur in the COPD patient. Therefore, it is important that oral corticosteroid use be minimized; only short "burst" therapy should be used if possible. If the patient requires extensive oral corticosteroid therapy, leukotriene inhibitors may be of value.

Mucokinetic Agents. Mucokinetic agents (organic iodide, acetylcysteine, etc.) have had little objective information published supporting their value in the treatment of COPD. Their use is far more accepted in Europe, where they are favored for their antioxidant effects in addition to their action of decreasing the viscosity of the mucus.

Antibiotics. In some COPD patients who experience recurrent bouts of acute bronchitis, prophylactic antibiotics may be of value. The decision is made clinically on the basis of local experience, sputum cultures, and local bacterial sensitivities. The major bacteria to be considered are *Streptococcus pneumonia, Hemophilus influenzae,* and *moraxella catarrhalis.* Older, less costly antibiotics should be used and the newer agents reserved for active treatment, so drugs such as tetracycline, doxycycline, amoxicillin, erythromycin, trimethoprim-sulfamethoxazole, and cephalexin will often be used in a monthly cycling regimen. The cycling is done to attempt to decrease possible resistance that might occur with overuse of any one antibiotic.

R ***α_1-Antitrypsin.*** α_1-Antitrypsin (α_1-AT) augmentation therapy is accomplished by administering **α_1 proteinase-inhibitor** (Prolastin). This therapy is appropriate in the nonsmoking, younger patient with severe α_1-AT deficiency and associated emphysema. This product is given by intravenous infusion and is considered safe for replacement therapy.

Oxygen. Oxygen therapy is often needed to maintain normal PaO_2 levels and to decrease the work of breathing associated with COPD. In addition, COPD causes associated cardiac stress, which oxygen therapy also helps to treat.

Step-by-Step Approach

Therapy of the patient with COPD is multifaceted. *The importance of smoking cessation cannot be overemphasized.* It is the single intervention that will slow the rate of decline in pulmonary function and improve the patient's quality of life. Additionally, therapy goals should include prevention of acute exacerbations, improvement in the chronic obstruction, reduction in the rate of progression of the disease, and improvement in both the physical and the psychological states of the patient.

Several therapeutic guidelines exist for the treatment of COPD: *American Thoracic Society (ATS) Statement on Standards for the Diagnosis and Care of Patients with COPD* (1995), *European Respiratory Society (ERS) Optimal Assessment and Management of COPD* (1995), and the *British Thoracic Society (BTS) Guidelines for the Management of COPD* (1997) are current and should be part of your reference stack for this disease.

There is good agreement among the various guidelines regarding the medical management of stable COPD. All three emphasize smoking cessation, and the ATS includes a smoking-cessation protocol. All three recommend influenza vaccination, but only the ATS recommends pneumococcal vaccination. All three recommend inhaled bronchodilators as first-line therapy, with the ERS and BTS offering no preference between drugs like ipratropium or β_2-agonists for initial therapy. The ATS suggests initial therapy with an anticholinergic if therapy will only be used on an as-needed basis; otherwise, ATS recommends β_2-agonists. All three state that the need for corticosteroids needs to be determined and documented before long-term use of oral or inhaled corticosteroids can be recommended, as airway inflammation is not always part of the disease. MDI dosage forms are recommended over nebulizers by all three guidelines, and mucokinetic agents are generally not recommended. α_1-AT replacement therapy is recommended for appropriate candidates in the ATS guidelines.

The ATS standard is the most current United States standard for COPD and provides guidance for the management for both acute and chronic COPD. Table 13-9 is from the ATS standard and provides a stepped approach to drug therapy for COPD.

Table 13-9   Step-by-Step Pharmacologic Therapy for COPD

1. For mild, variable symptoms:
   - Selective β_2-agonist MDI, 1–2 puffs every 2–6 hours as needed, not to exceed 8–12 puffs/24 hours
2. For mild to moderate continuing symptoms:
   - Ipratropium MDI, 2–6 puffs every 6–8 hours; not to be used more frequently
   PLUS
   - Selective β_2-agonist MDI, 1–4 puffs as required four times daily for rapid relief, when needed, or as regular supplement
3. If response to Step 2 is unsatisfactory, or there is a mild to moderate increase in symptoms:
   - Add sustained-release theophylline, 200–400 mg twice daily, or 400–800 mg at bedtime for nocturnal bronchospasm
   AND/OR
   - Consider use of sustained-release albuterol, 4–8 mg twice daily, or at night only
   AND/OR
   - Consider use of mucokinetic agent
4. If control of symptoms is suboptimal:
   - Consider course of oral corticosteroids (e.g., prednisone), up to 40 mg/day for 10–14 days
     ✓ If improvement occurs, wean to low daily or alternate-day dose (e.g., 7.5 mg)
     ✓ If no improvement occurs, stop oral corticosteroid
     ✓ If corticosteroid appears to help, consider possible use of MDI, especially if patient has evidence of airway hyperreactivity
5. For severe exacerbation:
   - Increase β_2-agonist dosage (e.g., if spacer not used before, use it now, and/or increase MDI dose to 6–8 puffs every 1/2 to 2 hours or use nebulizer or use subcutaneous administration of epinephrine or terbutaline 0.1 to 0.5 ml)
   AND/OR
   - Increase ipratropium dosage (e.g., MDI with spacer 6–8 puffs every 2–4 hours or inhalant solution of ipratropium 0.5 mg every 4–8 hours)
   AND
   - Provide theophylline dosage intravenously with calculated amount to bring serum level to 10–12 μ/ml
   AND
   - Provide methylprednisolone dosage intravenously, giving 50–100 mg immediately, then every 6–8 hours; taper as soon as clinically possible
   AND ADD
   - Antibiotic, if indicated
   - A mucokinetic agent if sputum is very viscous

Source: Adapted from the 1995 ATS Statement with permission of *American Journal of Respiratory and Critical Care Medicine.*

SUMMARY

Asthma and COPD include a spectrum of diseases characterized by cough, sputum production, dyspnea, airflow limitation, bronchospasm, airway hyperreactivity, and impaired gas exchange. Pharmacologic management of these symptoms and diseases begins with an awareness of risk factors and identification of at-risk patients. Once a disease is recognized, patients and families need education about the disease and how to control it. Smoking cessation is key to stop progression of this entire range of diseases. Appropriate drug therapy should be selected according to the patient's symptomatology and application of the accepted standards of care for the disease. Airway secretions and infections should be minimized, bronchodilation should be maximized, and anti-inflammatory drugs should be used where appropriate. In partnership with the patient, healthcare providers can help to improve the patient's quality of life and maximize their pulmonary function.

REVIEW QUESTIONS

1. Match the level of asthma with its definition:

mild	continuous symptoms with frequent exacerbations
moderate	daily symptoms with flare-ups affecting daily activity
severe	self-limited, brief symptoms up to twice a week

2. Check the category that describes the medication:

albuterol	__ quick relief
	__ long term
cromolyn	__ quick relief
	__ long term
prednisone	__ quick relief
	__ long term

3. Smoking is the most important initial screening that can clinically distinguish COPD from asthma.
   true__
   false__

4. The following are generally of less benefit to COPD patients than asthma patients:
   (a) oral steroids
   (b) inhaled steroids
   (c) cromolyn
   (d) all of the above
   (e) none of the above

5. Chronic bronchitis is characterized clinically by:
   (a) decreased FEV_1
   (b) common smoking history
   (c) minimal sputum
   (d) (a) and (b)
   (e) all of the above

6. Explain the difference between emphysema, asthma, and chronic bronchitis.

7. Describe some goals for an asthma patient, as recommended by the NAEPP2.

8. Discuss the role of an asthma action plan and what it may include.

9. Contrast the roles of MDIs versus spontaneous aerosol treatment of β_2-agonist delivery in emergent asthma exacerbations.

CASE STUDY

A 25-year-old male with a history of asthma and GERD presents to the emergency room with a chief complaint that when he woke up, he couldn't breathe. He reports breathing fine before he went to bed. On the way to the hospital, he was given albuterol nebs and SQ epinephrine.

Cimetidine 300mg BID
Atrovent 2 puffs QID
Albuterol 2 puffs BID prn

VS: 110/48, RR 28, P 132
Skin: no cyanosis
Chest: decreased breath sounds, bilateral wheezes

What other pharmacotherapy choices are available to treat this acute asthma attack?

What are short-term and long-term goals for this patient's pharmacotherapy?

What would you recommend for this patient on discharge?

GLOSSARY

asthma inflammatory process characterized by reversible airway narrowing and airway hyperreactivity.

chronic bronchitis productive cough, mucous gland enlargement, and hypertrophy of airway smooth muscle.

chronic obstructive pulmonary disease global term used to describe abnormal pulmonary conditions associated with cough, sputum production, dyspnea, airflow obstruction, and impaired gas exchange.

dyspnea labored or difficult breathing.

emphysema respiratory condition characterized by permanent, abnormal enlargement of airway spaces and destruction of alveolar wall.

long-term control type of asthma medications used to achieve and maintain control of persistent asthma.

quick-relief type of asthma medications used to provide rapid relief in treating asthma symptoms and exacerbations.

www.prenhall.com/colbert

Use the address above to access the free, interactive Companion Web site created specifically for this textbook. Enhance your studying by viewing videos and animations, answering practice quiz questions, and reviewing an audio glossary and much more related to Chapter 13.

CHAPTER 14

Pharmacologic Treatment of Respiratory Infectious Disease

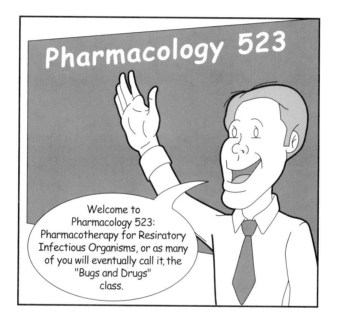

OBJECTIVES

Upon completion of this chapter you will be able to

- Discuss pathogens associated with and diagnosis of:
  community-acquired pneumonia
  hospital-acquired pneumonia
  otitis media
  sinusitis
  pharyngitis
  croup
  epiglottitis
  tuberculosis
  PCP pneumonia
  bronchitis
  bronchiolitis

- Describe goals of pharmacotherapy and monitoring parameters for:
  community-acquired pneumonia
  hospital-acquired pneumonia

Main contributing author Carla Frye

otitis media
sinusitis
pharyngitis
croup
epiglottitis
tuberculosis
PCP pneumonia
bronchitis
bronchiolitis

- Ask and find the answers to questions necessary to develop a therapeutic plan for an individual with a respiratory infectious disease
- Discuss controversies in pharmacological treatment of respiratory infectious disease

ABBREVIATIONS

CAP	community-acquired pneumonia	PaO$_2$	arterial partial pressure of oxygen
CMV	cytomegalovirus		
RSV	respiratory syncytial virus	DRSPTWG	Drug-Resistant *Streptococcus pneumoniae* Therapeutic Working Group
TB	tuberculosis		
CDC	Centers for Disease Control and Prevention		
		RNA	ribonucleic acid
PCP	*Pneumocystis carinii* pneumonia	DNA	deoxyribonucleic acid
HIV	human immunodeficiency virus	TMP-SMX	trimethoprim–sulfamethoxazole
ICU	intensive care unit		
HCW	healthcare worker		

INTRODUCTION

Respiratory tract infections are among the most common infectious diseases seen in healthcare today. Any area of the respiratory tract can become infected, and since it is a continuous system, disease can easily spread to other areas of the respiratory tract. Respiratory infections are generally differentiated on the basis of anatomy. Acute otitis media, sinusitis, and pharyngitis are the primary infectious processes of the upper airways, whereas bronchitis and pneumonia occur in the lower respiratory tract.

When treating these infections, several questions need to be answered. First and foremost, we need to consider whether an antibiotic is really necessary. Viral infections will not respond to antibiotics, and the use of antibiotics in viral syndromes negatively influences bacterial resistance patterns and puts the patient at unnecessary risk for the adverse effects that can be caused by antimicrobials. Second, if antimicrobial therapy is necessary, we need to consider what the likely infecting organisms are, how serious the infection is, and what the antibiotic susceptibility/resistance patterns in the locality are. We can hope to get cultures, but these are not always conclusive. Finally, we need to consider the patient. Will the antibiotic reach the site of infection? What drug(s), dose(s), administration route(s), and schedule(s) are best suited to the patient? What symptomatic treatment is necessary and when is prophylactic antibiotic therapy appropriate? This chapter will give you insight into these questions and the treatment of respiratory infectious diseases.

This chapter will present what seems like a host of organisms that cause respiratory infections, along with a corresponding host of antimicrobial agents to treat them. This may seem overwhelming, but reference tables will be presented when possible to simplify the material. While you received a basic foundation for learning anti-infective agents in Chapter 8, this chapter will build on it by integrating major respiratory infectious diseases with overall effective therapy. Keep in mind that most treatment ultimately depends on identifying the causative microorganism and then selecting an antimicrobial that is effective against that particular microorganism.

DEVELOPING A THERAPEUTIC PLAN FOR RESPIRATORY INFECTIOUS DISEASES

Empiric Treatment

To deliver effective therapy, you must develop a specific therapeutic plan. There are many steps to developing the therapeutic plan. You may be actively involved in several of these and not so involved in others. Here's a review of some of the things to consider for any respiratory infectious disease.

Much of the treatment of respiratory tract infections is **empiric,** meaning that antibiotic therapy is started without identification of the pathogenic organism or without a positive culture from a specimen. However, we do have knowledge of specific pathogens that are common in respiratory infections. In addition, we can empirically list antibiotics that have usually been effective against these suspected pathogens. We can then develop a table that lists the site of infection and suggested "best guess" antibiotic. See Table 14-1, which lists and matches the commonly suspected respiratory pathogens for the disease states covered in this chapter with their best-guess effective antibiotics. Of course if treatment of respiratory infectious disease were this easy, we could end this chapter right here; however, while this table does establish the background for this chapter, there is more to the story.

Local Resistance Patterns (the Antibiogram)

Once identification of the suspected common respiratory infection's pathogens and initial choice of antibiotics are determined, the next step is to customize that information for your

Table 14-1 Respiratory Infectious Diseases, Suspected Pathogens, and Initial Antimicrobial Recommendations

Disease	Suspected Pathogen	Intital Antimicrobial
Childhood otitis	*Streptococcus pneumoniae*	<3 yrs, amoxicillin or trimethoprim–sulfamethoxazole >3 yrs, cefuroxime or amoxicillin clavulanate
Sinusitis	*Streptococcus pneumoniae*	amoxicillin or trimethoprim–sulfamethoxazole
Pharyngitis	Group A *Streptococcus*	penicillin
Epiglottitis	*Haemophilus influenzae*	cefuroxime or cefotaxime or ceftriaxone
Croup	*Staphylococcus aureus, Haemophilus influenzae,* Parainfluenza, Group A *Streptococcus, Moraxella catarrhalis*	cefuroxime or cloxacillin and cefotaxime
Acute bronchitis	*Haemophilus influenzae*	azithromycin, erythromycin
Chronic bronchitis	Viral, *Mycoplasma pneumoniae,* chlamydia	macrolides
Bronchiolitis	RSV	ribavirin
Community-acquired pneumonia	*Streptococcus, Haemophilus influenzae*	see Table 14-7
Hospital-acquired pneumonia	Anaerobes, Gram-negative aerobic rods	see Table 14-7

particular healthcare setting and practice site. Some facilities may have different resistant strains, and the first- or second-choice drug may not be effective. Many factors must be considered in choosing empiric therapy, but a key element is understanding how effective antibiotics are against the likely infecting organisms in your local community or practice setting. Most healthcare systems will regularly provide something called an **antibiogram.** The antibiogram is a compilation of the culture results received by your local laboratory. It will give the type of organisms and numbers of strains, along with a comparison of the antibiotics that are both effective and noneffective in your particular institution. You can use this to make a "best guess" of which antibiotic to use for the suspected causative infecting organism.

www.prenhall.com/colbert

Got to the Web site to see an example of an antibiogram.

Individualizing Therapy

With the infectious process and likely pathogen identified, you are one step closer to empiric treatment. An antibiogram from your practice setting would help to narrow the antimicrobial choice. However, there are a few more steps that are necessary. You will need several more pieces of information before you'll know what, if any, antibiotic to use. Here are some further questions you will need to ask:

1. Is an antibiotic really necessary?
2. Does the patient have any allergies?
3. Are there any age restrictions for the antibiotic you wish to use?
4. How might the dosage form affect your choice of antibiotic?
5. Will the antibiotic reach the site of infection?

Is An Antibiotic Really Necessary? Many patients will present with respiratory symptoms and request treatment with antibiotics. A major question all clinicians must ask is whether the patient really needs antibiotics to treat the condition. Many of the conditions discussed in this chapter are viral in origin and will not respond to antibiotics. Patients who have previously gotten well after receiving an antibiotic will request antibiotics with their next illness; in fact, their main reason for seeing a healthcare provider may be to get an antibiotic.

Overuse of antibiotics has contributed to the rise in antibiotic resistance in the United States and throughout the world. Fortunately, this rise in resistance has been met with advances in antibiotic development. However, we have reached a point where new antibiotic discovery has slowed, and we could reach a point where the antibiotics we have will no longer be effective. It is also possible to cause the patient harm by overusing antibiotics. Our newer and more powerful antibiotics have the potential for more significant side effects and morbidity.

Does the Patient Have Any Allergies? Penicillin allergy is fairly common, and allergies to other antibiotics are becoming more common. We must also be aware of the incidence of **cross-allergenicity.** Cephalosporins and some other beta-lactam antibiotics frequently cause an allergic reaction in patients allergic to penicillins, so they should be avoided if possible in penicillin-allergic patients. You need to be certain of the description of the patient's allergic reaction, as that will give you an idea of the risk to the patient. The patient needs to be questioned about the time-course and symptoms of their allergic reaction, and this should be carefully documented in their medical record. Patients who have a history of rash to penicillin are less likely to react to the other beta-lactam antibiotics. Patients who have anaphylactic reactions, or even hives with one medication, are more likely to experience cross-allergenicity with chemically related compounds.

<u>CLINICAL PEARL</u>

There are always exceptions. Quinolone antibiotics, for example, are usually equally effective orally and intravenously.

Are There Any Age Restrictions for the Antibiotics You Wish to Use?

Children cannot be given all of the same antibiotics that adults can. Tetracyclines cause tooth staining and affect bone growth in developing children; thus they are contraindicated. Quinolones can also affect bone growth in children and thus should be avoided.

<CONTROVERSY>

The effects on bone growth relate to cartilage and are based on animal data from beagle dogs. In certain situations the benefit from using a quinolone in a child may outweigh the risk of cartilage damage.

How Might the Dosage Form Affect Your Choice of Antibiotic? If the patient is clinically ill and requiring hospitalization, you may wish to choose an intravenous dosage form. This is especially necessary if the patient is nauseated or otherwise unable to take a medication orally. In general, intravenous forms give higher, faster blood levels of the antibiotic and may work more quickly.

If a patient is acutely ill and in urgent need of an antibiotic, why is it still important to check the chart for medication allergies before antibiotic administration?

If the patient is a child, you might want a chewable or suspension form of the antibiotic if an oral dosage form is to be used. You may also want to see how these forms are flavored, as the taste of many antibiotics is very unpleasant.

Will the Antibiotic Reach the Site of Infection? Depending on the pharmacokinetic characteristics of the antibiotic, it might not reach the site of infection at an adequate concentration to eradicate the infecting organisms. This is especially problematic when treating pneumonia. Many antibiotics will not penetrate the pulmonary or pleural tissue very well, especially when the infectious process is affecting blood flow to the area. This doesn't necessarily preclude using the antibiotic, but it may mean that a higher than normal dose will be required.

Now that you know the questions to ask and the basics of developing a therapeutic plan, it's time to get more specific about different respiratory infectious diseases pertinent to the pulmonary system starting from the top anatomically and progressing to the lower respiratory tract.

UPPER AIRWAY INFECTIOUS DISEASES

Otitis Media

Although one may not consider ear infections pertinent to a discussion on respiratory infectious diseases, the ears' communication with the nasal passageways make them a common site for the spread of respiratory infections. **Otitis media** or inflammation of the middle ear is one of the most common causes of morbidity in infants and children, even with all of the antibiotic choices available. It is estimated that more than 60% of children will have at least one episode of acute otitis media by their first birthday, and about 75% will have had an episode by age 3.

Acute otitis media is most common in infancy and early childhood, peaking in incidence between the ages of 6 and 18 months. It is more common in males and in certain ethnic groups, including Native Americans and Alaskan and Canadian Eskimos. An estimated 3 to 4 billion dollars are spent annually on the medical and surgical treatment of otitis media in the United States. Table 14-2 lists the factors that increase the risk of acute otitis media in children.

Diagnosis and Treatment. The clinical course of otitis media may include nonspecific symptoms, particularly in young children. Typical symptoms include irritability, lethargy, anorexia, fever, and/or vomiting. These usually occur in a child who has had an upper respiratory tract infection for several days.

Diagnosis of acute otitis media is actually very difficult. Infants are not able to describe their symptoms, and visualization of the tympanic membrane is often difficult and not always conclusive. Since the infection is behind the tympanic membrane, it is also not possible to culture the middle ear fluid without perforating the membrane. Delay in appropriate treatment can lead to hearing loss, and therefore antibiotics are often given without a clear diagnosis. This has led to a divergence of opinion on when to start antibiotic therapy. Many clinicians are concerned that unnecessary antibiotic treatment of otitis media has led to the emergence of multidrug-resistant bacteria. Resistance of *Streptococcus pneumoniae* to a growing number of antibiotics has become a significant problem in the United States, providing evidence for this concern.

Symptomatic therapy and observation are appropriate measures in the treatment of acute otitis media; however, the question of when to give antibiotics is a difficult one to answer. The use of the conjugate polysaccharide *Haemophilus influenzae* type B vaccine has been very effective at decreasing the incidence of this organism as a pathogen for otitis media and gives us proof that prevention is important in this disease. Children with allergies, children of parents who smoke, and children regularly exposed to other sick children have a higher risk of recurrent otitis media. Therefore, measures should be taken to avoid exposure to allergens, irritants, and other sick individuals.

Table 14-2   Factors That Increase the Risk of Otitis Media in Children

Male gender
Sibling history of recurrent otitis media
Early age at onset of acute otitis media (before 4 mo of age)
Bottle feeding
Group day care
Exposure to tobacco smoke
Nationality—Native American and Alaskan and Canadian Eskimo
Family history of atopy

Table 14-3   Microbial Causes of Acute
Otitis Media

Pathogen	Percent of Cases
Streptococcus pneumoniae	~40%
Haemophilus influenzae	~20%
Moraxella catarrhalis	~10%
Streptococcus pyogenes	~3%
Staphylococcus aureus	~2%
Viral	~25%

Microbial Causes. Over the past several decades, the microbial causes of acute otitis media have remained relatively consistent. Table 14-3 lists the typical causes and their prevalence. Protection of the middle ear from microbial or viral invasion depends on the length of the eustachian tube, the pressure difference between the middle ear and the nasopharynx, and the angle of the eustachian tube opening. Infants are most likely to get otitis media, because their eustachian tubes are shorter and wider and are at a flatter angle relative to the nasopharynx than in older children or adults. Acute otitis media generally occurs when an infant develops a viral respiratory tract infection, which results in edema and congestion of the entire respiratory tract. Middle-ear secretions cannot be drained into the nasopharynx because of inflammatory obstruction of the eustachian tube. These accumulated secretions become an excellent environment for the growth of bacteria.

STOP

& REVIEW

What are some risk factors for development of otitis media?

<u>CLINICAL PEARL</u>

Do you know someone who has gotten "tubes put in their ears"? A frequent nonpharmacologic treatment for recurrent otitis media is myringotomy and insertion of tympanostomy tubes. This procedure reduces the recurrence of otitis media by approximately 50%. The insertion of tympanostomy tubes interrupts the cycle of recurrent infections and helps prevent hearing loss.

Pharmacologic Treatments. The first decision in the management of acute otitis media is whether to treat the patient with antibiotics. Children and adults with acute otitis media should receive therapy for associated symptoms; antihistamines and decongestants may be used for relief of symptoms of respiratory tract congestion. Topical corticosteroid therapy may help reduce the symptoms and the recurrence. However, these medications have not been shown to help hasten recovery from acute otitis media, nor do they help resolve effusions. Effusions are important, because they can result in hearing loss, which may also impair speech. Effusions are also relevant because presence of fluid in the ear decreases antibiotic penetration.

Analgesics and antipyretics such as acetaminophen, nonsteroidal anti-inflammatory agents (ibuprofen, naproxen, etc.), or aspirin are helpful in relieving the fever and ear pain often present. A significant percentage of children will recover from their acute episode of otitis media with symptomatic treatment only; however, oral antibiotic therapy continues to be the mainstay of therapy. Clinically, there is no way to know which patients will need antibiotics and which will spontaneously resolve; therefore, most patients with acute otitis media will receive antibiotics.

www.prenhall.com/colbert

Antibiotic costs are important, especially for uninsured children, for whom parents must often decide between food on the table and an antibiotic from the pharmacy. Go to the Web for an idea of the cost variations among differing dosing regimens of antibiotics used in respiratory tract infections.

Most cases of acute otitis media are treated empirically, and the causative organisms are not typically isolated. Therefore, as with many common infections, it is very important to know the likely pathogens and the local resistance patterns. If treatment fails, it is likely that the infection was caused by a virus, or else the bacterium is either resistant to the drug therapy or is one that does not typically cause otitis media. The development of resistance is rapidly becoming an all too common problem, and all healthcare providers must carefully evaluate the antibiotics to be used. An additional challenge is to use an antibiotic that will achieve a "killing" level in the fluid in the middle ear.

The three most common bacterial pathogens in acute otitis media are *Streptococcus pneumoniae, Haemophilus influenzae,* and *Moraxella catarrhalis.* Resistant strains of these bacteria have emerged and complicated the therapy choices for otitis as well as for other respiratory tract infections. There is no one preferred antimicrobial for all children or adults with acute otitis media. Amoxicillin or trimethoprim–sulfamethoxazole are usually used as first-line agents in young children. Amoxicillin achieves the highest concentrations in the middle ear effusions and should be the first choice in young children without penicillin allergy or recurrent infection. Older children are more likely to harbor resistant organisms, owing to their prior treatment with antibiotics and/or daycare attendance. First-line therapies in children over 3 years of age and adults include cefuroxime axetil (Ceftin), amoxicillin-clavulanate (Augmentin), cefpodoxime proxetil (Vantin) and cefprozil (Cefzil). These agents have good coverage against resistant pneumococcal infections.

Table 14-4 details the dosage and regimens that should be used with each of these antibiotics.

Sinusitis

Acute **sinusitis,** an inflammation of the mucosal lining of the paranasal sinuses, affects both children and adults. It is estimated to affect 31 to 35 million Americans per year and can

Table 14-4 First- and Second-Line Antibiotic Therapy for Acute Otitis Media

Antibiotic	Trade Name	Dosage Forms[a]	Dosage (for children)	Duration (days)	Cost ($)[b]
Amoxicillin	Many	c, ch, s	40 mg/kg/day in 3 divided doses	10	$
Trimethoprim–sulfamethoxazole	Bactrim, Septra	t, s	10 mg/kg/day (trimethoprim) in 2 divided doses	10	$
Amoxicillin clavulanate	Augmentin	t, ch, s	40 mg/kg/day (amoxicillin) in 3 divided doses or 45 mg/kd/day in 2 divided doses	10	$$$
Azithromycin	Zithromax	c, t, s	10 mg/kg on day 1, 5 mg/kg on days 2–5	5	$$
Cefpodoxime proxetil	Vantin	t, s	10 mg/kg/day in 1 or 2 divided doses	10	$$$
Cefprozil	Cefzil	t, s	30 mg/kg/day in 2 divided doses	10	$$$
Ceftriaxone	Rocephin	i	50 mg/kg IM × 1 dose	1	$$$
Cefuroxime	Ceftin	t, s	30 mg/kg/day in 2 divided doses	10	$$$
Clarithromycin	Biaxin	t, s	15 mg/kg/day in 2 divided doses	10	$$

[a]t = tablet, c = capsule, i = injectable, s = suspension, ch = chewable.

[b]Cost for treatment course: $ = less than $15, $$ = $15 to $30, $$$ = greater than $30.

exacerbate asthma attacks and trigger other pulmonary disease. Children experience an average of six to eight viral infections of the upper respiratory tract each year; adults experience two to three. Of these upper respiratory tract infections, approximately 0.5% will be complicated by acute sinusitis.

Sinusitis occurs when the mucociliary transport mechanism of the ciliary pseudocolumnar epithelium is impaired and pathogens are allowed to remain in the sinus cavities. Mucopurulent rhinorrhea (discharge from the nasal passages consisting of mucus and pus), postnasal drip, facial pain, maxillary toothache, cough, fever, nausea, and congestion preceded by an upper respiratory infection are typical complaints of patients with acute sinusitis. The persistence of nasal discharge and a cough for more than 10 days following an upper respiratory infection are indicative of sinusitis. Previously clear, thin nasal discharge may become mucoid or purulent, with an increase in both viscosity and quantity.

A poor response of these symptoms to decongestant medication gives clues that sinusitis may be the culprit. Headaches caused by sinusitis respond poorly to analgesics, and the pain usually corresponds directly to the sinuses affected. Adults typically experience the feeling of fullness or dull ache associated with an infection in the frontal sinuses.

Nasal allergies contribute to the edema and swelling of the nasal mucosa, but little evidence is available to actually link allergy to acute sinusitis. Barotrauma from deep-sea diving and airplane travel are also recognized precipitating factors for sinusitis. Chemical irritants such as chlorine may impair secretion clearance and thus foster development of sinusitis.

Diagnosis and Treatment. A computerized tomography (CT) scan is considered the "gold standard" for evaluating sinusitis but is a very expensive diagnostic tool. Sinus puncture is the only definitive way of determining the presence of infection. Sinus X-rays can help the physician detect mucosal thickening, air-fluid level, or sinus opacification. However, a normal sinus X-ray does not rule out sinusitis, and sinus films have high false-positive and false-negative rates. Transillumination of the frontal and maxillary sinuses is a simple and inexpensive test that is done in a darkened room with a high-intensity light source. The presence of an opacified sinus can be detected in this fashion and would be diagnostic of acute sinusitis in a patient with previously normal sinuses.

Microbial Causes. As noted in Table 14-5, the most common bacterial cause of sinusitis in both children and adults is *Streptococcus pneumoniae.* Empiric antibiotic coverage is generally focused on that organism. Patients in the intensive care unit are more likely to have Gram-negative organisms. If the sphenoid sinuses are infected, *Staphylococcus aureus* is more common.

Are streptococcus pneumoniae and staphylococcus aureus Gram-positive or Gram-negative organisms?

Pharmacological Treatment. The treatment of sinusitis is most effective when the cause is clearly identified. Therapies for chronic sinusitis are focused on control of symptoms, whereas antibiotics will be required for acute bacterial sinusitis. The medications used for symptomatic relief have not been proven to reduce the duration of the illness, but at least they can make you feel better until it is resolved. Intranasal cromolyn, antihistamines, intranasal corticosteroids, and topical decongestants are all used to treat or prevent symptoms. Intranasal cromolyn can help to protect the sinus mucosa from an allergic response

Table 14-5   Etiology of Acute Sinusitis

| Microbial Agent | | Average Percent of Cases | |
Type	Species	Adults	Children
Bacteria	Streptococcus pneumoniae	34	41
	nontypical Haemophilus influenzae	25	29
	Moraxella catarrhalis	2	26
	anaerobic bacteria	6	—
	Staphylococcus aureus	4	—
	Staphylococcus pyogenes	2	—
	Gram-negative bacteria	9	—
Virus	rhinovirus	10	—
	influenza virus	5	—
	parainfluenza virus	3	2
	adenovirus	—	2

that would contribute to the sinusitis. Antihistamines can also help prevent an allergic response but should be used cautiously, as they can make the nasal secretions more viscous, interfering with the clearance of purulent mucous secretions. Intranasal corticosteroids are very effective for allergic rhinitis and may help control chronic sinusitis symptoms. The topical decongestants (phenylephrine and oxymetazoline) may facilitate nasal drainage but should only be used for less than 72 hours, because they induce tolerance and rebound congestion. Irrigation of the nasal cavity with a saline solution is also effective at providing symptomatic relief, especially when the nasal mucosa are dry.

Antimicrobial therapy has been shown to shorten the course of acute sinusitis. Empiric therapy must be directed at the common organisms *Streptococcus pneumoniae* and *Haemophilus influenzae*. In sinusitis, many antibiotics are effective, but we must always consider bacterial resistance and choose therapies that are effective without inducing resistance. Amoxicillin and trimethoprim–sulfamethoxazole have long been the first-line therapies for acute sinusitis, but as the number of beta-lactamase-producing and/or penicillin-resistant pathogens increases, amoxicillin has a diminished role. *S. pneumoniae* has also developed significant resistance to trimethoprim–sulfamethoxazole. Therefore, many other agents have become part of the therapy for this infection.

If the patient does not respond in 72 hours to amoxicillin or trimethoprim–sulfamethoxazole, antibiotic therapy should be changed to an agent less likely to have developed bacterial resistance. Usually this means changing to amoxicillin clavulanate, a second- or third-generation cephalosporin (cefuroxime axetil, loracarbef, cefixime, cefaclor), or a quinolone (levofloxacin is generally the preferred quinolone, as ciprofloxacin and ofloxacin have poor *S. pneumoniae* activity). Macrolides (azithromycin and clarithromycin) are also effective against the common pathogens and are rapidly becoming the drugs of choice. Table 14-6 describes the antibiotics generally used for acute sinusitis.

Pharyngitis

Pharyngitis (sore throat) is an inflammation of the pharynx and surrounding lymphoid tissue that may be of bacterial or viral cause. The evaluation, diagnosis, and treatment of patients with pharyngitis is a common problem in primary care. The occurrence of a sore throat is associated with more than 10% of physician office visits, while less than 20% of those patients who experience a sore throat actually seek care.

CLINICAL PEARL

Rebound congestion occurs when topical decongestants are used for more than three consecutive days in a row. Use beyond the recommended time frame makes the congestion worse, not better. The fancy medical term for this is rhinitis medicamentosa.

CLINICAL PEARL

All of the antimicrobial regimens should be continued for at least 10 days, and preferably 14 to 21 days, as blood flow and antibiotic penetration into the infected sinuses are generally very poor.

Table 14-6 Antimicrobial Regimens for Acute Sinusitis

Antimicrobial Agent	Brand Name	Oral dose in Adults
Ampicillin	various	500 mg q 6 hours
Amoxicillin	various	500 mg q 6 hours
Amoxicillin clavulanate	Augmentin	250–500 mg q 8 hours or 875 mg q 12 hours
Azithromycin	Zithromax	250 mg q day
Cefaclor	Ceclor	250–500 mg q 8 hours
Cefixime	Suprax	500 mg day 1, 250 mg daily thereafter
Cefuroxime	Ceftin	250 mg q 12 hours
Clarithromycin	Biaxin	250–500 mg q 12 hours
Levofloxacin	Levaquin	500 mg q 24 hours
Loracarbef	Lorabid	400 mg q 12 hours
Trimethoprim–sulfamethoxazole	Bactrim, Septra	1 DS tablet q 12 hours

Microbiological Causes. Viruses cause most pharyngitis; they are generally the same ones that cause the common cold (rhinovirus, coronavirus, adenovirus, and parainfluenza virus). Other viral causes include herpes simplex virus, influenza virus, coxsackievirus, Epstein–Barr virus, and cytomegalovirus (CMV). However, some pharyngitis (10% to 30%) is the result of bacterial infection, most commonly with Group A beta-hemolytic streptococci such as *Streptococcus pyogenes*. Acute bacterial pharyngitis can also be caused by group C and G streptococci such as *Arcanobacterium hemolyticum* and, possibly, *Mycoplasma pneumoniae* or *Chlamydia pneumoniae*.

Diagnosis and Treatment. Most often, pharyngitis is self-limiting, lasting from 2 to 7 days. The major symptom is sore throat, with or without associated dysphagia (difficulty swallowing). Fever is typically present. Examination usually reveals erythema and possible exudate (white patches), and mucosal congestion is present. The presence of an exudate with fever usually suggests a bacterial infection, but a culture or rapid antigen detection test (quick strep test) should be obtained to confirm the causative organism. The rapid antigen detection test allows the diagnosis of Group A beta-hemolytic streptococcus infection within 5 minutes. This test is very specific for Group A beta-hemolytic streptococcus, and patients with a positive test can be treated immediately without waiting for culture results.

Complications of untreated pharyngitis include spread of the infection to the tonsils, retropharyngeal abscess, cervical lymphadenitis, otitis media, sinusitis, and mastoiditis. Other complications include acute rheumatic fever (common before the second half of the twentieth century and the advent of antibiotics) and acute glomerulonephritis. The most serious of the sequelae of acute rheumatic fever is heart valve damage.

Pharmacological Treatment. Penicillin has long been the antibiotic of choice for pharyngitis. Even with the development of antimicrobial resistance, Group A *Streptococcus* remains susceptible to penicillin, and penicillin remains the drug of choice for this infection. Children younger than 12 years of age should receive 250 mg twice daily of penicillin V for 10 days, or an injection of benzathine penicillin 25,000 to 50,000 U/kg IM as a single dose. For adolescents and adults, penicillin V 500 mg twice daily for 10 days should be given. In the penicillin-allergic patient, erythromycin estolate 20–40 mg/kg/d in two to four divided doses for 10 days is a suitable alternative. See Figure 14-1 for a protocol for treating pharyngitis.

Question the patient:

- Absence of cough?
- Exudate present?
- History of fever >38°C or >100°F?
- Swollen, tender anterior cervical nodes?

Number of Criteria Met	Likelihood of Group A Beta-Hemolytic *Streptococcus*	Suggested Action
0 1	2% – 3% 3% – 7%	No culture indicated and no antibiotics required
2 3	8% – 16% 19% – 34%	Culture, treat if culture is positive
4	41% – 61%	Culture, treat with antibiotics if clinically indicated regardless of culture results[a]

[a]If patient has a high fever, is clinically unwell, and presents early in disease course.

Figure 14-1 Protocol for Treating Pharyngitis

STOP & REVIEW

Why might it be appropriate for you, the healthcare worker, to encourage a patient with a history of respiratory disease and a sore throat to see a physician?

OTHER UPPER AIRWAY INFECTIONS

Epiglottitis

Epiglottitis is an airway emergency whereby *Haemophilus influenzae* type B causes acute airway obstruction. It is most prevalent in children ages 2 to 6 and requires rapid recognition and treatment.

LEARNING HINT

Respiratory distress, drooling, dysphagia, and dysphonia are the four Ds that are signs of this dangerous disease, epiglottitis.

Diagnosis and Treatment. Its onset is fast, and fever is usually the first symptom. It is nonseasonal, and recurrence is rare. Respiratory distress, inspiratory stridor, loss of voice, and intercostal retractions are common manifestations.

Microbiologial Causes. Airway maintenance is the mainstay of treatment with antibiotic therapy empirically selected against *H. influenzae* type B.

Pharmacological Treatment. The preferred treatments are cefuroxime (50–100 mg/kg/day), cefotaxime (150–225 mg/kg/day), or ceftriaxone (80–100 mg/kg/day).

Croup

Croup is different from epiglottitis but also results from infections of the laryngeal area. It too can cause airway obstruction and is characterized by noisy breathing, especially on inspiration.

Microbiological Causes. Croup can be viral or bacterial. Bacterial causes include: *Staphylococcus aureus,* group A beta-hemoplytic streptococci, *Haemophilus influenzae* B, *Moraxella catarrhalis,* and pneumococci. Parainfluenza types I and II cause viral croup.

Diagnosis and Treatment. Croup progresses slowly, usually at night. Fever is uncommon. It is most common in late spring and late fall. Children less than 3 years old most commonly get croup. It is characterized by stridor and no drooling. Treatment consists of air humidification and oxygen.

Pharmacological Treatment. Pharmacological therapy may include epinephrine or corticosteroids to decrease swelling and inflammation. If a laryngotracheitis develops, antibiotic treatment for the bacteria may be necessary with cefuroxime, cloxacillin, cefotaxime, or vancomycin and an aminoglycoside.

Now that we've discussed the upper respiratory tract infections, we will move down to lower respiratory tract infections, including bronchitis, bronchiolitis, pneumonia, and tuberculosis.

LOWER RESPIRATORY TRACT INFECTIONS

Acute Bronchitis and Bronchiolitis

Acute **bronchitis** and **bronchiolitis** are inflammatory conditions of the large and small airways of the tracheobronchial tree. They are usually associated with a respiratory infection. The inflammatory/infectious process in these two conditions does not extend to the alveoli. The treatment of chronic bronchitis was covered in the previous chapter, as it is primarily an inflammatory process. Acute bronchitis occurs in all ages and is seen most commonly in the winter months, following a pattern very similar to that of other acute respiratory tract infections. Damp, cold climates, the presence of respiratory pollutants in the air, or cigarette smoke can precipitate acute attacks. Bronchiolitis is the term for this disease in infants.

Diagnosis and Treatment. Acute bronchitis is usually a self-limiting illness and rarely leads to further complications. In general, infection in the trachea and bronchi leads to increased bronchial secretions and may affect bronchial mucociliary function. The secretions may become thick and tenacious, further affecting mucociliary activity. Acute bronchitis generally begins in the upper airways, and patients present with nonspecific complaints including headache, malaise, and sore throat.

The cough may develop slowly or rapidly and the symptoms persist despite resolution of the preceding nasal symptoms or sore throat. The cough usually progresses, becoming productive, with mucopurulent sputum. Fever is not usually present. The chest exam may reveal rhonchi and coarse crackles bilaterally, and the chest X-ray is usually normal. Cultures are usually not valuable, as it is difficult to sort out the normal nasopharyngeal flora from pathogens.

Most infants will have symptoms suggestive of an upper respiratory tract infection for 2 to 7 days prior to the onset of bronchiolitis. Infants are usually irritable and restless, with a mild fever. Again, the most common clinical sign is cough. As the infection progresses, the infant may experience vomiting, diarrhea, noisy upper airway breathing, and an increased respiratory rate. Infants who require hospitalization will have noisy, labored breathing, with tachypnea and tachycardia. Many of the infants will have a mild conjunctivitis, and 5% to 10% may also have otitis media. Because of their increased work of breathing and coughing, combined with fever, the infants are frequently dehydrated. Diagnosis is made according to clinical symptoms and history. There are several other diseases in infants (asthma, foreign body obstruction, gastroesophageal reflux, etc.) that can present with similar clinical symptoms.

In the adult, acute bronchitis is almost always self-limiting, and the goals of therapy should be to provide comfort to the patient and, in the unusually severe case, to provide antibiotic therapy and supportive therapy if needed. In the well infant, bronchiolitis is also usually a self-limiting disease, and all that is necessary is to wait for the underlying viral infection to resolve. Hospitalization will be necessary for the child suffering from respiratory failure or dehydration.

Microbiological Causes.

Viruses are the most common infectious agents causing bronchitis. The common cold viruses, influenza virus, adenovirus, respiratory syncytial virus (RSV), and coronavirus are most often involved. In infants and children, the same pathogens are usually involved. Bacterial causes usually tend to be *Mycoplasma pneumoniae, Chlamydia pneumoniae,* and *Bordetella pertussis.*

Bronchiolitis is an acute viral infection of the lower respiratory tract of infants. The peak attack age for children is between the ages of 2 and 10 months. Incidence spikes in the winter months and persists through the spring. Bronchiolitis is one of the major reasons that infants under the age of 6 months require hospitalization. RSV is the most common cause of bronchiolitis, accounting for over 50% of cases. Certain times of the year can bring almost epidemic incidence of RSV, with over 80% of bronchiolitis cases during those times caused by the virus. Parainfluenza virus types 1, 2, and 3 cause most of the rest of the cases of bronchiolitis. Bacteria only rarely cause this disease.

Pharmacological Treatment.

Acute Bronchitis. The most common medications used will be for symptomatic therapy. Analgesics/antipyretics such as aspirin or acetaminophen will be helpful in reducing the malaise, lethargy, and fever in adults. Patients with acute bronchitis will frequently self-medicate with over-the-counter cough and cold remedies, although there is no evidence that any of these various combination therapies will be effective.

Persistent cough may require nighttime suppression with dextromethorphan. More severe cough may require intermittent treatment with codeine-containing cough mixtures. One should avoid suppressing a productive cough except when it is persistent enough to disrupt sleep. Use of expectorants has not generally provided clinically effective results and thus can be left to patient preference.

CLINICAL PEARL
Patients should be cautioned not to use any of the over-the-counter combinations that might dry secretions (mostly those containing antihistamines), as they could aggravate the condition and prolong the recovery time.

Bronchiolitis. Aerosolized β-adrenergic therapy has been used to treat bronchiolitis. It is probably best used in the child who has shown some symptoms of bronchospasm. Inhaled or systemic corticosteroids have not been shown to be conclusively beneficial. Since bacteria rarely cause bronchiolitis, antibiotics should not be routinely used. Ribavirin may offer benefit to a small number of bronchiolitis cases. This agent is effective against a variety of RNA and DNA viruses, including influenza, parainfluenza, and RSV. Use of the aerosolized drug requires special nebulizer equipment (small-particle aerosol generator) and specifically trained personnel for administration via an oxygen hood or mist tent. Special care must

⟨ **CONTROVERSY** ⟩

Routine use of antibiotics for acute bronchitis is not recommended. However, if patients have symptoms for more than 4 to 6 days and are febrile, bacterial infection may be present. Antibiotic therapy should be directed at the most common pathogens (*Mycoplasma pneumoniae, Chlamydia pneumoniae,* and *Bordetella pertussis*). The macrolides (azithromycin, erythromycin, and clarithromycin) should be effective.

be taken to avoid drug particle deposition and clogging of respiratory tubing and valves in mechanical ventilators.

Most experts recommend reserving ribavirin for severely ill patients, especially those with serious underlying disorders such as bronchopulmonary dysplasia, congenital heart disease, prematurity, or immunodeficiency disorders.

Pneumonia

Pneumonia is the sixth leading cause of death in the United States as well as one of the most common causes of hospitalization. It is defined as an inflammation of the lung tissue and may be caused by bacteria, viruses, or even noninfectious agents such as drugs or chemicals. The principal site of infection is in the alveoli and surrounding interstitial tissue.

Individuals with pneumonia classically present with high white blood cell counts ($> 10,000$) and high fevers, crackles, rhonchi, bronchial breath sounds, and dullness to percussion over the involved areas of the lung. Patients with pneumonia may have pleural effusions, and their chest X-rays usually reveal infiltrates or signs of consolidation. Patients with pneumonia are far more likely to experience complications such as hypoxia, cardiopulmonary failure, local abscesses or empyemas, and possible spread of infection to other organs by way of the bloodstream. There are several well-defined categories of pneumonia that help to define appropriate therapy, and we will review this disease according to these subclassifications.

Community-Acquired Pneumonia. **Community-acquired pneumonia (CAP)** is an infection of the lung tissue that, in its purest definition, is contracted outside of the institutional setting (institutional meaning nursing homes, hospitals, or any other place that might encourage the transmission of bacteria between compromised individuals). This definition by setting has evolved to be more a description of the likely pathogens than a delineation of where the disease was contracted. *Streptococcus pneumoniae, Haemophilus influenzae,* and *Moraxella catarrhalis* account for the majority of cases of bacterial CAP, with *S. pneumoniae* responsible for 50% to 90% of the cases of acute CAP. Gram-negative bacteria do not commonly cause this disorder. However, over the last 20 years, an increasing proportion of CAP is being caused by "atypical" organisms, and the incidence of *S. pneumoniae* as a cause is changing.

The most significant problem in the treatment of CAP is not the rise of atypical causes; effective therapy is available for most of these. The real problem with CAP in the new millennium is the growing resistance of *Streptococcus pneumoniae* to most antimicrobials. This increasing resistance, combined with the much wider variety of organisms causing the disease, has made diagnosis and treatment a much greater therapeutic challenge.

Atypical Pneumonia. The term **"atypical pneumonia"** has been in use in the medical literature for over a century but perhaps should be abandoned in this new millennium. It is a difficult term to define and even more difficult to correlate to bacterial cause and antibiotic therapy.

www.prenhall.com/colbert

The term atypical pneumonia has an interesting story, which begins in the late 1800s with Louis Pasteur. Go to the Web site for this historical perspective.

Over the years, many other organisms, including viruses and fungi, have been found to cause pneumonia. All of these causes other than *S. pneumoniae, M. catarrhalis,* and *H. influenzae* were lumped into the classification of atypical pneumonia. Prior to the outbreak and identification of a new organism, *Legionella pneumophila,* at the 1976 Philadelphia convention of the American Legion, and the increasingly common incidence of *Chlamydia pneumoniae* and *Mycoplasma* infections, atypical pneumonia was generally mild and self-limiting, with very low mortality. These new atypical pneumonias were much more deadly and made the "atypical" classification very imprecise. Physicians had to rethink the diagnosis and treatment of community-acquired pneumonia to allow for the presence of these atypical organisms.

Mycoplasma pneumoniae infections tend to follow epidemic patterns, with outbreaks every 4 to 8 years making it hard to define its true incidence. *Legionella* tends to infect older and more immunocompromised patients. It also has a more seasonal occurrence, tending to break out in the spring, when air conditioning is started. *Chlamydia* tends to infect young people such as college students and military recruits.

When you analyze the signs, symptoms, and chest X-rays of patients infected with these three atypical pathogens, very little difference can be seen between atypical and typical pneumonia. The only real difference between the atypical organisms—*Chlamydia, Legionella,* and *Mycoplasma*—and the typical pneumonia organisms—*S. pneumoniae, M. catarrhalis,* and *H. influenzae*—is that the atypical organisms cannot be cultured with standard microbiologic media or techniques, and they do not respond to treatment with penicillins or other antibiotics classically used for typical pneumonia.

Whereas "typical" pneumonia tends to affect patients with some other chronic illness and who are greater than 50 years of age, atypical pneumonia tends to affect young adults with no underlying illness. Typical pneumonia tends to have a rapid onset and high fever, while atypical pneumonia may be more insidious in onset. However, it has become very difficult to distinguish atypical infections from typical infections clinically as the atypical organisms have become more virulent and *S. pneumoniae* has become more resistant to therapy. Current recommendations from the American Thoracic Society for the treatment of CAP recommend that empiric therapy should cover both the "typical" and "atypical" causative organisms.

Therapy Recommendations for Community-Acquired Pneumonia (CAP) and Atypical Pneumonias.
In the past, antibiotic therapy for CAP was fairly simple. It was quite likely that *S. pneumoniae* was the causative organism, and the pneumococcus responded very well to treatment with penicillin. However, as early as 1967, resistant pneumococcus began to show up. We are now faced with 20% to 40% of *S. pneu-*

moniae strains showing resistance to penicillin. *S. pneumoniae* still accounts for the majority of CAP cases, but other organisms are creeping up in incidence. It is believed that *Mycoplasma pneumoniae* now accounts for up to 20% of all acute bacterial pneumonias. Since eradication of the offending organism is one of our major treatment goals in pneumonia, appropriate empiric antibiotic therapy is a major challenge. Therapy should minimize any associated morbidity and not cause any drug-induced side effects or organ dysfunction.

The first priority in the treatment of pneumonia is to evaluate the patient's respiratory function and treat any problems symptomatically. Patients may require intravenous fluids, oxygen, bronchodilators, chest physiotherapy with postural drainage, or even mechanical ventilation. The second priority is to obtain cultures of the sputum and to use other diagnostic procedures to determine the microbiologic cause of the acute disease. Assessing the patient's clinical setting can help the choice of empiric therapy once you understand what pathogens are likely in specific patient populations. Table 14-7 can help you consider these circumstances.

The empiric antibiotic choices for the treatment of community-acquired pneumonia are no longer very simple. In the past, all patients with the clinical picture of a pneumonia were started on penicillin, since *S. pneumoniae* was the most likely and the most aggressive of the likely organisms causing the infection. As *S. pneumoniae* continues to become more resistant to penicillin and other "atypical" organisms are becoming more predominant,

Table 14-7 Empiric Antibiotic Choices for Adult Pneumonias

Patient	*Likely Infecting Organisms*	*Empiric Antibiotic Choices*
Elderly patient, from nursing home or other care facility	*Streptococcus pneumoniae, Mycoplasma pneumoniae*	ticarcillin clavulanate, piperacillin tazobactam, second- or third-generation cephalosporins, imipenem–cilastin or meropenem
History of chronic bronchitis	*Streptococcus pneumoniae,* Gram-negative bacilli (such as *Klebsiella pneumoniae), Staphylococcus aureus, Haemophilus influenzae*	amoxicillin, tetracycline, trimethoprim–sulfamethoxazole, cefuroxime, cefprozil, amoxicillin clavulanate, clarithromycin, erythromycin, azithromycin, levofloxacin
Alcoholic	*Streptococcus pneumoniae, Klebsiella pneumoniae, Staphylococcus aureus, Haemophilus influenzae,* possibly anaerobes from the oral cavity	ticarcillin clavulanate, piperacillin tazobactam, plus aminoglycoside; imipenem–cilastatin or meropenem
Previously healthy, ambulatory patient	*Streptococcus pneumoniae, Mycoplasma pneumoniae*	clarithromycin, erythromycin, or azithromycin; tetracyclines
Aspiration pneumonia community-acquired hospital-acquired	Anaerobes from the oral cavity Anaerobes from the oral cavity, *Staphylococcus aureus,* Gram-negative enteric organisms	penicillin or clindamycin clindamycin, ticarcillin clavulanate, piperacillin tazobactam, plus aminoglycoside
Nosocomial pneumonia	Gram-negative bacilli such as *Klebsiella pneumoniae, Enterobacter* sp., *Pseudomonas aeruginosa, Staphylococcus aureus*	ticarcillin clavulanate, piperacillin tazobactam, imipenem–cilastatin or meropenem, or expanded-spectrum cephalosporins such as ceftazidime or cefepime plus an aminoglycoside

it is very difficult to pick one antibiotic as the best choice. The prescriber must carefully consider the patient's clinical setting, their prior exposure to antibiotics, their clinical condition, their chest X-ray, the local susceptibility patterns, and the patient's underlying state of health.

Guidelines for the treatment of CAP continue to be revised, and the clinician must be careful to review current literature for the most up-to-date recommendations. The Drug-Resistant *Streptococcus pneumoniae* Therapeutic Working Group (DRSPTWG), convened by the Centers for Disease Control, published their recommendations in May of 2000. They recommend macrolides (erythromycin, clarithromycin, or azithromycin) or doxycycline (or tetracycline) for children aged 8 years or older, or an oral beta-lactam with good antipneumococcal activity (cefuroxime axetil, amoxicillin, amoxicillin clavulanate) as the first-line therapies for CAP. An oral fluoroquinolone with improved activity against *S. pneumoniae* (levofloxacin, or sparfloxacin) may be used for the treatment of adults for whom one of these regimens has already failed, or who are allergic to the alternative agents, or who have a documented infection with a highly drug-resistant pneumococcus. The fluoroquinolones should not be used in children, and sparfloxacin has a fairly high incidence of phototoxicity. For children younger than 5 years in whom atypical pathogens are uncommon and for whom doxycycline and fluorquinolone should be avoided, beta-lactams are the best choice.

Nosocomial Pneumonia.

Pneumonia is the second most common nosocomial (hospital-acquired) infection in the United States and is associated with substantial morbidity and mortality. Most patients who have **nosocomial pneumonia** are persons who have severe underlying disease, are immunosuppressed, are comatose, or are otherwise incapacitated and who have cardiopulmonary disease. In addition, some nosocomial pneumonia patients are persons who have had thoracic or abdominal surgery. Although patients receiving mechanical ventilation do not represent a major proportion of patients who have nosocomial pneumonia, they are at highest risk for acquiring the infection.

Pneumonias caused by *Legionella* sp., *Aspergillus* sp., and influenza virus are often caused by inhalation of contaminated aerosols. RSV infection usually occurs after viral inoculation of the conjunctivae or nasal mucosa by contaminated hands. Traditional preventive measures for nosocomial pneumonia include taking precautions to decrease aspiration by the patient, preventing cross-contamination or colonization via hands of personnel, appropriate disinfection or sterilization of respiratory-therapy devices, use of available vaccines to protect against particular infections, and education of hospital staff and patients. Figure 14-2 describes the pathogenesis of nosocomical pneumonia.

Recent epidemiologic studies have identified other subsets of patients at high risk for acquiring nosocomial bacterial pneumonia. Such patients include persons older than 70 years; persons who have endotracheal intubation and/or mechanically assisted ventilation, a depressed level of consciousness (particularly those with closed-head injury), or underlying chronic lung disease; and persons who have previously had an episode of a large-volume aspiration. Other risk factors include 24-hour ventilator-circuit changes, hospitalization during the fall or winter, stress-bleeding prophylaxis with cimetidine (either with or without antacid), administration of antimicrobials, presence of a nasogastric tube, severe trauma, and recent bronchoscopy.

Nosocomial pneumonia has been associated with high fatality rates. Mortality rates of 20% to 50% have been reported. Patients receiving mechanically assisted ventilation have higher mortality rates than patients not receiving ventilation support; however, other factors (e.g., the patient's underlying disease and organ failure) are stronger predictors of death in patients who have pneumonia.

CLINICAL PEARL

Because intubation and mechanical ventilation alter first-line patient respiratory defenses, they greatly increase the risk for nosocomial bacterial pneumonia.

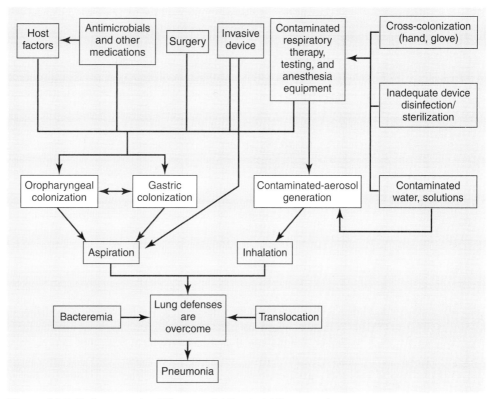

Figure 14-2 Pathogenesis of Nosocomial Bacterial Pneumonia

The high incidence of Gram-negative bacillary pneumonia in hospitalized patients might result from factors that promote colonization of the pharynx by Gram-negative bacilli and the subsequent entry of these organisms into the lower respiratory tract. Although aerobic Gram-negative bacilli are recovered infrequently or are found in low numbers in pharyngeal cultures of healthy persons, the likelihood of colonization substantially increases in comatose patients, in patients treated with antimicrobial agents, and in patients who have hypotension, acidosis, azotemia, alcoholism, diabetes mellitus, leukocytosis, leukopenia, pulmonary disease, or nasogastric or endotracheal tubes in place.

Bacteria also can enter the lower respiratory tract of hospitalized patients through inhalation of aerosols generated primarily by contaminated respiratory-therapy or anesthesia–breathing equipment. Outbreaks related to the use of respiratory-therapy equipment have been associated with contaminated nebulizers. When the fluid in the reservoir of a nebulizer becomes contaminated with bacteria, the aerosol produced may contain high concentrations of bacteria that can be deposited deep in the patient's lower respiratory tract. Contaminated aerosol inhalation is particularly hazardous for intubated patients, because endotracheal and tracheal tubes provide direct access to the lower respiratory tract.

Several large studies have examined the potential risk factors for nosocomially acquired bacterial pneumonia. Although specific risk factors have differed among study populations, they can be grouped into the following general categories: (a) host factors (e.g., extremes of age and severe underlying conditions, including immunosuppression); (b) factors that enhance colonization of the oropharynx and/or stomach by microorganisms (e.g., administration of antimicrobials, admission to an ICU, underlying chronic lung disease, or coma);

(c) conditions favoring aspiration or reflux (e.g., endotracheal intubation, insertion of a nasogastric tube, or supine position); (d) conditions requiring prolonged use of mechanical ventilatory support with potential exposure to contaminated respiratory equipment and/or contact with contaminated or colonized hands of healthcare workers (HCWs); and (e) factors that impede adequate pulmonary toilet (e.g., undergoing surgical procedures that involve the head, neck, thorax, or upper abdomen, or being immobilized as a result of trauma or illness).

www.prenhall.com/colbert

The United States Centers for Disease Control and Prevention give recommendations on staff education, surveillance, interrupting transmission of microorganisms, and precautions in patient care to minimize nosocomial infections. Go to the Web site for a detailed description of these guidelines.

By sorting out these risk categories, the clinician can better define the likely pathogens and then choose the most appropriate empiric antibiotic therapy. Each patient will be different, and individual analyses must be made. Table 14-7 on page 281 showed some of the likely pathogens in nosocomial pneumonia and the general antibiotic choices. Most of these antibiotics would be considered the "big guns" of the antibiotic world. They are costly, require parenteral therapy, have significant toxicities, and will require close monitoring. In general, the antibiotic selection for the patient with nosocomial pneumonia will require an antibiotic to cover Gram-negative pathogens as well as the more common pneumonia pathogens. Most patients will require more than one antibiotic to cover the entire spectrum of likely organisms. If a culture is obtained and the pathogenic organisms are isolated, the antibiotic regimen may be simplified or narrowed to specifically cover the isolated organisms.

Antibiotic Therapy Recommendations for the Treatment of Nosocomial Pneumonia.

Patients with nosocomial pneumonia will require many supportive and symptomatic therapies. They may be mechanically ventilated, they may be in the intensive care unit, and they may be very sick. It is not possible to go over all of their potential therapies in detail; you will need to use your clinical knowledge of respiratory illness to help the prescriber know what symptomatic therapies will be needed. We will focus on the antibiotic therapies at this point.

The DRSPTWG recommends that moderately ill patients with pneumonia receive an intravenous beta-lactam, such as cefotaxime or ceftriaxone, and an intravenous macrolide, such as erythromycin or azithromycin. Alternatively, intravenous ceftriaxone or cefotaxime and a fluoroquinolone with improved activity against *S. pneumoniae* may be used for critically ill adults. A fluoroquinolone with improved anti-pneumococcal activity may be used alone, but caution should be exercised, because the efficacy of the new fluoroquinolones as monotherapy for critically ill patients with pneumococcal pneumonia has not been determined.

Vancomycin is NOT routinely recommended for the treatment of CAP but may be necessary in nosocomial pneumonia, especially if bacterial meningitis is also suspected. Vancomycin is reserved for resistant or severe infections, not routine treatment. Additionally, vancomycin may be appropriate for selected critically ill children with CAP. If vancomycin therapy is begun, it should be promptly discontinued if a subsequent culture indicates that the drug is not needed.

Aspiration Pneumonia.

Aspiration pneumonia can be either chemical (exposure to stomach acid) or bacterial. Bacteria can invade the lower respiratory tract by aspiration of oropharyngeal organisms, inhalation of aerosols containing bacteria, or, less frequently, by hematogenous spread from a distant body site. In addition, bacterial translocation from the gastrointestinal tract has been hypothesized recently as a mechanism for infection. Of these routes, aspiration is believed to be the most important for both nosocomial and community-acquired pneumonia.

Aspiration pneumonia brings a different set of possible pathogens. If the pneumonia is due to the acid exposure, antibiotics won't help. Only symptomatic therapy can be used as the lungs heal. Empiric antibiotic therapy generally consists of agents with anaerobic and Gram-negative coverage in their spectrums of activity.

Patients who develop aspiration pneumonia in the community setting should be treated with an antibiotic that is effective against Gram-positive anaerobes. Such antibiotics include clindamycin or penicillins. If the patient aspirated while hospitalized or is significantly debilitated by coexisting disease, broader-spectrum therapy should be used to expand the coverage to Gram-negative pathogens. Generally clindamycin or a penicillin combined with a beta-lactamase inhibitor (such as piperacillin–tazobactam) plus an aminoglycoside (tobramycin, gentamicin, or amikacin) should be used.

Why would Gram-negative pathogenic bacteria be more common in aspiration?

Therapeutic Guidelines.

Because care of patients with pneumonia is quite common, therapeutic guidelines are published and updated frequently for the care of pneumonia patients. It is important to stay updated with the current recommendations. The American Thoracic Society (1993), the British Thoracic Society (1993), the Canadian Infectious Disease Society (1993), and the Infectious Disease Society of America (1998) are all recently published sets of guidelines, and each of those societies updates them regularly. Individual institutions may have guidelines as well.

Pneumocystis carinii pneumonia.

Pneumocystis carinii pneumonia (PCP) is a complication of HIV infection. It should be noted that it can also occur in non-HIV-infected patients. Like TB, *Pneumocystis* can be asymptomatic and latent.

Treatment and Diagnosis.

Symptoms, when present, can include fever, cough, tachypnea, and dyspnea. Treatment is divided into acute and chronic. Arterial blood gases are one of the key factors in therapy decisions. The disease can be classified as mild, moderate, or severe on the basis of oxygenation.

Factors to consider when starting drug therapy for PCP are whether it is a first episode, arterial blood gases, history of drug reaction, and route of therapy. Drugs used for acute treatment are intravenous trimethoprim–sulfamethoxazole (TMP–SMX) or parenteral pentamidine. These drugs are toxic. For example, more than 50% of patients receiving trimethoprim–sulfomethoxazole may develop rash, fever, leukopenia, hepatitis, or thrombocytopenia. Pentamidine can cause azotemia, pancreatitis, hypocalcemia, or leukopenia, to name a few. Corticosteroids have a role in patients with acute, moderate-to-severe PCP, and calculation of PaO_2 gradient can guide their use.

Cystic Fibrosis and Pneumonia.

Cystic fibrosis is a genetic disease of exocrine gland secretions. Recurrent respiratory infections play a big role in this chronic pulmonary disease. At different times during the course of the disease, different pathogens are found. It's common to have multiple bacterial isolates that have different antibiotic sensitivities. Systemic antibiotics are used to treat pulmonary infections in cystic fibrosis, frequently in combination therapy. Common agents are an aminoglycoside combined with an extended-spectrum penicillin or third-generation cephalosporin.

Because antibiotics penetrate poorly in lung tissue, aerosolized antibiotics have been utilized with some success. One of the limiting factors in aerosol antibiotic administration is the bronchospasm that can result from aerosolized antibiotics. The role of aerosol antibiotics in cystic fibrosis infection treatment, prophylaxis, and resistance remains to be determined.

Tuberculosis

No respiratory infectious disease chapter would be complete without a short discussion of **tuberculosis.** Tuberculosis (TB) is a chronic disease caused by *Mycobacterium tuberculosis.* Although it can affect any part of the body, it most commonly affects the lungs. While there has been a gradual decline in the number of active cases over the years, there are still millions of people with TB infection that haven't progressed to active TB. TB is spread by microscopic droplets and is an airborne disease. It can be spread when an infected person coughs or sneezes. Once the droplet is inhaled, it becomes encapsulated, and the infection is latent.

Diagnosis and Treatment.

When the infection droplets called bacilli escape, the disease becomes active. Symptoms of active TB can range from none to weight loss, fever, night sweats, or bloody sputum. Diagnosis is made with a skin test, sputum sample, and chest X-ray. Drug therapy of TB is aimed at preventive therapy for latent infection or treatment of active TB disease.

Pharmacological Treatment.

Preventive therapy is usually with isoniazid for 6–12 months, which will decrease the risk the infection will progress to disease. Research is always in progress to determine the easiest yet most effective method of prophylaxis. Certain people are at a higher risk for developing TB; this group includes people who are in close contact with others with TB, people with a chest X-ray suggesting previous TB that hasn't been treated, persons with HIV, and people who are substance abusers, for example. Patients on corticosteroids also may be at increased risk of disease progression.

www.prenhall.com/colbert

For the most recent risk factors for TB and treatment regimens, go to the Web site.

Treatment of TB takes 6 to 24 months. Drug treatment must be in combination, since resistance is a problem. Drugs used are isoniazid, rifampin, pyrazinamide, ethambutol, and streptomycin. Because of resistance, adherence to the drug regimen is the key point for TB.

SUMMARY

Respiratory infections are the major cause of morbidity and mortality from acute illness in the United States. The majority of these infections follow colonization of the upper respiratory tract with potential pathogens. Less commonly, the pathogen may gain access to the lungs via the blood, or by inhalation of infected aerosol particles. The patient's own immune status will have much to do with their susceptibility to a respiratory tract infection.

Appropriate therapy for respiratory tract infections is a multifaceted decision. The clinician must consider the patient's history, the physical examination, chest X-ray, culture results, and local pathogen incidence and resistance patterns. The most common pathogen in respiratory illness is *S. pneumoniae,* but this is changing. Other pathogens are becoming more virulent and deadly, and *S. pneumoniae* has changed significantly in its resistance to antimicrobial therapy.

REVIEW QUESTIONS

1. A usual first-line antibiotic agent for children with acute otitis media is:
   (a) tetracycline (Achromycin)
   (b) metronidazole (Flagyl)
   (c) amoxicillin (Amoxil)
   (d) cefaclor (Ceclor)
   (e) any of the above

2. Most cases of acute sinusitis develop from what causative organism?
   (a) anaerobic bacteria
   (b) *Streptococcus pneumoniae*
   (c) *E. coli*
   (d) influenza virus

3. The treatment of choice for pharyngitis is:
   (a) penicillin
   (b) tetracycline
   (c) cephalexin
   (d) erythromycin

4. A patient presents with a high white blood cell count, fever, bronchial breathing, and rhonchi on auscultation. What type of infectious process do you suspect?
   (a) otitis media
   (b) sinusitis
   (c) croup
   (d) pneumonia

5. Gram-negative bacteria are frequently colonized in:
   (a) healthy persons
   (b) hypertensive patients
   (c) patients with nasogastric tubes
   (d) patients with community-acquired pneumonia
   (e) all of the above

6. What is empiric therapy? What are some of the questions that need to be answered when treating infections?

7. Can you give an example of an indication when an antibiotic may not be appropriate?

8. Why does an ear or sinus infection have respiratory implications?

9. What is community-acquired pneumonia, and what are some problems with its treatment?

10. A 62-year-old male presents to the walk-in clinic with a chief complaint of headache, sore throat, and cough. A sputum sample isolates *Streptococcus* and *Haemophilus.* The physician is debating whether to treat the patient with an antibiotic. What would you recommend?

11. A child is brought to the emergency department in respiratory distress, and the mother states she has difficulty swallowing and has been drooling for the last three hours. What infection would you suspect, and what antibiotic therapy would be indicated? What respiratory intervention may be needed?

GLOSSARY

antibiogram hospital compilation of microbiological culture results from the laboratory.

bronchiolitis inflammatory condition of the small airways usually associated with respiratory infection.

bronchitis inflammatory condition of the large airways usually associated with respiratory infection.

community-acquired pneumonia infection of lung tissue that is contracted outside of the institutional setting.

cross-allergenicity drug allergy reactions with one antibiotic class that cross over and present with another antibiotic class as well.

croup infection of the respiratory tract that can cause airway obstruction; it usually affects small children.

culture lab testing process that involves growing microorganisms to determine which drugs might fight the infection.

empiric therapy antibiotic therapy initiated before the causative microorganism is detected.

epiglottitis infection usually caused by *H. influenzae* type B that causes airway obstruction in children.

nosocomial pneumonia pneumonia that develops in hospitalized patients as a result of conditions there that predispose to the pathogenesis.

otitis media middle ear inflammation common in children.

pharyngitis inflammation of the pharynx and surrounding tissue; pharyngitis may be bacterial or viral.

pneumonia inflammation of lung tissue in the alveoli and interstitial tissue.

sinusitis inflammation of the mucosal lining of the paranasal sinuses.

www.prenhall.com/colbert

Use the address above to access the free, interactive Companion Web site created specifically for this textbook. Enhance your studying by viewing videos and animations, answering practice quiz questions, and reviewing an audio glossary and much more related to Chapter 14.

CHAPTER 15

Pharmacology for Advanced Cardiac Life Support

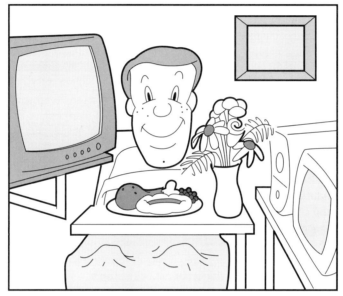

A patient's dream of "advanced LIFE SUPPORT"

OBJECTIVES

Upon completion of this chapter you will be able to

- Define key terms related to advanced cardiac life support (ACLS)

- Identify the conduction pathway for a normal heartbeat

- Describe the pharmacological effects of the drugs commonly used in the treatment of AMI, cardiac arrest, cardiogenic shock, and the various arrhythmias

- Review algorithms for treatment of cardiac arrest and arrhythmias

ABBREVIATIONS

ACLS	advanced cardiac life support	mV	milivolt
CO$_2$	carbon dioxide	SA	sino-atrial
TCP	transcutaneous pacemaker	AV	atrio-ventricular
CPR	cardio-pulmonary resuscitation	TPA	tissue plasminogen factor
PEA	pulseless electrical activity	CHF	congestive heart failure

Main contributing author Terri Price

INTRODUCTION

A variety of healthcare practitioners participate in the emergency treatment of patients who have suffered **acute myocardial infarctions,** cardiogenic shock, **cardiac arrest,** and **stroke.** The American Heart Association offers courses in advanced cardiac life support (ACLS) to help healthcare practitioners recognize important signs and symptoms and treat patients accordingly. These courses emphasize the skills and knowledge necessary to ensure that members of the resuscitation team will be prepared to act quickly and efficiently to treat and resuscitate the cardiac arrest victim. Some of these practitioners may have the primary responsibility of administering medications, while others may be more concerned with airway management and support of circulation. Regardless of the specific role, to be truly prepared for emergencies, members of the resuscitation team need to be knowledgeable about the entire process and be prepared to act.

In this chapter, we will introduce the reader to some of the drugs and treatment algorithms used for serious, life-threatening **arrhythmias** and acute myocardial infarction. You will no doubt recognize many of these drugs from previous chapters, but in this chapter we will be looking at their specific roles in the context of the emergency setting. This chapter is not intended to be a substitute for the American Heart Association's *Textbook for Advanced Cardiac Life Support,* but rather a brief overview of its basic components.

In order for any discussion of the pharmacologic agents used in ACLS to be meaningful, the reader should have a general understanding of rhythm disturbances. We will begin with an overview of some common arrhythmias, and you may also want to refer back to the cardiac section of Chapter 9. Then we will discuss pharmacologic treatment for serious arrhythmias and cardiac arrest. Finally we will review several examples of treatment algorithms to show how the pharmacology fits into the complete management of the patient. Remember that an algorithm provides practitioners with a systematic approach to treat the victim of a cardiac emergency. It is intended to help guide and standardize treatment. Algorithms should not limit the physician from implementing alternate therapy based on assessment of each individual patient or situation.

NORMAL CONDUCTION AND ARRHYTHMIAS

Electrophysiology

The heart's conduction network coordinates organized muscle contraction. The conduction cells transmit impulses by depolarization. In its resting or polarized state, the cell has about –90 mV of stored energy. This charge is maintained by differences in concentrations of sodium and potassium ions. An electrical, chemical, or mechanical stimulation causes this stored energy to be released by opening cell membrane channels and allowing a rapid influx of Na+ ions into the cell, reversing the polarity to about +20 mV. This is called depolarization and causes muscle contraction. Calcium also begins to enter the cell to aid in muscle contraction.

The depolarized cell now needs to repolarize before it can conduct another impulse. During repolarization the sodium channels close and potassium channels open thereby restoring the membrane potential back to the resting level of –90 mV. In the late phase of repolarization, sodium ions are actively extruded from the cell while potassium re-enters. See Figure 15-1.

Normal Conduction

Normally, the electrical impulses begin in the SA node. The wave of depolarization spreads through the atria, then to the AV node, where there is a brief pause (.1 second). The pause allows time for the atria to contract and the blood from the atria to flow into the ventricles.

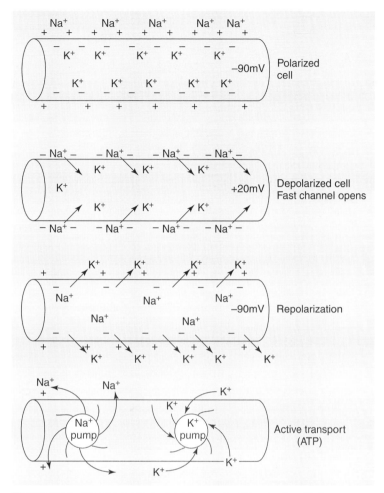

Figure 15-1 Depolarization of a Myocardial Conduction Cell

Now that the ventricles are fully loaded, the impulse travels to the AV bundle, or bundle of His, to the right and left bundle branches. The bundle branches terminate in Purkinje fibers. The numerous fibers of the Purkinje system serve to rapidly transmit the impulse to the contractile ventricles, so that they depolarize and contract in unison (see Figure 15-2).

Myocardial Infarction

The heart contracts with amazing regularity. It also manages to compensate for a variety of pathological conditions. But in spite of this, heart disease remains the leading cause of death in the United States. High fat/high calorie diets, a sedentary lifestyle, cigarette smoking, and high blood pressure are just a few of the contributing factors in heart disease. High levels of cholesterol in the bloodstream build up, narrowing the walls of the arteries. Smoking causes constriction of the arteries, which can further reduce oxygen delivery to the heart. High blood pressure and narrowed arteries make the heart work harder and consume more oxygen as it pumps blood and oxygen to the rest of the body. When the heart is no longer getting the full supply of oxygen it needs, the myocardial cells become more irritable. The patient may begin to experience chest pain, which is referred to as angina. If the interruption in the supply of oxygen continues, tissue damage occurs, and the damaged myocardium becomes electrically unstable. The ability of the myocardial cells to depolarize and repolarize normally may be affected, and abnormal beats can then develop. If the oxygen supply

LEARNING HINT

Beats that begin anywhere outside of the normal conduction system are called ectopic beats. Ectopic beats can be further defined as premature if they come earlier than a normal beat would, or as escape beats if they come late.

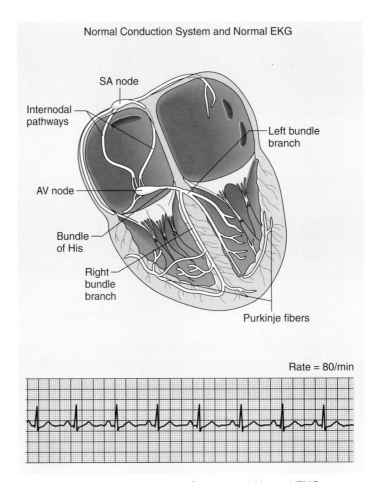

Figure 15-2 Normal Conduction System and Normal EKG

is not reestablished quickly, myocardial cells will die. Death of myocardial cells is irreversible, and this is what is known as myocardial infarction.

Bradycardia

Bradycardia simply means a slow heart rate. The SA node is called the pacemaker of the heart, and it normally fires 60 to 100 times per minute. Various conditions such as increased parasympathetic tone, profound hypoxia, and damage to the conduction system of the heart (heart block) may result in a rate that is too slow for the patient (normally less than 60). When the heart rate becomes too slow, the cardiac output decreases, and the patient's blood pressure drops. Oxygen delivery to the tissues may also be compromised. This can cause serious signs and symptoms, such as chest pain and loss of consciousness.

How might damage to the heart's conduction system affect cardiac output and tissue perfusion?

Figure 15-3 gives an algorithm for the treatment of bradycardia. The drugs discussed in the algorithm and the ones to follow will be individually discussed in the later part of this chapter. Again, most were also covered in Chapters 9 and 10.

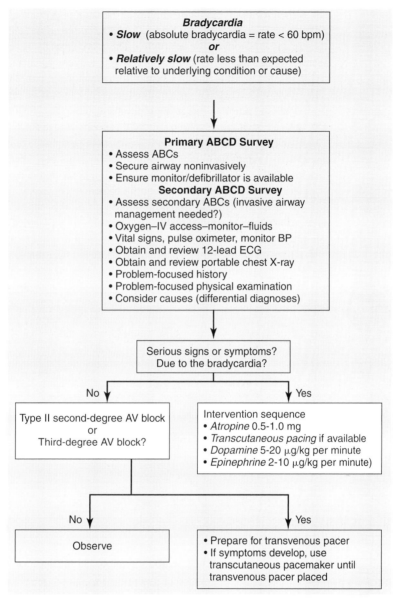

Figure 15-3 Bradycardia Algorithm (with the patient not in cardiac arrest)
Source: Used with permission of the American Heart Association, Dallas, Texas.

Tachycardia

Tachycardia (fast heart) is when the heart rate increases above 100 beats per minute. The increased heart rate increases the cardiac output and blood pressure. In sinus tachycardia, the heart rate ranges between 100 and less than 130. This is usually an appropriate physiologic response to stress, fever, exercise, hypovolemia, or hypoxemia. Heart rates faster than 130 are usually due to some type of pathologic arrhythmia, such as another pacemaker or pacemakers that override the SA node, an electrical short circuit called reentry, or they may be due to increased irritability in the myocardial cells.

Fast heart rates may actually compromise the heart's function. The heart may not get enough oxygen or the ventricles may not have enough time to fill, and the cardiac output and blood pressure begin to drop. Heart rates that are extremely fast (greater than 150) are usually so compromising that they require direct current countershock.

When the tachycardia originates in the atria or AV node, the QRS complexes are usually narrow, as on the normal EKG. These are called supraventricular tachycardias, because they originate "above" the ventricles. There are actually several different supraventricular tachycardias with narrow complexes (atrial tachycardia, atrial fibrillation, and atrial flutter, to name a few), but it is not critical to initially differentiate them in the emergency setting. They are grouped together as supraventricular tachycardias, and their treatment is the same.

When the impulses originate *in* the ventricles, the QRS complexes take on a wide, tall, and bizarre appearance. When we see these very unusual QRS complexes on the EKG, we can *usually* assume that they are originating from the ventricles. There are some important exceptions to this rule, but we will not get into that now. Ventricular tachycardia is a very serious rhythm, because some patients with it do not have a pulse. It is important to assess the patient's pulse quickly and treat the patient accordingly.

Patients with either tachycardia should be quickly evaluated to determine whether they are stable or having serious signs and symptoms, and whether it is a ventricular or supraventricular rhythm. If the patient is stable, then they would be treated pharmacologically. Unstable patients need electrical countershock (defibrillation or cardioversion). Figures 15-4a and b shows the atrial and ventricular tachycardia, respectively.

Stop and Review: How can you tell where a tachycardia is originating?

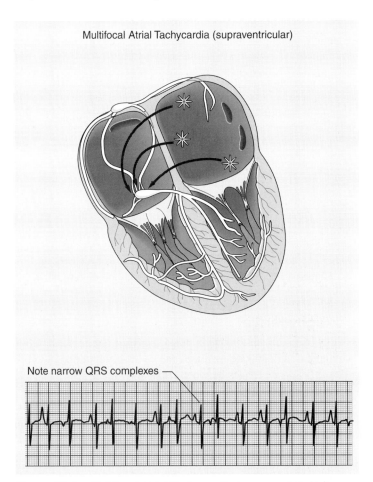

Figure 15-4a Multifocal Atrial Tachycardia (supraventricular)

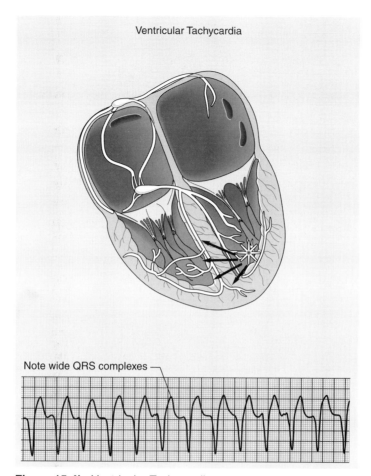

Figure 15-4b Ventricular Tachycardia

Figure 15-5 is the narrow-complex tachycardia algorithm. It may seem complicated, but the several branches are needed, owing to the various types of tachyarrythmias that can exist. Identification of the type of tachycardia and the amount of compromise in heart function it causes is key to following the correct pathway for treatment. While the scope of this textbook does not allow us to cover all aspects of the algorithms, it does show where and when the medications are indicated.

Ventricular Fibrillation

Ventricular fibrillation occurs when there are multiple rapid ventricular pacemakers firing. The patient's heart will not be contracting. Instead, the ventricles quiver, or fibrillate. This is a very serious rhythm, in which the patient never has a pulse. The treatment for ventricular tachycardia and ventricular fibrillation are exactly the same. CPR must be initiated while defibrillation and appropriate drug therapy are provided. Please see Figure 15-6, which illustrates ventricular fibrillation, and Figure 15-7 (on p. 298), which shows the ventricular fibrillation algorithm.

What is the relationship between a fibrillating heart and cardiac output? What is the main treatment for fibrillation?

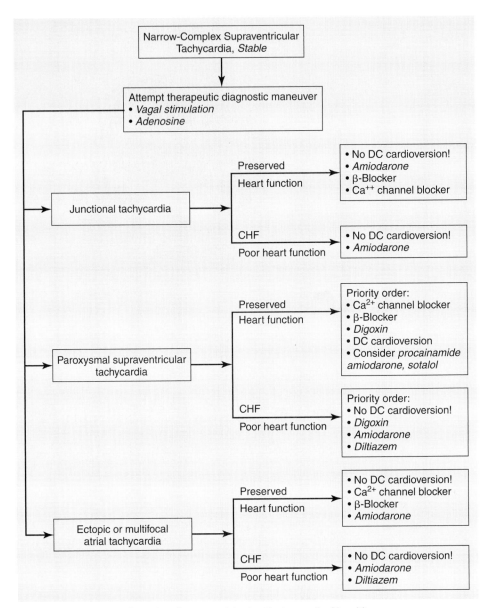

Figure 15-5 Narrow-Complex Supraventricular Tachycardia Algorithm
Source: Used with permission of the American Heart Association, Dallas, Texas.

Asystole

Asystole means without rhythm. The heart is electrically silent. Of course the patient is pulseless, and CPR needs to be initiated. Epinephrine and atropine are the key drugs in the treatment of asystole. In addition, an artificial pacemaker should be considered, to provide the electrical stimulation needed to initiate depolarization of the heart.

Pulseless Electrical Activity (PEA)

PEA is the presence of some type of electrical activity (other than ventricular tachycardia or ventricular fibrillation) although the patient has no pulse. Treatment of this condition requires rapid assessment to determine the cause of the pulselessness. The patient can be supported with CPR and some general pharmacological agents, but ultimately, successful resuscitation will depend on correcting the underlying problem. Causes include severe

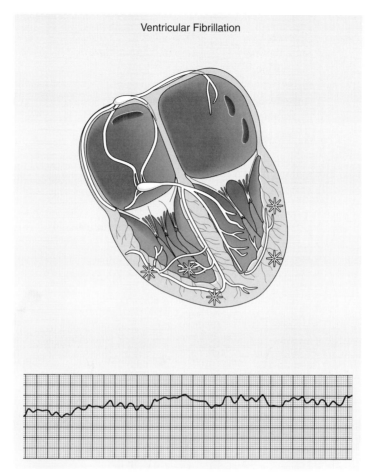

Figure 15-6 Ventricular Fibrillation

hypovolemia, tension pneumothorax, cardiac tamponade, hypoxia, hypothermia, massive pulmonary embolism, some types of drug overdose, hyperkalemia, acidosis, and massive acute myocardial infarction. Epinephrine is the key drug administered to treat PEA; however, atropine may be given if there is bradycardia.

Asystole and PEA both do not have a pulse. What is the difference in recognition and treatment?

PHARMACOLOGIC AGENTS FOR ADVANCED LIFE SUPPORT

Categories of ACLS Drugs

The drugs used in advanced cardiac life support are divided into two groups. The drugs in the Pharmacology I category are used in the algorithms for full cardiac arrest. These include:

oxygen
epinephrine
atropine

the antiarrhythmic agents:

lidocaine	procainamide
amiodarone	verapamil and diltiazem
adenosine	

miscellaneous

magnesium	sodium bicarbonate
morphine	calcium chloride

The Pharmacology II category includes agents used to treat acute myocardial infarction and its complications: hypertension, hypotension, and cardiogenic shock. Cardiogenic shock is described as a systolic BP below 80–90 mm Hg, or a drop of 70 mm Hg or more.

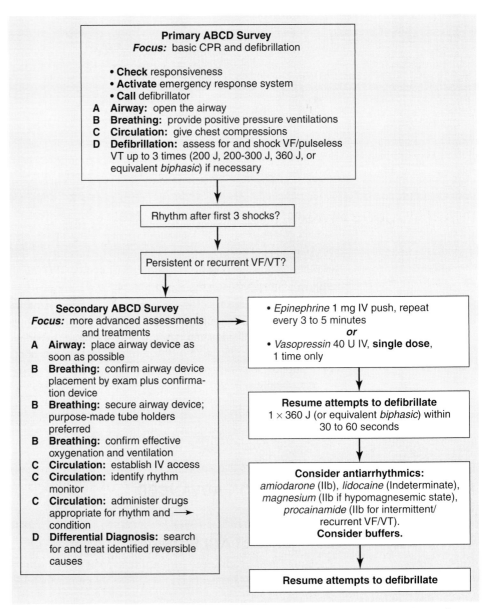

Figure 15-7 Algorithm for Ventricular Fibrillation and Pulseless Venricular Tachycardia
Source: Used with permission of the American Heart Association, Dallas, Texas.

Shock results in poor tissue perfusion, as evidenced by oliguria, decreased mental status or loss of consciousness, and pulmonary congestion.

Category II agents include:

inotropic vasoactive agents (Chapters 9 and 10):
    epinephrine   norepinephrine
    dopamine   dobutamine
    isoproterenol   amrinone
    digoxin
vasodilators (Chapter 10):
    sodium nitroprusside
    nitroglycerin
beta blockers (Chapters 9 and 10):
    propranolol   metoprolol
    atenolol   esmolol
diuretics (Chapters 9 and 10):
    furosemide
thrombolytics (Chapter 10):
    plasminogen activator complex
    streptokinase
    tissue plasminogen activator (TPA)

PHARMACOLOGY I AGENTS

Oxygen

Oxygen is a key component in resuscitation and emergency cardiac care, yet it is frequently taken for granted or overlooked as a drug. The atmosphere that we breathe contains 21% oxygen. This is enough to maintain a partial pressure in the blood (PaO_2) of 80–100 mm Hg. In healthy individuals, this keeps the red blood cells saturated with oxygen. During mouth-to-mouth or mouth-to-mask ventilation, the breath exhaled by the rescuer to the victim contains only 16% to 17% oxygen. In addition, the cardiac output of the victim during CPR is only about 25% to 30% of normal. Low perfusion makes it necessary for the body to extract much more oxygen than usual from the blood. In turn, the venous blood will be extremely depleted of oxygen, and 21% oxygen may not be enough to resaturate the blood of the cardiac arrest victim. Administering 100% oxygen as quickly as possible is critical in preventing organ damage in the cardiac arrest victim.

Indications. Oxygen is indicated for all patients with acute chest pain due to cardiac **ischemia,** hypoxemia of any cause, and victims of cardiac arrest.

Dosage. Oxygen delivery devices for spontaneously breathing patients are in Chapter 12, Therapeutic Medical Gases. Patients who are not breathing on their own must have their breathing assisted with positive pressure ventilation or with a manual resuscitator bag and 100% oxygen.

Precautions. Problems associated with the overuse of oxygen depend on the concentration and the duration of exposure. This should never be a concern during short-term exposure to oxygen during resuscitation.

Epinephrine

Epinephrine is a natural catecholamine with both α and β effects. It plays a critical role in cardiac arrest. In fact, if you look at the algorithms for cardiac arrest, you will see that it is the first drug administered in all of them. The reason is that the primary beneficial effect is to produce peripheral vasoconstriction, which leads to improved myocardial and cerebral perfusion. This is important because, as we said before, cardiac output is low during CPR.

Epinephrine appears to improve cerebral blood flow more than other adrenergic agents. It also makes the heart more susceptible to direct countershock, improving the likelihood of converting ventricular fibrillation and ventricular tachycardia to rhythms with spontaneous circulation. Epinephrine increases the rate and force of myocardial contraction. This tends to increase the oxygen consumption of the heart, which could increase ischemia of the myocardial tissue. During cardiac arrest, it is felt that the beneficial effects of epinephrine outweigh any potential risk of cardiac ischemia.

Indications. Indications include cardiac arrest of any kind (ventricular fibrillation, pulseless ventricular tachycardia, pulseless electrical activity, and asystole). It can also be considered for treatment of profoundly symptomatic bradycardia.

Dosage. The standard dose of epinephrine is 1 mg (not based on body weight) given intravenously every 3 to 5 minutes. When given to improve the blood pressure in patients who are not in cardiac arrest, the dose is 1.0 μg/min, titrated to achieve the desired blood pressure.

Precautions. Epinephrine should not be mixed in alkaline solutions (including sodium bicarbonate). Its positive inotropic and chronotropic effects can increase myocardial ischemia. Large doses in patients who are not in cardiac arrest can cause hypertension. It can also cause ventricular ectopy, especially in patients receiving digitalis.

Atropine

Atropine sulfate is a parasympatholytic drug. Patients with advanced heart disease frequently have increased parasympathetic tone. As you may recall, one of the effects of the parasympathetic nervous system is to slow the heart rate, and the result can be bradycardia or even asystole. Atropine increases the heart rate by increasing the automaticity of the sinus node and conduction through the AV node.

Indications. Atropine is indicated for treatment of symptomatic bradycardia and relative bradycardia. Symptomatic bradycardia is a slow heart rate accompanied by serious signs and symptoms such as chest pain, shortness of breath, decreased level of consciousness, very low blood pressure, and acute congestive heart failure. Relative bradycardia is the term used for a heart rate in the "normal range" of 60–100 when a tachycardia would be more appropriate for the patient's condition. For example, tachycardia is a normal physiologic response to hypotension. A patient with a blood pressure of 80/40 and a heart rate of 70 is not "normal;" the heart rate needs to be faster to maintain adequate circulation.

Dosage. For patients who have symptomatic bradycardia but still have a pulse, .5 to 1.0 mg of atropine is administered IV. The dose can be repeated at 5 minute intervals until the patient's heart rate is up to 60 beats per minute or greater, or until the signs and symptoms subside. The total dose should not exceed 2–3 mg (.03–.04 mg/kg). If the bradycardia is recurrent, an electrical pacemaker may be used to keep the heart rate up.

For patients in cardiac arrest due to bradycardia and asystole, 1 mg of atropine is administered by IV. The dose can be repeated in 3–5 min up to a maximum of 3 mg (.04 mg/kg).

Precautions. Particularly in the setting of cardiac arrest, hazards may seem to be of little consequence, but there are still a few things to keep in mind when administering atropine. Tachycardia may occur, and this tends to increase myocardial oxygen consumption, increasing incidence of ischemia and risk of myocardial infarction. Ventricular tachycardia and fibrillation have also occurred. Excessive doses of atropine can cause an anticholinergic syndrome that may include delirium, tachycardia, coma, flushed hot skin, ataxia, and blurred vision. Finally, doses of less than .5 mg can produce paradoxical worsening of bradycardia.

Lidocaine (Xylocaine)

Lidocaine is said to decrease automaticity, increase the fibrillation threshold, and decrease the defibrillation threshold. This means that it makes the heart more resistant to fibrillation and more responsive to defibrillation. Lidocaine does not usually affect myocardial contractility, blood pressure, or atrial arrhythmias.

Indications. Lidocaine has long been considered the gold standard in antiarrhythmics, and although it is still considered to be clinically useful, it is no longer the first-line antiarrhythmic drug used to treat ventricular tachycardia and ventricular fibrillation. Premature ventricular contractions and wide complex PSVT may also be treated with lidocaine.

Dosage. For ventricular fibrillation and pulseless ventricular tachycardia that has not responded to epinephrine and defibrillation, the initial lidocaine dose is 1.0 to 1.5 mg/kg. When ventricular fibrillation persists after defibrillation and administration of epinephrine, the 1.5 mg/kg dose is recommended. If necessary, .5 to 1.5 mg/kg of lidocaine can be given every 3 to 5 minutes until the total loading dose of 3 mg/kg has been reached. Patients in cardiac arrest are given lidocaine by **bolus.** After the return of a spontaneous pulse, an **IV infusion** can be started at a rate of 2.0 to 4.0 mg/kg.

Precautions. Excessive doses and prolonged administration of lidocaine can result in toxicity. The dosage may need to be reduced in patients over 70, those with hepatic dysfunction, and those with low cardiac output states. Signs of toxicity include slurred speech, drowsiness, disorientation, decreased hearing ability, paresthesia, and muscle twitching. The most severe toxicity can cause grand mal seizures.

Amiodarone

Amiodarone is an antiarrhythmic that is useful in treating both atrial and ventricular tachycardias and for ventricular fibrillation. Its actions are complex. It effects sodium, potassium, and calcium channels. It also has α- and β-adrenergic blocking properties. Its ability to block the AV node makes it useful in the treatment of supraventricular tachycardias. Its effectiveness is comparable to procainamide and magnesium. Other AV nodal blocking agents include sotalol, propafenone, and flecainide.

Indications. Amiodarone is indicated for supraventricular tachycardia, ventricular tachycardia, ventricular tachycardia without a pulse, and ventricular fibrillation. It is not indicated for torsade de pointes (a specific sub type of ventricular tachycardia that is treated with magnesium sulfate).

Dosage. 150 mg of amiodarone is given over 10 minutes, followed by a 1 mg/min infusion for 6 hours and then .5 mg/min. Supplementary infusions at the higher dose can be repeated if necessary for recurrance of the arrhythmia, but the maximum recommended daily dose is 2 grams.

Precautions. Major adverse effects are hypotension and bradycardia, which can be prevented by slowing the rate of drug infusion and giving fluid, vasopressor, or chronotropic agents.

Procainamide (Pronestyl)

Procainamide suppresses a variety of ectopic arrhythmias. It is particularly useful for ventricular ectopy because it decreases automaticity in the ventricular muscle and Purkinje fibers. This slows intraventricular conduction. It can be effective even when lidocaine has failed to suppress ventricular ectopic rhythms. It has also been shown to be useful in some types of supraventricular rhythms.

Indications

- Procainamide is indicated for suppressing PVCs and ventricular tachycardia with a pulse.
- It is acceptable and probably helpful in ventricular fibrillation and pulseless ventricular tachycardia when lidocaine and bretyllium have failed. However, it is rarely used in this instance, because it takes a long time to administer (rapid infusion exacerbates hypotension).
- Procainamide can also be used to treat wide-complex supraventricular tachycardias (though not as a first-line drug).

Dosage. For PVCs and V-tach, the dose is 20–30 mg/min by infusion, until:

- the rhythm is suppressed
- hypotension develops
- the QRS complex widens by 50% of its original width
- 17 mg/kg has been administered

The maintenance dose is an IV infusion of 1–4 mg/min.

Precautions. The most common problem with procainamide is that it can cause hypotension, especially if given too rapidly, or if blood levels get too high. When the QRS widens by more than 50%, it can cause heart blocks or even cardiac arrest. The patient needs to be carefully monitored, and blood levels of the drug should be monitored in patients receiving continuous infusions and those with cardiac or renal failure.

Magnesium Sulfate

Magnesium plays a role in several important enzymatic reactions, such as the sodium–potassium ATPase pump, and it is a physiologic calcium-channel blocker. Low magnesium increases the incidence of cardiac arrhythmias and sudden cardiac death.

Indications. Magnesium is the drug of choice for the treatment of torsades de pointes. IV magnesium decreases the complication of arrhythmias following acute MI.

Dosage. For ventricular tachycardia, the dose is 1–2 g of magnesium sulfate (2–4 ml of 50% solution, diluted in 10 ml of 5% dextrose solution given intravenously over 1–2 minutes). In ventricular fibrillation, the same dose is pushed in more rapidly (IV push).

For torsades de pointes, the dose is higher (up to 5–10 g have been used with success), but the optimal dose has not been clearly established by clinical research.

Precautions. When magnesium is given too fast to patients who have a pulse, hypotension and even asystole can occur. However, actual toxicity is rare.

℞ Sodium Bicarbonate

Sodium bicarbonate is a buffer (base) that combines with acid (in effect neutralizing the acid). In the process, carbon dioxide and water are produced, and of course the carbon dioxide is excreted by the lungs. Sodium bicarbonate is indicated in situations where there has been a bicarbonate-responsive metabolic acidosis prior to arrest, hyperkalemia, or some drug overdoses.

During CPR, cardiac compressions produce only about 25% to 30% of the normal cardiac output. This low perfusion may mean that insufficient amounts of oxygen are delivered to the tissues. This results in anaerobic metabolism and production of lactic acid. The decreased blood flow to the lungs also decreases carbon dioxide excretion by the lungs, further contributing to the acidosis. Since administration of sodium bicarbonate increases the amount of CO_2 in the blood and CO_2 removal is compromised, bicarbonate must be used very judiciously during cardiac arrest. Increased amounts of carbon dioxide in the blood also lower the pH of the blood, and this leads to a respiratory acidosis.

Indications. Sodium bicarbonate is primarily indicated when the patient was known to have metabolic acidosis prior to the cardiac arrest, or when the patient has been in cardiac arrest for a prolonged period of time. It is also helpful when there is hyperkalemia or tricyclic antidepressant or phenobarbital overdose, and as indicated by the treatment algorithms, it should follow defibrillation, CPR, intubation, and more than one dose of epinephrine.

Dosage. 1 mEq/kg can be given IV bolus as an initial dose, followed by half of this dose every 10 min. Administration of bicarbonate should be guided by arterial blood gas analysis to monitor the patient's acid–base status. Inducing alkalosis should always be avoided.

Precautions. Sodium bicarbonate rapidly combines with acid to produce carbon dioxide, so good ventilation is essential to eliminate the carbon dioxide, or the patient will remain acidotic because of the excess carbon dioxide. Administration of bicarbonate can cause alkalosis, increased serum sodium, and hyperosmolality. It also compromises oxygen release at the tissues, which further endangers survival.

CALCIUM-CHANNEL BLOCKERS

Calcium-channel blockers are drugs that inhibit the slow-channel activity of the cardiac and vascular smooth muscle. The slow channels, as you may recall, allow for the influx of calcium and sodium ions. This results in several effects that can be clinically useful, and as you will see, the effects of the following two calcium-channel blockers are somewhat different from each other. Diltiazem has fewer hemodynamic effects than verapamil, but they both dilate coronary arteries and slow conduction through the AV node, which makes them useful in terminating supraventricular tachycardias that are due to reentry pathways at the AV node. They also slow the ventricular response rate in atrial fibrillation.

Verapamil (Calan, Isoptin)

Verapamil has potent negative chronotropic and negative inotropic effects. It is highly effective for the treatment and prevention of supraventricular tachycardias. Slowing the flux of calcium and sodium ions by way of the slow channels decreases the rate and force of contraction. This results in reduced myocardial oxygen consumption and less ischemia. The drug's negative inotropic effect would tend to reduce the patient's stroke volume and cardiac output, but it is counterbalanced by a concurrent reduction in systemic vascular resistance secondary to vasodilation.

Indications. Verapamil is indicated in paroxysmal supraventricular tachycardia, atrial fibrillation, and atrial flutter when the ventricular rate is too fast.

Dosage. Verapamil dose is 2.5 to 5.0 mg IV bolus, given over 1 to 2 minutes. The peak effect is achieved within 3 to 5 minutes of the bolus injection. If this dose is not adequate, a second dose of 5 to 10 mg can be given 15 to 30 minutes after the initial dose, or a 5-mg bolus can be given every 15 minutes until the desired response is achieved. The total dose should not exceed 30 mg.

Precautions. A transient decrease in blood pressure due to vasodilation should be expected, particularly in patients with severe left ventricular dysfunction. Pretreatment with calcium can help prevent this problem. Verapamil should be avoided or used with great caution in patients with tachycardia that is due to Wolf–Parkinson–White syndrome, as their heart rate may actually speed up and cause ventricular fibrillation. Verapamil is not effective for most types of ventricular tachycardia, and it may induce severe hypotension and ventricular fibrillation.

Diltiazem (Cardizem)

Diltiazem has potent negative chronotropic effects, with only mild negative inotropic action. It produces less mycordial depression than verapamil, particularly in patients with left ventricular dysfunction. It is highly effective in controlling the ventricular response rate in patients with atrial fibrillation.

Dose. The initial bolus dose is .25 mg/kg (about 20 mg for the average-sized patient), which can be followed with an IV infusion that is titrated to achieve the desired rate.

Precautions. Although it is less likely to occur with diltiazem than with verapamil, hypotension can still occur, and pretreatment with calcium should be considered. The use of IV beta blockers with IV calcium-channel blockers (verapamil or diltiazem) is contraindicated, because their hemodynamic effects may be synergistic. Even if the beta blockers are given orally, calcium-channel blockers should only be used with great caution.

Adenosine

Adenosine has taken the place of verapamil as the drug of choice for treating supraventricular tachycardia. It also slows conduction through the AV node and interrupts reentry pathways at the AV node. It can convert PSVT (including that associated with Wolff–Parkinson–White syndrome) to a normal sinus rhythm. Adenosine will not terminate atrial fibrillation, atrial flutter, or ventricular tachycardia, because they are caused by the rapid firing of atrial ectopic foci rather than a reentry mechanism. There are also some atrial tachycardias that are not due to reentry, so adenosine will not convert them but may produce a transient AV block. However, adenosine is still indicated, because the response to adenosine may help to clarify the diagnosis. Adenosine has a very short duration of action, owing to rapid uptake by the red blood cells. It has a half-life of only 10 seconds.

Dosage. The initial dose is usually a 6-mg bolus given rapidly over 1 to 3 seconds. It is common for a long pause to occur (up to 15 seconds) in the heart rhythm after administration of adenosine. Be careful—this can be very scary and your own heart may want to skip a beat, too! A second dose of 12 mg can be given if there has been no response within 1 to 2 minutes after the first dose.

Precautions. Side effects of adenosine are quite common, but they usually only last 1 or 2 minutes. They include flushing, dyspnea, and chest pain. Sinus bradycardia and ventricular ectopy are also common. Also, it should be noted that therapeutic levels of methylxanthines block the action of adenosine by blocking its receptors.

β-ADRENERGIC BLOCKERS

When a patient has an acute myocardial infarction, their body responds to the stress by releasing a lot of endogenous catecholamines. You should recall that this increases the patient's heart rate and force of contraction, which increases blood pressure and increases the heart's demand for oxygen. The result can be more ischemia and injury to the heart muscle. Beta blockers inhibit the action of circulating catecholamines by blocking the adrenergic receptor sites. This results in decreased heart rate and decreased contractility, decreased blood pressure, and reduced myocardial oxygen consumption. It may also prevent recurrent episodes of ventricular tachycardia and fibrillation when these arrhythmias are caused by myocardial ischemia. In emergency situations, rapid action is critical, so once again using the IV preparations of these drugs is indicated. This would include atenolol (Tenormin), metoprolol (Lopressor), propanolol (Inderal), and esmolol.

The effects of these agents vary slightly depending on their degree of β_1 and β_2 specificity. Propranolol is nonspecific; it blocks both β_1 and β_2 receptors, which results in decreased heart rate, decreased force of contraction, and bronchospasm. Metoprolol, atenolol, and esmolol are β_1 specific at low doses but may still cause bronchoconstriction when used at higher doses.

Propanolol and metoprolol sustain their effects for 6 to 8 hours following IV administration. Esmolol is β_1 selective and has a short duration (15 to 20 minutes), which makes it safer.

Indications. In emergency cardiac care, beta blockers are indicated for control of recurrent ventricular tachycardia, recurrent ventricular fibrillation, and supraventricular tachycardias that are refractory to other therapies. Thes drugs are most effective when these arrhythmias are being caused by β-adrenergic stimulation or myocardial ischemia.

Dosing and Precautions. Each of the drugs mentioned in this category has its own specific loading dose, interval for repeat dose, and IV drip rate. There are many good references for these specifics, including the ACLS manual, but for our purposes, it is important to simply note that any of these agents can precipitate hypotension, congestive heart failure (CHF), and/or bronchospasm. Administering beta blockers is particularly hazardous when cardiac function is already depressed. Beta blockers are contraindicated in patients with bradycardia and AV heart blocks. When it does occur, CHF can be managed with diuretics and vasodilators, and of course bronchospasm would require treatment with bronchodilators. As was mentioned before, adverse effects increase when beta blockers are combined with calcium-channel blockers, antihypertensive agents, and antiarrhythmic agents.

LEARNING HINT

Remember the Learning Hint in Chapter 5 that you have 1 heart and 2 lungs, corresponding to β_1 effects in the heart and β_2 effects in the lungs? A nonselective beta-blocking agent may also block the β_2 receptors in the lungs, causing bronchoconstriction in susceptible individuals.

POSITIVE INOTROPIC DRUGS

Digoxin

Positive inotropic drugs increase the force of contraction of the heart. This in turn increases cardiac output, blood pressure, and tissue perfusion. They depress the sodium pump, which increases intracellular sodium and calcium. Calcium increases the force of the heart's contraction. There is also a decrease in heart rate and decreased conduction through the AV node. The decrease in heart rate and the slower conduction are beneficial, because they allow for more ventricular filling time, coupled with a more efficient ventricular contraction.

Digoxin has little to contribute to the management of acute heart failure but has proven to be very useful in the chronic treatment of congestive heart failure (CHF). It is also useful as an antiarrhythmic for atrial fibrillation or flutter.

Amrinone

Amrinone is a phosphodiesterase inhibitor. It has a positive inotropic effect and a vasodilating effect, which decreases afterload. Together, these effects result in an increased cardiac output. It is also used in the treatment of CHF.

Epinephrine

This was discussed previously in this chapter and falls in both Pharmacology I and Pharmacology II classifications.

Isoproterenol

Isoproterenol has almost pure β-adrenergic activity. It has potent β_1 effects that increase heart rate and force of contraction (positive chronotrope and inotrope). Isoproterenol certainly can increase cardiac output despite a decrease in blood pressure, owing to vasodilation. However, it does this at the expense of significantly increased oxygen consumption. It can be used for temporary control of symptomatic bradycardia, but atropine and use of artificial pacemakers are preferred. The major indication is for treatment of bradycardia in patients with denervated, transplanted hearts.

Dopamine

Dopamine is a chemical precursor of norepinephrine. Its effects are dose dependant. Low doses (1–2 μg/kg per min) stimulate the dopaminergic receptors to produce cerebral, renal, and mesenteric vasodilation, but overall venous tone is increased because of concurrent α-adrenergic effect. This dose is sometimes used to increase renal perfusion and urine output.

When administered at 2 to 10 μg/kg per min, dopamine stimulates the β_1 and α receptors. The main effect is to increase cardiac output. At doses of greater than 10 μg/kg per min, dopamine's α-adrenergic effect predominates. There is marked vasoconstriction (arterial and venous), which increases preload, afterload, and blood pressure. This effect may be useful when there is hypotension or shock without hypovolemia. If the dose of dopamine exceeds 20 μg/kg per min, it produces a potent α-adrenergic effect and increases systemic vascular resistance, similar to norepinephrine.

Explain why dopamine is considered a dosage-dependent cardiovascular medication.

Dobutamine (Dobutrex)

This is a synthetic catecholamine that stimulates β_1 receptors. It has a strong positive inotropic effect, with less chronotropic effect than dopamine. It does not increase peripheral vascular resistance and renal vasoconstriction, as dopamine does. Dopamine and dobutamine are often used together in the treatment of cardiogenic shock. It is used in conjunction with nitroprusside to improve cardiac output and decrease afterload.

www.prenhall.com/colbert

ACLS standards are updated regularly, so please visit the Web for changes in currently administered drugs as well as new ones that may be added as new research becomes available.

REVIEW QUESTIONS

1. Which of the following would be indicated for any patient who is in cardiac arrest?
   (a) atropine
   (b) dopamine
   (c) amrinone
   (d) epinephrine

2. A patient is experiencing chest pain that radiates down his left arm. Which of the following would you do first?
   (a) administer oxygen by nasal cannula
   (b) give a bolus of lidocaine
   (c) start an infusion of lidocaine
   (d) defibrillate

3. In which of the following heart rhythms would the patient be most likely to have a pulse?
   (a) ventricular fibrillation
   (b) atrial tachycardia
   (c) atrial fibrillation
   (d) asystole

4. Which of the following are precautions associated with amiodarone?
   (a) hypotension and bradycardia
   (b) nausea and vomiting
   (c) vasoconstriction
   (d) AV node block

5. Magnesium sulfate would best be used to treat:
   (a) ventricular tachycardia
   (b) atrial tachycardia

   (c) ventricular fibrillation
   (d) pulseless electrical activity

6. What percentage of oxygen should be administered to a victim in cardiac arrest?
   (a) 16% to 17%
   (b) 21%
   (c) 25% to 30%
   (d) 100%

7. Which of the following is indicated for a patient in ventricular tachycardia who is seriously hypotensive and having chest pain?
   (a) sodium bicarbonate
   (b) amiodarone
   (c) epinephrine
   (d) defibrillation

8. Describe how medications can be given to a cardiac arrest victim when no IV can be established.

9. List three antiarrhythmic drugs that could be used to treat a patient in ventricular tachycardia.

10. Explain why it may be hazardous to administer epinephrine to a bradycardic patient who is having an acute myocardial infarction. What drug would you suggest?

CASE STUDY

A 67-year-old female is brought to the emergency department by her husband. She is complaining of chest pain that radiates to her left arm and jaw, and she is short of breath. She is being placed on a heart monitor and a nurse is getting set up to start her on IV. What else needs to be done immediately?

Ten minutes later the patient becomes bradycardic. Her heart rate is 35 and her blood pressure is 40/0. What drug should be administered?

What dose?

An hour later, her heart rate is 78 and her blood pressure is 120/80, but she is exhibiting frequent PVCs (premature ventricular contractions). What would you now recommend?

GLOSSARY

acute myocardial infarction   new or recent onset of a cardiac event that leads to the death of myocardial tissue; this process is irreversible.

arrhythmia   technically an absence of rhythm, but the term is also used to refer to an abnormal rhythm.

automaticity   characteristic of cardiac cells that allows them to spontaneously depolarize without innervation from the central nervous system.

bolus   a large dose of medication that is usually pushed manually into an IV for rapid effect.

cardiac arrest   absence of breathing and pulse.

defibrillate   to apply direct countershock to the heart in order to depolarize the myocardial cells simultaneously.

infusion   medication or fluid that is given gradually and continuously into an IV by an infusion pump, often used to maintain the effect achieved by bolus administration of the drug.

ischemia   a decrease in perfusion to an organ or body part that may result in pain and organ dysfunction.

www.prenhall.com/colbert

Use the address above to access the free, interactive Companion Web site created specifically for this textbook. Enhance your studying by viewing videos and animations, answering practice quiz questions, and reviewing an audio glossary and much more related to Chapter 15.

References

CHAPTER 1

Benet LZ, Kroetz DL, Sheiner LB. Pharmacokinetics: The dynamics of drug absorption, distribution, and elimination. In: Goodman and Gilman's *The Pharmacological Basis of Therapeutics*, 9th ed. Hardman JG, et al. (editors). McGraw-Hill, 1996.

Committee on Drugs, American Academy of Pediatrics. The transfer of drugs and other chemicals into human milk. *Pediatrics* 1994;93:137–150.

deShazo RD, Kemp SF. Allergic reactions to drugs and biologic agents. *JAMA* 1997;278:1895–1906.

Dunn TL, Gerber MJ, Shen AS, et al. The effect of topical ophthalmic instillation of timolol and betaxolol on lung function in asthmatic subjects. *Am Rev Respir Dis* 1986;133:264–268.

Eisenberg DM. Advising patients who seek alternate medical therapies. *Ann Intern Med* 1997;127:61–69.

Erstad BL. Oxygen transport goals in the resuscitation of critically ill patients. *Ann Pharmacother* 1994;28:1273–1284.

Fingerhut LA, Cox CS. Poisoning mortality. *Public Health Rep* 1998;113:218–233.

Fisher HK. Drug-induced asthma syndromes. In: Weiss EB, Segal MS, Stein M, eds. *Bronchial Asthma: Mechanisms and Therapeutics.* 2nd ed. Boston: Little, Brown, 1985;938–949.

Leape LL. Error in medicine. *JAMA* 1994;272:1851–1857.

Lee WM. Drug-induced hepatotoxicity. *N Engl J Med* 1995;333:1118–1127.

Parker BM, Cusack BJ, Vestal RE. Pharmacokinetic optimisation of drug therapy in elderly patients. *Drugs Aging* 1995;7:10–18.

Shulman SR, Hewitt P, Manocchia M. Studies and inquiries into the FDA regulatory process: A historical review. *DIJ* 1995;29:385–413.

Sivan SK, Bennett WM. Drug dosing guidelines in patients with renal failure. *West J Med* 1992;156:633–638.

Suresh Babu K, Salvi S. Aspirin and Asthma. *Chest* 2000;118(5):1470–1476.

Uchegbu IF, Florence AT. Adverse drug events related to dosage forms and delivery systems. *Drug Saf* 1996;14:39–67.

Young LR, Wurtzbacher JD, Blankenship CA. Adverse drug reactions: A review for healthcare practitioners. *Am J Managed Care* 1997;3:1884–1906.

CHAPTER 2

Doucette L. *Basic Mathematics for the Health-Related Professions.* Philadelphia: W. B. Saunders Company, 2000.

Meyer R. *Master Guide for Passing Respiratory Care Credentialing Exams,* 4th ed. New Jersey: Prentice Hall, 2000.

CHAPTER 3

Aquilonius S-M, Hartvig P. Clinical pharmacology of cholinesterase inhibitors. *Clin Pharmacokinet* 1986;11:236.

Barnes PJ, Minette P, Maclagan J. Muscarinic receptor subtypes in airways. *Trends Pharmacol Sci* 1988;9:412.

Goyal RK. Muscarinic receptor subtypes. Physiology and clinical implications. *N Engl J Med* 1989;321:1022.

Goyal RK, Hirano I. The enteric nervous system. *N Engl J Med* 1996;334:1106.

Insel PA. Seminars in medicine of the Beth Israel Hospital, Boston. Adrenergic receptors: Evolving concepts and clinical implications. *N Engl J Med* 1996;334:580.

Ruffolo RR Jr, et al. Pharmacologic and therapeutic applications of α_2-adrenoceptor subtypes. *Annu Rev Pharmacol Toxicol* 1993;32:243.

CHAPTER 4

British Thoracic Society. Current best practices for nebulizer treatment. *Thorax* 1997;52(suppl 2):S1–S106.

Consensus Statement: Aerosols and delivery devices. *Respir Care* 2000;45:589–596.

Dolvich M. Influence of inspiratory flow rate, particle size, and airway caliber on aerosolized drug delivery to the lung. *Respir Care* 2000;45:597–608.

Fink J. Metered-dose inhalers, dry powder inhalers, and transitions. *Respir Care* 2000;45:623–635.

Hess D. Nebulizers: Principles and performance. *Respir Care* 2000;45:609–622.

Suarez S, Hickey A. Drug properties affecting aerosol behavior. *Respir Care* 2000;45:652–666.

CHAPTER 5

Barnes PJ. Theophylline in the management of asthma: Time for a reappraisal? *Eur Respir J* 1994;7:579–591.

Kelly HW, Murphy S. Beta-adrenergic agonists for acute, severe asthma. *Ann Pharmacother* 1992;26:81–91.

Mullen M, Mullen B, Carey M. The association between β-agonist use and death from asthma: A meta-analytic integration of case-control studies. *JAMA* 1993;270:1842–1845.

Nelson HS. β-Adrenergic bronchodilators. *N Engl J Med* 1995;333:499–506

CHAPTER 6

Anzueto A, Jubran A, Ohar JA, et al. Effects of aerosolized surfactant in patients with stable chronic bronchitis. *JAMA* 1997;278:1426–1481.

Jobe AH. Pulmonary surfactant therapy. *N Engl J Med* 1993;328:861–868.

Kresch MJ, Lin WH, Thrall RS. Surfactant replacement therapy. *Thorax* 1996;51:1137–1154.

MacIntyre N. Aerosolized medications for altering lung surface active properties. *Respir Care* 2000;45:676–683.

Pramanik AK, Holtzman RB, Merritt TA. Surfactant replacement therapy for pulmonary diseases. *Pediatr Clin North Am* 1993;40:913–936.

Watling SM, Yanos J. Acute respiratory distress syndrome. *Ann Pharmacother* 1995;29:1002–1009.

CHAPTER 7

Baker JR Jr, Zylke JW, eds. Primer on allergic and immunologic diseases-4th ed. *JAMA* 1997;278:1804–1814, 1815–1822, 1842–1848, 1881–1887.

Ballow M, Nelson R. Immunopharmacology: Immunomodulation and immunotherapy. *JAMA* 1997;278(22):2008–2017.

Baranuik JN. Pathogenesis of allergic rhinitis. *J Allergy Clin Immunol* 1997;99(2 Pt 2): 763–772.

Busse WW, Rachelefsky GS. 21st century management of upper respiratory allergic diseases: A focus on allergy and asthma. *J Allergy Clin Immunol* 1998;101(2 Pt 2):345–392.

Creticos PS. The consideration of immunotherapy in the treatment of allergic asthma. *J Allergy Clin Immunol* 2000;105:S559–S574.

DuBuske LM. Clinical comparison of histamine H one-receptor antagonist drugs. *J Allergy Clin Immunol* 1996;98(6 Pt 3):307–318.

Henderson WR. The role of leukotrienes in inflammation. *Ann Intern Med* 1994;141:684–697.

Holgate ST, Bradding P, Sampson AP. Leukotriene antagonists and synthesis inhibitors: New directions in asthma therapy. Review. *J Allergy Clin Immunol* 1998;98:1–13.

Jatulis DE, Meng Y-Y, Elashoff RM, et al. Preventive pharmacologic therapy among asthmatics. Five years after publication of guidelines. *Ann Allergy, Asthma, Immunol* 1998;81:82–88.

Johnson M. Pharmacodynamics and pharmacokinetics of inhaled glucocorticoids. *J Allergy Clin Immunol* 1996;97:169–176.

Joint Task Force on Practice Parameters. Practice parameters for allergen immunotherapy. *J Allergy Clin Immunol* 1996;98(6 Pt 1):1001–1011.

Kelly HW. Comparison of inhaled corticosteroids. *Ann Pharmacother* 1998;32:220–232.

Knorr B, Matz J, Bernstein JA, et al. Montelukast for chronic asthma in 6- to 14-year-old children. A randomized, double-blind trial. *JAMA* 1998;279:1181–1186.

Selroos O, Pietinalho A, Lofroos A, Riska H. Effect of early vs late intervention with inhaled corticosteroids in asthma. *Chest* 1995;108:1228–1234.

Szefler SJ, Nelson HS. Alternative agents for anti-inflammatory treatment of asthma. *J Allergy Clin Immunol* 1998;102(suppl):S23–S35.

CHAPTER 8

Chysky V, Kapla M, Hullman R, et al. Safety of ciprofloxacin in children: World wide clinical experience based on compassionate usage. *Infection* 1991;19:289–296.

Cunha BA. Antimicrobial therapy I. *Med Clin North Am* 1995;75:463.

File TM Jr. Overview of resistance in the 1990s. *Chest* 1999;115:3S–8S.

Gleckman RA. Antibiotic concerns in the elderly. *Infect Dis Clin North Am* 1995;9:575–589.

Hessen MT, Kaye D. Principles of selection and use of antimicrobial agents. *Infect Dis Clin North Am* 1995;9:531–545.

Isenberg DH. Antimicrobial susceptibility testing: A critical evaluation. *J Antimicrob Chemother* 1988;22(suppl A):73–86.

Jacoby GA. Prevalence and resistance mechanisms of common bacterial respiratory pathogens. *Clini Infect Dis* 1993;18:951.

Korzeniowski OM. Antibacterial agents in pregnancy. *Infect Dis Clin North Am* 1995;9:613–639.

Nightingale CH, Quintiliani R. Cost of oral antibiotic therapy. *Pharmacother* 1997;17:302–307.

Smaldone G, Palmer L. Aerosolized antibiotics: Current and future. *Respir Care* 2000;45:667–675.

Virk A, Steckelberg JM. Clinical aspects of antimicrobial resistance. *Mayo Clin Proc* 2000;75:200–214.

CHAPTER 9

Abrams J. The role of nitrates in coronary heart disease. *Arch Intern Med* 1995;155:357–364.

Ackerman MJ, Clapham DE. Ion channels—Basic science and clinical disease. *N Engl J Med* 1997;336:1575–1586.

Ambrose J, Dangas G. Unstable angina: Current concepts of pathogenesis and treatment. *Arch Int Med* 2000;160:25–37.

American College of Cardiology/American Heart Association Task Force on Practice Guidelines. Guidelines for the evaluation and management of heart failure. *Circulation* 1995;92:2764–84.

Brater DC. Diuretic resistance: Mechanisms and therapeutic strategies. *Cardiology* 1994;84(suppl 2):57–67.

Braunwald E, Jones RH, Mark DB, et al. Diagnosing and managing unstable angina. Agency for Health Care Policy and Research. *Circulation* 1994;90:613–622.

Francis GS. The relationship of the sympathetic nervous system and the renin-angiotensin system in congestive heart failure. *Am Heart J* 1989;118:642.

Lastini R, Maggion AP, Flather M, Sleight P, Tognoni G. ACE-inhibitor use in patients post myocardial infarction: Summary of evidence from clinical trials. *Circulation* 1995;92:3132–3137.

Law MR, Frost CD, Wald NJ. Analysis of data from trials of salt reduction. *Br Med J* 1991;302:819.

Packer M, Bristow MR, Cohn JN, et al. The effect of carvedilol on morbidity and mortality in patients with chronic heart failure. *N Engl J Med* 1996;334:1349–1355.

Parmley WW. Optimal treatment of stable angina. *Cardiology* 1997;88:27–31.

Roden DM. Risks and benefits of antiarrhythmic therapy. *N Engl J Med* 1994;331:785.

Sebastian JL, McKinney WP, Kaufman J, et al. Angiotensin converting enzyme inhibitors and cough: Prevalence in an outpatient medical clinic population. *Chest* 1991;99:36–39.

Simon SR, Black HR, Moser M, Berland WE. Cough and ACE inhibitors. *Arch Intern Med* 1992;152:1698–1700.

Tisdale JE, Patel R, Webb CR, et al. Electrophysiologic and proarrhythmic effects of intravenous inotropic agents. *Progr Cardiovasc Dis* 1995;38:167–180.

Vaughan Williams EM. A classification of antiarrhythmic actions reassessed after a decade of new drugs. *J Clin Pharmacol* 1984;24:129–147.

Yeghiazarians Y, Braunstein J, Askari A, Stone P. Unstable angina pectoris. *N Engl J Med* 2000;342:101–114.

CHAPTER 10

Anon. The Sixth Report of the Joint National Committee on Prevention, Detection, Evaluation, and Treatment of High Blood Pressure. *Arch Intern Med* 1997;157:2413–2446.

Clagett GP, Anderson FA Jr, Geerts W, et al. Prevention of venous thromboembolism. *Chest* 1998;114(suppl):531S–560S.

Dalen JE, Hirsh J, eds. Fifth ACCP Consensus Conference on Antithrombotic Therapy. *Chest* 1998;114(suppl 5):439S–769S.

Gourlay SG, Benowitz NL. Is clonidine an effective smoking cessation therapy? *Drugs* 1995;50:197.

Hirsh J, Warkentin TE, Raschke R, Granger C, Ohman EM, Dalen JE. Heparin and low-molecular-weight heparin: mechanisms of action, pharmacokinetics, dosing considerations, monitoring, efficacy, and safety. *Chest* 1998;114(suppl):489S–510S.

Hyers TM, Agnelli G, Hull RD, et al. Antithrombotic therapy for venous thromboembolic disease. *Chest* 1998;114(suppl):561S–578S.

Kaplan NM. *Clinical Hypertension*, 7th ed. Baltimore: Williams and Wilkins, 1998.

CHAPTER 11

Acello B. Meeting JCAHO standards for pain control. *Nursing* 2000;40(3):52–54.

American Society of Anesthesiologists: Practice guidelines for sedation and analgesia by non-anesthesiologists. *Anesthesiology* 1996;84:459–471.

Atherton DP, Hunter JM. Clinical pharmacokinetics of the newer neuromuscular blocking. *Clin Pharmacokinet* 1999;36:169–189.

Bevan DR. Recovery from neuromuscular block and its assessment. *Anesth Analg* 2000;90:S7–S13.

Bevan DR, Donati F, Kopman AF. Reversal of neuromuscular blockade. *Anesthesiology* 1992;77:785–805.

Brody H, Campbell ML, Faber-Langendoen K, Ogle KS. Withdrawing extensive life-sustaining treatment—recommendations for compassionate clinical management. *N Engl J Med* 1997;336:652–657.

Brookoff D. Chronic pain:2. The case for opioids. *Hosp Pract* 81-4 2000;35(9):69–72.

Donati F. Neuromuscular blocking drugs for the new millenium: Current practice, future trends—comparative pharmacology of neuromuscular blocking drugs. *Anesth Analg* 2000;90:S2–S6.

Hunter JM. New neuromuscular blocking drugs. *N Engl J Med* 1995;332:1691–1699

Jadad AR, Cepeda MA. Evidence-based emergency medicine. Ten challenges at the intersection of clinical research, evidence-based medicine, and pain relief. *Annals of Emerg Med* 2000;36(3):247–252.

Rushton C, Terry PB. Neuromuscular blockade and ventilator withdrawal: Ethical controversies. *Am J Crit Care* 1995;4:112–115.

Sjostrom B, Dahlgren LO, Halijamach. Strategies used in post-operative pain assessment and their clinical accuracy. *Journ of Clin Nurs* 2000;9(1):111–118.

Sottile FD. Managing dying patients and paralytic agents. *Chest* 1995;108:887.

Watling SM, Dasta JF. Prolonged paralysis in intensive care unit patients after the use of neuromuscular blocking agents: A review of the literature. *Crit Care Med* 1994;22:884–893.

CHAPTER 12

Adams PF, Marano MA. Current estimates from the National Health Interview Survey, 1994. *Vital Health Stat* 1995;10:94.

Alkins SA, O'Malley P. Should health-care systems pay for replacement therapy in patients with alpha$_1$-antitrypsin deficiency: A critical review and cost-effectiveness analysis. *Chest* 2000;117:875–880.

American Thoracic Society. Standards for the diagnosis and care of patients with chronic obstructive pulmonary disease. *Am J Respir Crit Care Med* 1995;152(5 Pt 2):77S–121S.

Badgett RG, Tanaka DF, Hunt DK, et al. Can moderate chronic obstructive pulmonary disease be diagnosed by historical and physical findings alone? *Am J Med* 1993;94(2):188–196.

BTS guidelines for the management of chronic obstructive pulmonary disease: The COPD Guideline Group of the Standards of Care Committee of the BTS. *Thorax* 1997:52(suppl 5):S1–S28.

Buist SA. Smoking and other risk factors. In: Murray JF and Nadel JA, eds. *Textbook of Respiratory Medicine*, 2nd ed. Philadelphia: W. B. Saunders, 1994, 1259–1287.

Centers for Disease Control and Prevention. Prevention of pneumococcal disease: Recommendations of the Advisory Committee on Immunization Practices (ACIP). *MMWR* 1997;46:1–24.

Dale LC, Hurt RD, Hays JT. Drug therapy to aid in smoking cessation. *Postgrad Med* 1998;104:75–84.

Expert Panel Report 2, National Heart, Lung, and Blood Institute and World Health Organization. Clinical Practice Guidelines: Guidelines for the diagnosis and management of asthma. Bethesda, MD: National Institutes of Health; 1997 (Publication No. NIH 97-4051).

Ferguson GT. Recommendations for the management of COPD. *Chest* 2000;117:23S–28S.

Ferguson GT, Cherniack RM. Management of chronic obstructive pulmonary disease. *NEJM* 1993;328(14):1017–1022.

Fiore MC, Bailey WC, Cohen SJ, et al. Smoking cessation. Clinical practice guideline No. 18. Rockville, MD: US Dept of Health and Human Services, Public Health Service, Agency for Health Care Policy and Research; Washington, D.C.: Centers for Disease

Control and Prevention, April 1996: AHCPR Publication No. 96-0692. Available at: http://www.ahcpr.gov.

Gadek JE, Crystal RG. Alpha 1-antitrypsin deficiency. In Stanbury JB, Wyngarrden JB, Frederickson DS, et al., eds. The metabolic basis of inherited disease, 5th ed. New York: McGraw-Hill, 1983;1450–1467.

Global Initiative for Asthma. Pocket guide for asthma management and prevention. U.S. Dept. of Health and Human Services, Public Health Service, National Institutes of Health, National Heart Lung and Blood Institute; Washington, D.C.: December 1995; NIH Publication No. 96-3659B.

Heatherton TF, Kozlowski LT, Frecker RC, et al. The Fagerstrom test for nicotine dependence: A revision of the Fagerstrom tolerance questionnaire. *Br J Addic* 1991;86: 1119–1127.

Higgins MW, Thom T. Incidence, prevalence, and mortality: intra- and inter-county differences. In Hensley MJ and Saunders NA, eds. *Clinical Epidemiology of Chronic Obstructive Pulmonary Disease*. New York: Marcel Dekker, 1990;23–43.

Kollef MH, Shapiro SD, Clinkscale D, et al. The effect of respiratory therapist-initiated treatment protocols on patient outcomes and resource utilization. *Chest* 2000;117: 467–475.

Kottke TE, Battista, RN, DeFriese GH, et al. Attributes of successful smoking cessation interventions in medical practice: A meta-analysis of 39 controlled trials. *JAMA* 1988;259: 2883–2889.

Larsen GL. Asthma in children. *N Engl J Med* 1992;326:1540–1545.

Lieberman J, Winter B, Sastre A. Alpha 1-antitrypsin P-types in 965 COPD patients. *Chest* 1986;89:370–373.

Löwhagen O. Asthma and asthma-like disorders. *Respir Med* 1999;93:851–855.

McGinnis JM, Foege WH. Actual causes of death in the United States. *JAMA* 1993;270:2207–2212.

National Asthma Education and Prevention Program Coordinating Committee, National Heart, Lung, and Blood Institute and World Health Organization. Global Initiative for Asthma. Bethesda (MD): National Institute of Health; 1995 (Publication No. NIH 95-3659).

NHLBI morbidity and mortality chartbook, 1998. Available at www.nhlbi.nih.gov/resources/doc/cht-book.htm.

Patel AM, Axen DM, Bartling SL, Guarderas JC. Practical considerations for managing asthma in adults. *Mayo Clin Proc* 1997;72:749–756.

Pierce JA. Alpha$_1$-antitrypsin augmentation therapy (editorial). *Chest* 1997;112:872–874.

Sherrill DL, Lebowitz MD, Burrows B. Epidemiology of chronic obstructive pulmonary disease. *Clin Chest Med* 1990;11:375–388.

Siafakas NM, Vermeire P, Price NB, et al. Optimal assessment and management of chronic obstructive pulmonary disease (COPD): The European respiratory society task force. *Eur Respir J* 1995;8:1398–1420.

Stoller JK. Clinical features and natural history of severe alpha$_1$-antitrypsin deficiency. *Chest* 1997;111:123S–128S.

Sullivan SD, Ramsey SD, Lee TA. The economic burden of COPD. *Chest* 2000;117:5S–9S.

Warner GO, Goetz M, Landau LI, et al. Management of asthma: A consensus statement. *Arch Dis Child* 1989;64:1065–1079.

Weiss EB, Stein M, eds. *Bronchial Asthma: Mechanisms and Therapeutics*, 3rd ed. Boston; Little, Brown, 1993.

White S, Leff A. The relationship of COPD to asthma. In: Cherniack NS, ed. *Chronic Obstructive Pulmonary Disease: Philadelphia: Saunders, (1991), 307–316.*

CHAPTER 13

Otitis Media

Bartelds AIM, Bowers P, Bridges-Webb C. et al. Acute otitis media in adults: A report from the international primary care network. *J Am Board Fam Pract* 1993;6:333–339.

Berman S. Otitis media in children. *NEJM* 1995;332:1560–1565.

Drake AF. Modern management of otitis media. *Hospital Medicine* June 1993;99–120.

Hoppe HL, Johnson CE. Otitis media: focus on antimicrobial resistance and new treatment options. *Am J Health-Syst Pharm* 1998;55:1881–1897.

Institute for Clinical Systems Improvement. *Postgrad Med* 2000;107:239–247.

Swanson JA, Hoecker JL. Otitis media in young children. *Mayo Clin Proc* 1996;71:179–183.

Sinusitis

Ferguson B. Acute and chronic sinusitis. *Postgrad Med* 1995;97:45–57.

Guarderas JC. Rhinitis and sinusitis: Office management. *Mayo Clin Proc* 1996;71:882–888.

Halpern M, Schmier J, Richner R, Togias A. Antimicrobial treatment patterns, resource utilization and charges associated with acute sinusitis in asthma patients. *Am J Health-Syst Pharm* 2000;57:875–881.

Haugen JR, Ramlo JH. Serious complications of acute sinusitis. *Postgrad Med* 1993;93:115–125.

Institute for Clinical Systems Integration. Acute sinusitis in adults. *Postgrad Med* 1998;103:154–168.

Kankum CG, Sallis R. Acute sinusitis in adults. *Postgrad Med* 1997;102:253–258.

Oppenheimer RW. Sinusitis. *Postgrad Med* 1992;91:281–292.

Pneumonia

Chien JW, Johnson JL. Viral pneumonias. *Postgrad Med* 2000;107:41–52.

Gleckman RA. Oral empirical treatment of pneumonia. *Postgrad Med* 1994;95:165–172.

Kohler RB. Severe pneumonia, when and why to hospitalize. *Postgrad Med* 1999;105:117–129.

Community-Acquired Pneumonia

File TM, Tan JS, Plouffe, JF. Community-acquired pneumonia. *Postgrad Med* 1996;99:95–107.

Institute for Clinical Systems Improvement. Community-acquired pneumonia (algorithm for treatment). *Postgrad Med* 2000;107:246–253.

Rubins JB, Janoff EN. Community-acquired pneumonia. *Postgrad Med* 1997;102:45–62.

Atypical Pneumonia

Cunha BA, Ortega A. Atypical pneumonia. *Postgrad Med* 1996;99:123–132.

Sarosi GA. Atypical Pneumonia: Why this term may be better left unsaid. *Postgrad Med* 1999;105:131–138.

Nosocomial Pneumonia

Broughton WA, Foner BJ, Bass JB. Nosocomial pneumonia, trying to make sense of the literature. *Postgrad Med* 1996;99:221–242.

Aerosolized Antibiotics

Wood GC, Boucher BA. Aerosolized antimicrobial therapy in acutely ill patients. *Pharmacotherapy* 2000;20:166–181.

Therapeutic Guidelines

Bartlett JG, Breiman RF, Mandell LA, et al., for the Infectious Diseases Society of America. Community-acquired pneumonia in adults: Guidelines for management. *Clin Infect Dis* 1998;26:811–838.

Guidelines for Prevention of Nosocomial Pneumonia. MMWR 46(RR-1);1–79 Publication January, 1997.

Heffelfinger JD, Dowell SF, Jorgensen JH, et al. Management of community-acquired pneumonia in the era of pneumococcal resistance. A report from the drug-resistant streptococcus pneumoniae therapeutic working group. *Arch Intern Med* 2000;160: 1399–1408.

Niederman MS, Bass JB, Campbell GD, et al. Guidelines for the initial management of adults with community-acquired pneumonia: Diagnosis, assessment of severity, and initial antimicrobial therapy. Official statement of the American Thoracic Society. *Am Rev Respir Dis* 1993;148(5):1418–1426.

Stool SE, Berg AO, Berman, et al. Managing otitis media with effusion in young children. Quick Reference Guide for Clinicians. *AHCPR Publication* 94-0623. Rockville, MD: Agency for Health Care Policy and Research, Public Health Service, U.S. Department of Health and Human Services, July 1994.

CHAPTER 14

Ashutosh, Phadke K, Jackson JF, Steele D. Use of nitric oxide inhalation in chronic obstructive pulmonary disease. *Thorax* 2000;55:109–113.

Barnes PJ. NO or no NO in asthma? *Thorax* 1996;51:218–220.

Moncada S, et al. Nitric oxide: Physiology, pathophysiology, and pharmacology. *Pharmacol Rev* 1991;43:109.

Tarpy SP, Celli BR. Long-term oxygen therapy. *N Engl J Med* 1995;333:710–714.

Zapol WM, Rimar S, Gillis N, et al. Nitric oxide and the lung. *Am Rev Respir Crit Care Med* 1994;149:1375–1380.

CHAPTER 15

Supplement to Circulation 2000;102(8): Guidelines 2000 for Cardiopulmonary Resuscitation and Emergency Cardiovascular Care International Consensus on Science, American Heart Association.

Web sites

National Institute of Allergy and Infectious Diseases, *www.niaid.nih.gov/publications/allergens/infor.htm*

American Academy of Allergy, Asthma and Immunology, *www.nhlbi.hih.gov/nhlbi/lung/asthma/prof/asthhc.htm*

American Academy of Allergy, Asthma and Immunology, *www.aaaai.org*

"Facts About Asthma," Centers for Disease Control and Prevention Fact Sheet, *www.cdc.gov/od/oc/media/fact/asthma.htm* Accessed November 11, 1999.

Medscape Resource Center, *www.medscape.com/resource/asthma*

Asthma in America™ Survey Project, *www.asthmainamerica.com*

Asthma Management Model System, *www.nhlbisupport.com/asthma/*

American Medical Association (AMA) Asthma Information Center, *www.ama-assn.org/special/asthma/asthma.htm*

Allergy and Asthma Network/Mothers of Asthmatics, Inc. (AANMA), *www.aanma.org/*

National Institute of Allergy and infectious Diseases (NIAID), *www.niaid.nih.gov/*

Drug List

BRAND NAMES

Following are the drugs listed in this book. More information may be found on our Web site.

Abbokinase (urokinase)
Accolate (zafirlukast)
Activase (alteplase)
Adenocard (adenosine)
Aerobid (flunisolide)
Afrin (oxymetazoline)
Aggrastat (tirofiban)
Aldactone (spironolactone, potassium sparing)
Allegra (fexofenadine)
Alupent (metaproterenol)
Alveofact (bovine surfactant)
Amikin (amikacin)
Amoxil (amoxicillin)
Anaprox (naproxen sodium)
Anbesol (benzocaine)
Ancef (cefazolin)
Anectine (succinylcholine)
Anexsia (hydrocodone plus acetaminophen)
Antabuse (disulfuram)
Apresoline (hydralazine)
Arduan (pipecuronium)
AsthmaNefrin (epinephrine)
Atrovent (ipratropium bromide)
Azactam (aztreonam)
Augmentin (amoxicillin clavulanate)
Azmacort (triamcinolone)

Bactrim (sulfamethoxazole trimethoprim)
Beclovent (beclomethasone dipropionate)
Beconase (beclomethasone dipropionate)
Benadryl (diphenhydramine)
Betapace (sotalol)
Biaxin (clarithromycin)
Brethaire (terbutaline)
Brethine (terbutaline)
Bretylol (bretylium)
Brevibloc (esmolol)
Brevital (methohexital)
Bricanyl (terbutaline)
Bronkometer (isoetharine)

Bronkosol (isoetharine)
Bumex (bumetanide)

Calan (verapamil)
Calciparine (heparin sodium)
Capoten (captopril)
Carbocaine (mepivacaine)
Cardizem (diltiazem)
Cardura (doxazosin)
Cartrol (carteolol)
Catapres (clonidine)
Ceclor (cefaclor)
Cefobid (cefoperazone)
Ceftin (cefuroxime)
Cefzil (cefprozil)
Chlor-Trimeton (chlorpheniramine)
Cipro (ciprofloxacin)
Claritin (loratidine)
Clinoril (sulindac)
Combivent (ipratropium plus albuterol)
Compazine (prochlorperazine)
Cordarone (amiodarone)
Coreg (carvedilol)
Cortef (hydrocortisone)
Coumadin (warfarin sodium)
Cozaar (losartan)
Curosurf (porcine surfactant)

Dantrium (dantrolene)
Darvon (propoxyphene)
Decadron (dexamethasone)
Demerol (meperidine)
Depakote (divalproex sodium)
Depo-Provera (medroxyprogesterone)
Desyrel (trazodone)
Diflucan (fluconazole)
Dilaudid (hydromorphone)
Dimetane (brompheniramine)
Diovan (valsartan)
Diprivan (propofol)
Diuril (chlorothiazide; a thiazide diuretic)
Dobutrex (dobutamine)
Dolophine (methadone)
Dopram (doxapram)
Duragesic (fentanyl)
Dynapen (dicloxacillin)
Dyrenium (triamterene)

Elavil (amitriptyline)
Elixophyllin (theophylline)
Empirin (aspirin plus codeine)

E-mycin (erythromycin)
Ethmozine (moricizine)
Ethrane (enflurane)
Exosurf (colfosceril palmitate)

Famvir (famciclovir)
Feldene (piroxicam)
Flagyl (metronidazole)
Flexeril (cyclobenzaprine)
Flonase (fluticasone propionate)
Flovent (fluticasone)
Flumadine (rimantadine)
Fluothane (halothane)
Forane (isoflurane)
Fortaz (ceftazidime)
Fungizone (amphotericin B)

Gantanol (sulfamethoxazole)
Gantrisin (sulfisoxazole)
Garamycin (gentamicin)

Habitrol (nicotine)
Hismanol (astemizole)
Hyperstat (diazoxide)
Hytrin (terazosin)

Inderal (propranolol)
Indocin (indomethacin)
Infasurf (calf lung surfactant)
INH (isoniazid)
Inocor (amrinone)
Intal (cromolyn)
Integrilin (eptifibatide)
Isoptin (verapamil)
Isuprel (isoproterenol)
Isuprel Mistometer (isoproterenol)

Keflex (cephalexin)
Ketalar (ketamine)

Lamictal (lamotrigine)
Lasix (furosemide)
Levaquin (levofloxacin)
Levatol (penbutolol)
Levo-Dromoran (levorphanol)
Librium (chlordiazepoxide)
Loniten (minoxidil)
Lopressor (metoprolol)
Lorabid (loracarbef)
Lortab (hydrocodone plus acetaminophen)
Lotensin (benazepril)

Lovenox (enoxaparin)
Lozol (indapamide)

Marcaine (bupivacaine)
Maxair (pirbuterol)
Maxipime (cefepime)
Medihaler-Iso (isoproterenol)
Mefoxin (cefoxitin)
Merrem (meropenem)
Metaprel (metaproterenol)
Mexitil (mexiletene)
microNefrin (epinephrine)
Midamor (amiloride)
Minipress (prazosin)
Minocin (minocycline)
Mivacron (mivacurium)
Monistat (miconazole)
Motrin (ibuprofen)
Mucomyst (acetylcysteine)
Mucosil (acetylcysteine)
Myambutol (ethambutol)
Mycostatin (nystatin)

Nalfon (fenoprofen)
Naprosyn (naproxen HCl)
Narcan (naloxone)
Nasacort (triamcinolone)
Nasalcrom (cromolyn)
Nasalide (flunisolide)
Nasonex (mometasone furoate)
NegGram (nalidixic acid)
Nebcin (tobramycin)
Neo-Synephrine (phenylephrine)
Neurontin (gabapentin)
Nicoderm
Nicorette
Nicotrol
Nimbex (cisatracurium)
Nipride (nitroprusside)
Nitropress (nitroprusside)
Nizoral (ketoconazole)
Norcuron (vecuronium)
Norflex (orphenadrine)
Norpramin (desipramine)
Norvasc (amlodipine)
Novocain (procaine)
Numorphan (oxymorphone)
Nuromax (doxacurium)

Omnipen (ampicillin)
Orudis (ketoprofen)

Pamelor (nortriptyline)
Parafon Forte (chlorzoxazone)
Pavulon (pancuronium)
Paxil (paroxetine)
Penthrane (methoxyflurane)
Pentothal (thiopental)
Percocet (oxycodone plus acetaminophen)
Percodan (oxycodone plus aspirin)
Persantine (dipyridamole)
Phenergan (promethazine)
Pipracil (piperacillin)
Plavix (clopidogrel)
Pneumactant (artificial lung-expanding compound)
Pontocaine (tetracaine)
Primacor (milrinone)
Primatene Mist (epinephrine)
Primaxin (imipenem)
Pronestyl (procainamide)
Proscar (finasteride)
Prostep (nicotine)
Proventil (albuterol)
Prozac (fluoxetine)
Pulmicort Turbuhaler (budesonide)
Pulmozyme (dornase alfa)

Quibron (theophylline and guaifenesin)
Quinaglute (quinidine)

Raplon (rapacuronium)
Relenza (zanamivir)
Respbid (theophylline)
Retavase (reteplase)
Rhinocort (budesonide)
Rhythmol (propafenone)
Rimactane (rifampin)
Robaxin (methocarbamol)
Rocephin (ceftriaxone sodium)
Rogaine (minoxidil)
Roxicodone (oxycodone)

Sectral (acebutolol)
Septra (sulfamethoxazole trimethoprim)
Serevent (salmeterol)
Seromycin (cycloserine)
Sinequan (doxepin)
Singulair (montelukast)
Slo-Bid (theophylline)
Slo-Phyllin (theophylline)
SoluMedrol (methylprednisolone)
Stadol (butorphanol)
Sublimaze (fentanyl)

Sudafed (pseudoephedrine)
Suprax (cefixime)
Surfacten (surfactant-TA)
Surfaxin (sinapultide)
Survanta (beractant)
Streptase (streptokinase)
Symmetrel (amantadine)
Synercid (dalfopristin/quinupristine)

Tagamet (cimetidine)
Tambocor (flecainide)
Tamiflu (oseltamivir)
Targocid (teicoplanin)
Tebrazid (pyrazinamide)
Tegretol (carbamazepine)
Tenex (guanfacine)
Tenormin (atenolol)
Tensilon (edrophonium)
Theobid (theophylline)
Theo-Dur (theophylline)
Theolair (theophylline)
Theostat (theophylline)
Ticar (ticarcillin)
Ticlid (ticlopidine)
Tilade (nedocromil)
Tofranil (imipramine)
Tonocard (tocainide)
Toradol (ketorolac)
Tornalate (bitolterol mesylate)
Tracrium (atracurium)
Trecator-SC (ethionamide)
Tylenol (acetaminophen)
Tylox (oxycodone plus acetaminophen)

Ultram (tramadol)
Unasyn (ampicillin sulbactam)
Unipen (nafcillin)

Valium (diazepam)
Vancenase (beclomethasone dipropionate)
Vanceril (beclomethasone dipropionate)
Vancocin (vancomycin)
Vantin (cefpodoxime proxetil)
Vaponefrin (epinephrine)
Vasotec (enalapril)
Veetids (penicillin G)
Ventolin (albuterol)
Versed (midazolam)
Vibramycin (doxycycline)
Vicodin (hydrocodone plus acetaminophen)
Vicoprofen (ibuprofen plus hydrocodone)

Virazole (ribavirin)
Vivactyl (protriptyline)

Wellbutrin (bupropion)
Wytensin (guanabenz)

Xanax (alprazolam)
Xopenex (levalbuterol)
Xylocaine (lidocaine)

Zaditen (ketotifen)
Zemuron (rocuronium)
Zinacef (cefuroxime)
Zithromax (azithromycin)
Zoloft (sertraline)
Zosyn (piperacillin-tazobactam)
Zovirax (acyclovir)
Zyban (bupropion)
Zyflo (zileuton)
Zyrtec (cetirizine)
Zyvox (linezolid)

GENERIC NAMES

acebutolol (Sectral)
acetylcysteine (Mucomyst, Mucosil)
adenosine (Adenocard)
albuterol (Proventil, Ventolin)
alprazolam (Xanax)
amikacin (Amikin)
amiloride (Midamor)
aminophylline (Truphylline)
amiodarone (Cordarone)
amitriptyline (Elavil)
amlodipine (Norvasc)
amoxicillin (Amoxil)
amoxicillin clavulanate (Augmentin)
amphotericin B (Fungizone)
amrinone (Inocor)
acetaminophen (Tylenol)
aspirin (Bayer, etc.)
atenolol (Tenormin)
atracurium (Tracrium)
atropine sulfate
azithromycin (Zithromax)

beclomethasone dipropionate (Beclovent, Beconase, Vancenase)
benazepril (Lotensin)
benzocaine (Anbesol)
bethanechol (Urecholine)
bitolterol mesylate (Tornalate)

bretylium (Bretylol)
budesonide (Rhinocort)
bumetanide (Bumex)
bupivacaine (Marcaine)
bupropion (Zyban)
butorphanol (Stadol)

caffeine
captopril (Capoten)
carbamazepine (Tegretol)
carteolol (Cartrol)
cefaclor (Ceclor)
cefepime (Maxipime)
cefixime (Suprax)
cefotaxime (Claforan)
cefpodoxime proxetil (Vantin)
cefprozil (Cefzil)
ceftazidime (Fortaz)
ceftriaxone sodium (Rocephin)
cefuroxime (Ceftin)
cephalexin (Keflex)
chlordiazepoxide (Librium)
chlorothiazide (Diuril)
chlorzoxazone (Parafon Forte)
cimetidine (Tagamet)
cisatracurium (Nimbex)
clarithromycin (Biaxin)
clindamycin (Cleocin)
clonidine (Catapres)
cloxacillin (Tegopen)
carvedilol (Coreg)
clonidine (Catapres)
clopidogrel (Plavix)
cocaine
codeine
cortisone (Cortone)
cromolyn sodium (Intal)
cyclobenzaprine (Flexeril)

dantrolene (Dantrium)
desipramine (Norpramin)
dexamethasone (Decadron)
diazepam (Valium)
diazoxide (Hyperstat)
digoxin (Lamoxim)
diltiazem (Cardizem)
dipyridamole (Persantine)
divalproex sodium (Depakote)
dobutamine (Dobutrex)
dopamine (Intropin)
dornase alfa (Pulmozyme)
doxacurium (Nuromax)

doxapram (Dopram)
doxazosin (Cardura)
doxepin (Sinequan)

enalapril (Vasotec)
enflurane (Ethrane)
enoxaparin (Lovenox)
epinephrine (AsthmaNefrin, microNefrin, Vaponefrin)
eptifibatide (Integrilin)
erythromycin (E-mycin)
esmolol (Brevibloc)
ethanol

fenoprofen (Nalfon)
fentanyl (Sublimaze, Duragesic)
finasteride (Proscar)
flecainide (Tambocor)
flunisolide (Nasalide)
fluoxetine (Prozac)
fluticasone (Flovent)
furosemide (Lasix)

gabapentin (Neurontin)
gentamicin (Garamycin)
guanabenz (Wytensin)
guanfacine (Tenex)

halothane (Fluothane)
heparin (Calciparine)
hydralazine (Apresoline)
hydrocodone
hydrocodone plus acetaminophen (Anexsia, Vicodin, Lortab)
hydrocortisone
hydromorphone (Dilaudid)

ibuprofen (Motrin)
imipenem-cilastatin (Primaxin)
imipramine (Tofranil)
indapamide (Lozol)
indomethacin (Indocin)
ipratropium bromide (Atrovent)
ipratropium plus albuterol (Combivent)
isoetharine (Bronkometer, Bronkosol)
isoflurane (Forane)
isoniazid (INH)
isoproterenol (Isuprel Mistometer)

ketamine (Ketalar)
ketoprofen (Orudis)
ketorolac (Toradol)

lamotrigine (Lamictal)
levalbuterol (Xopenex)
levofloxacin (Levaquin)
levorphanol (Levo-Dromoran)
lidocaine (Xylocaine)
loracarbef (Lorabid)
losartan (Cozaar)

magnesium
medroxyprogesterone (Depo-Provera)
meperidine (Demerol)
mepivacaine (Carbocaine)
meropenem (Merrem)
metaproterenol (Alupent, Metaprel)
methadone (Dolophine)
methocarbamol (Robaxin)
methohexital (Brevital)
methoxyflurane (Penthrane)
methylprednisolone
metoprolol (Lopressor)
metronidazole (Flagyl)
mexiletene (Mexitil)
midazolam (Versed)
milrinone (Primacor)
minoxidil (Rogaine, Loniten)
mivacurium (Mivacron)
montelukast (Singulair)
moricizine (Ethmozine)
morphine (Duramorph)

naloxone (Narcan)
naproxen HCl (Naprosyn)
naproxen sodium (Anaprox)
nedocromil sodium (Tilade)
neostigmine (Prostigmin)
nitroglycerin
nitroprusside (Nipride, Nitropress)
nitrous oxide
nortriptyline (Pamelor)

orphenadrine (Norflex)
oxycodone (Roxicodone)
oxycodone plus acetaminophen (Tylox, Percocet)
oxycodone plus aspirin (Percodan)
oxygen
oxymetazoline (Afrin)
oxymorphone (Numorphan)

pancuronium (Pavulon)
paroxetine (Paxil)
penicillin

pentamidine (Nubupent)
phenylephrine (Neo-Synephrine)
pilocarpine (Zosyn)
pipecuronium (Arduan)
piperacillin tazobactam
pirbuterol (Maxair)
piroxicam (Feldene)
prazosin (Minipress)
prednisolone (Delta-Cortef)
prednisone (Delta-Zone)
procainamide (Pronestyl)
procaine (Novocain)
prochlorperazine (Compazine)
promethazine (Phenergan)
propafenone (Rhythmol)
propofol (Diprivan)
propoxyphene (Darvon)
propranolol (Inderal)
protamine
protriptyline (Vivactyl)
pyridostigmine (Mestinon)

quinidine (Quinaglute)

rapacuronium (Raplon)
reteplase (Retavase)
ribavirin (Virazole)
rifampin (Rimactane)
rocuronium (Zemuron)

salmeterol (Serevent)
sertraline (Zoloft)
sotalol (Betapace)
spironolactone (Aldactone)
streptokinase (Streptase)
streptomycin
succinylcholine (Anectine)
sulindac (Clinoril)

terazosin (Hytrin)
terbutaline (Brethaire, Bricanyl)
tetracaine (Pontocaine)
tetracycline (Timentin)
theophylline (Respbid, Slo-Phyllin, Theobid, Theo-Dur, Theolair)
thiopental (Pentothal)
ticarcillin clavulanate (Timentin)
ticlopidine (Ticlid)
tirofiban (Aggrastat)
tobramycin (Nebcin)
tocainide (Tonocard)
tramadol (Ultram)

trazodone (Desyrel)
triamcinolone (Azmacort)
triamterene (Dyrenium)
trimethoprim–sulfamethoxazole (Bactrim, Septra)

urokinase (Abbokinase)

valsartan (Diovan)
vancomycin (Vancocin)
vecuronium (Norcuron)
verapamil (Calan, Isoptin)

warfarin (Coumadin)

zafirlukast (Accolate)
zileuton (Zyflo)

Index

In this index, page numbers in *italic* designate figures; page numbers followed by the letter "t" designate tables. *See also* cross-references designate related topics or detailed subtopic breakdowns. Drugs are indexed under both generic names and trade names when available.